Myositis and You

A Guide to Juvenile Dermatomyositis for Patients, Families, and Healthcare Providers

Edited by

Lisa G. Rider, MD
Lauren M. Pachman, MD
Frederick W. Miller, MD, PhD
Harriet Bollar

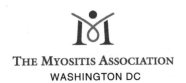

THE MYOSITIS ASSOCIATION
WASHINGTON DC

1st printing 2007 • 2nd printing 2016

ATTENTION CORPORATIONS, UNIVERSITIES, COLLEGES, AND PROFESSIONAL ORGANIZATIONS: Quantity discounts are available on bulk purchases of this book for educational, gift purposes, or as premiums for increasing magazine subscriptions or renewals. Special books or book excerpts can also be created to fit specific needs. For information, please contact The Myositis Association, 1233 20th Street NW, Suite 402, Washington DC 20036 or tma@myositis.org.

Publisher's Cataloging-in-Publication data

Rider, Lisa G.
    Myositis and you : a guide to juvenile dermatomyositis for patients, families, and healthcare providers / Lisa G. Rider, MD, Lauren M. Pachman, MD, Frederick W. Miller, MD PhD, and Harriet Bollar.
    p. cm.
    Includes index.
    ISBN 0-9785225-3-2
    ISBN 13 978-0-9785225-3-7

1. Myositis. 2. Dermatomyositis. 3. Pediatric rheumatology. 4. Polymyosis. 5. Rheumatic Diseases—Child. 6. Autoimmune Diseases. I. Pachman, Lauren. II. Miller, Frederick W, 1951-. III. Bollar, Harriet. IV. Title.

RC935.M9 R53 2006
616.74421—dc22   2006925755

Acknowledgments

We thank the many health professionals who have dedicated their time, expertise, and wisdom to helping children with myositis and to writing these chapters. The authors thank the children with myositis and their families who were the inspiration for this book. Their heartfelt concerns are reflected in the quotations at the beginning of every chapter. We are especially indebted to Kathryn Spooner from The Myositis Association who devoted countless hours to helping us interface with all of the contributors to the book, editing, and keeping us on track, and to Shari Weber who assembled a large number of valuable resources, assisted in organizing and editing the project's final stages, and whose committee provided helpful feedback on the text. We are grateful to our copy editor, Lisa Maroski, for making the text approachable for families and to Adrienne Woodworth for illustrations and organizational support. We appreciate the helpful feedback from field testers, who included parents, patients, and health professionals. We are grateful to The Myositis Association and Cure JM Foundation for their vision in supporting the development and publication of this first book dedicated solely to helping families of children with myositis. We thank our families, Ben and Simon, Mark, Lori, and Leo, for their help and support to enable us to devote more than three years to this task.

Dedication

To the children with myositis and their families:
May you find your strength on the path to recovery.

To Amanda and Parker, whose courage and determination
to overcome juvenile dermatomyositis
inspired their families to take up the fight against it,
which ultimately led to the funding and inspiration for this book.

Myositis and You

A Guide to Juvenile Dermatomyositis for Patients, Families, and Healthcare Providers

Editors and Contributors viii

Introduction 1

Section 1: What Is Juvenile Myositis?

Chapter 1 **What Is Juvenile Myositis?** 9
Lisa G. Rider and Frederick W. Miller

Chapter 2 **Explaining Juvenile Myositis: A Kid's Guide** 23
Lauren M. Pachman

Chapter 3 **The Pathways to Juvenile Myositis** 31
Lauren M. Pachman and Ann M. Reed

Section 2: At the Beginning

Chapter 4 **First Signs of Illness** 43
Lauren M. Pachman and Carol B. Lindsley

Chapter 5 **Finding Help** 53
Janalee Taylor, Sandra Parker, Miriam S. Granger, and Murray H. Passo

Chapter 6 **Tests Your Child's Doctor Might Order** 63
Richard S. Finkel, Kevin E. Bove, and Lauren M. Pachman

Chapter 7 **Treatment Possibilities in the Beginning** 77
Bianca A. Lang, Ann M. Reed, Peter N. Malleson, and Lauren M. Pachman

Section 3: Coping with Juvenile Myositis

Chapter 8 **Adapting to Physical Limitations** 95
Kristi Whitney-Mahoney, Dorothy P. I. Ho, and Susan M. Maillard

Chapter 9 **Coping with Myositis As a Family** 109
Miriam S. Granger, Ilona S. Szer, and Arlette Lefebvre

Section 4: Following Your Child's Progress

Chapter 10 **Charting Your Child's Progress** 127
Lisa G. Rider, Clarissa M. Pilkington, Nicolino Ruperto, and David A. Isenberg

Chapter 11 **Assessing Muscle Strength, Endurance, and Function** 139
Adam M. Huber, Robert M. Rennebohm, and Susan M. Maillard

Section 5: Treatment Options

Chapter 12 **Possible Medicines During the Course** 153
Lisa G. Rider, Clarissa M. Pilkington, Bianca A. Lang, and Peter N. Malleson

Chapter 13 **Rehabilitation of the Child with Myositis** 173
Minal S. Jain, Michaele R. Smith, and Jeanne E. Hicks

Chapter 14 **Complementary and Alternative Approaches
to Juvenile Myositis** 191
Lori A. Love

Chapter 15 **New Therapies on the Horizon** 207
Frederick W. Miller and Daniel J. Lovell

Section 6: Important Issues on the Road to Recovery

Chapter 16 **Skin Rashes and Sun Protection** 217
Victoria R. Barrio, Jeffrey P. Callen, and Amy S. Paller

Chapter 17 **Calcinosis** 231
Lauren M. Pachman and Lisa G. Rider

Chapter 18 **Swallowing and Other Digestive Problems** 241
Barbara C. Sonies, Margaret A. Marcon, and Lisa F. Imundo

Chapter 19 **Nutrition and Your Child's Weight** 253
Carol J. Henderson and Barbara E. Ostrov

Chapter 20 **Growth and Development** 261
Aida N. Lteif, Wendy J. Brickman, and Patricia Woo

Chapter 21 **Maintaining Flexibility: Joints and Other Considerations** 269
Brian M. Feldman and Angelo Ravelli

Chapter 22 **Taking Care of the Bones** 275
Emily von Scheven, Rolando Cimaz, and Kelly A. Rouster-Stevens

Chapter 23 **Tune to Your Voice** 283
Beth Solomon

Chapter 24 **When Children Have Difficulty Breathing** 291
Fernanda Falcini, Susanna A. McColley, and Rolando Cimaz

Chapter 25 **Attention to Sugar and Fat Metabolism** 297
Jean-Pierre Chanoine and Barbara S. Adams

Chapter 26 **Too Much Body Fat Loss** 305
Barbara S. Adams and Elif Arioglu Oral

Chapter 27 **Eye Health** 313
Janine A. Smith and Manuel B. Datiles, III

Chapter 28 **When Your Child Has More Than One Autoimmune Disease** . . 321
Clarissa M. Pilkington and Ann M. Reed

Chapter 29 **Vaccines and Infection Protection** 327
Laura J. Mirkinson, Judy A. Beeler, and Ildy M. Katona

Section 7: Hopes of Recovery

Chapter 30 **The Clinical Course and Outcome of Juvenile Myositis** 341
Robert M. Rennebohm, Brian M. Feldman, Adam M. Huber,
Charles H. Spencer, Robert P. Sundel, and Lisa G. Rider

Chapter 31 **Planning for the Future** 351
Patience H. White and Patricia A. Rettig

Chapter 32 **Approaching Adolescence** 361
Cynthia J. Mears

Chapter 33 **Pregnancy and Fertility** 367
Ann M. Reed and Chester V. Oddis

Section 8: Resources and Opportunities

Chapter 34 **Protecting Your Child's Rights** 377
Ann Kunkel, Susan J. Wright, Carol B. Lindsley, and Jane G. Schaller

Chapter 35 **Insurance and Medical Expenses** 383
Carolyn L. Yancey, Donna LaRue, and Marisa S. Klein-Gitelman

Chapter 36 **School Issues** 395
Renee Thomas, Nancy Y. Olson, Susan J. Wright, and Laurie Ebner-Lyon

Chapter 37 **Summer Camps** 411
Ann S. Christiano, Dana Driesman-Klover, Megan Perron,
Joyce L. Sundberg, and Ilona S. Szer

Chapter 38 **Searching the Internet for Reliable Information** 419
Ann Kunkel, Susan J. Wright, Carol B. Lindsley, and Jane G. Schaller

Chapter 39 **How We Learn About Juvenile Myositis** 423
Daniel J. Lovell and Frederick W. Miller

Chapter 40 **How You Can Help: Raising Awareness
and Funds for Research** 435
Harriet Bollar, Patience H. White, Marco Herrera, and Bob Goldberg

Color Plates 227

Glossary of Terms 441

Resource Appendix 449
Kathryn A. Spooner, Harriet Bollar, and Clarissa M. Pilkington, Editors
with contributing authors

Index 461

Editors

Lisa G. Rider, MD, is a pediatric rheumatologist at the National Institutes of Health, where she sees a number of juvenile myositis (JM) patients. Her JM research spans more than twelve years, in which she has led several national collaborative studies and established a JM registry of over four hundred patients. She is co-chair of the International Myositis Assessment and Clinical Studies Group (IMACS), a coalition of healthcare providers working toward developing standards for conducting and reporting adult and juvenile myositis studies and collaborating on international research studies. She serves as an advisor to a number of rheumatology-related organizations, including as a longstanding member and Vice Chair of The Myositis Association's Medical Advisory Board. She has been recognized by the U.S. Public Health Service with a number of awards for her research on JM and her regulatory accomplishments in promoting the development of new treatments for children with pediatric rheumatic diseases. She is recognized as a top physician in the United States.

Lauren M. Pachman, MD, a Professor of Pediatrics at Northwestern University's Feinberg School of Medicine, founded the Immunology/Rheumatology Division at The Children's Memorial Hospital, where she cares for more than three hundred children with inflammatory myopathy. As Director of the Molecular and Cellular Pathobiology Program at the Children's Memorial Research Center, the focus of her research is the pathogenesis and therapy of juvenile dermatomyositis. She received the Clinical Research Award from the American College of Rheumatology, as well as the Master of Rheumatology Award and an Award of Distinction from the American Academy of Pediatrics, Pediatric Rheumatology Sub-section. She serves on the boards of many rheumatology-related organizations, including the Medical Advisory Board of The Myositis Association.

Frederick W. Miller, MD, PhD, is a rheumatologist and immunologist who evaluates adult and juvenile myositis patients and their families at the National Institutes of Health in Bethesda MD. His work in the field of myositis research spans more than two decades and involves many aspects of the study and treatment of persons with these diseases. He has been Vice Chair and a longstanding member of The Myositis Association's Medical Advisory Board and represented this group on the TMA Board of Directors. He is co-chair of the International Myositis Assessment and Clinical Studies Group (IMACS), a coalition of healthcare providers working toward developing standards for the conduct and reporting of myositis studies.

Harriet Bollar is Co-Founder and Chairman of the Cure JM Foundation, which was established to help families face the challenges of JM and to raise awareness and funds for juvenile myositis research. She is a Cure JM family support representative and volunteer member of Team JM. Her efforts have been inspired by her granddaughter's determination to overcome juvenile dermatomyositis.

Contributors

Barbara S. Adams, MD, Professor, University of Michigan School of Medicine; Director, Pediatric Rheumatology and Co-Director, Pediatric Rheumatology/Nephrology Clinic, University of Michigan Health System, Ann Arbor MI

Victoria R. Barrio, MD, Assistant Clinical Professor of Pediatrics and Medicine (Dermatology), University of California San Diego School of Medicine; Pediatric and Adolescent Dermatology, Rady Children's Hospital and Health Center, San Diego CA

Judy A. Beeler, MD, Medical Officer, Division of Viral Products, Office of Vaccines Research and Review, Center for Biologics Evaluation and Research, U.S. Food and Drug Administration, Department of Health and Human Services (DHHS), Bethesda MD

Harriet Bollar, Co-Founder and Chairman, Cure JM Foundation, Encinitas CA

Kevin E. Bove, MD, Professor, Pathology and Pediatrics, University of Cincinnati College of Medicine; Staff Pathologist, Cincinnati Children's Hospital Medical Center, Cincinnati OH

Wendy J. Brickman, MD, Assistant Professor, Northwestern University's Feinberg School of Medicine; Attending Physician, Endocrinology, Children's Memorial Hospital, Chicago IL

Jeffrey P. Callen, MD, Professor of Medicine (Dermatology), Chief, Division of Dermatology, University of Louisville School of Medicine, Louisville KY

Jean-Pierre Chanoine, MD, PhD, Clinical Professor and Head, Endocrinology and Diabetes Unit, British Columbia's Children's Hospital, University of British Columbia, Vancouver BC Canada

Ann S. Christiano, MS, ARNP, Pediatric Endocrinology, Dartmouth-Hitchcock Medical Center, Lebanon NH

Rolando Cimaz, MD, Department of Pediatrics, Fondazione Policlinico Mangiagalli, Milano Italy; Department of Pediatrics, Hopital Eduard Herriot and Université Claude Bernard Lyon 1, Lyon France

Anne M. Connolly, MD, Associate Professor, Departments of Neurology and Pediatrics, Washington University School of Medicine, St. Louis MO

Manuel B. Datiles, III, MD, Medical Officer and Chief, Cataract Section, National Eye Institute, National Institutes of Health, DHHS, Bethesda MD

Peter B. Dent, MD, Professor Emeritus, Pediatrics, Immunology/Rheumatology, McMaster University, Hamilton ON Canada

Dana Driesman-Klover, BSc OT, OT Reg. Ont., Occupational Therapist, Bloorview MacMillan Children's Centre, Toronto ON Canada

Laurie Ebner-Lyon, RN, APN.C., Advanced Practice Nurse, Pediatric Rheumatology, The Joseph M. Sanzari Children's Hospital, Hackensack University Medical Center, Hackensack NJ

Fernanda Falcini, MD, Associate Professor of Pediatrics, Rheumatology, A. Meyer Hospital, University of Florence, Florence Italy

Brian M. Feldman, MD, MSc, FRCPC, Associate Professor of Paediatrics, Health Policy Management & Evaluation, University of Toronto; Staff Rheumatologist, The Hospital for Sick Children, Toronto; Clinical Chief, Arthritis Team, Bloorview MacMillan Children's Centre, Toronto ON Canada

Richard S. Finkel, MD, Director, Neuromuscular Program, The Children's Hospital of Philadelphia; Clinical Professor in Neurology and Pediatrics, The University of Pennsylvania School of Medicine, Philadelphia PA

Bob Goldberg, Executive Director, The Myositis Association, Washington DC

Miriam S. Granger, MSW, RSW, Social Worker, Division of Rheumatology, The Hospital for Sick Children, Toronto ON Canada

Carol J. Henderson, PhD, RD, Epidemiologist, Hatton Institute for Research and Education, Good Samaritan Hospital, Cincinnati OH

Marco Herrera, Legislative Chair, Southern Nevada Chapter, The Juvenile Diabetes Research Foundation, Las Vegas NV

Jeanne E. Hicks, MD, Consultant, Medical Consultant Services, Charlotte NC; Past Deputy Chief, Rehabilitation Medicine Department, WG Magnuson Clinical Center, National Institutes of Health, DHHS, Bethesda MD

Dorothy P. I. Ho, PT, Physical Therapist, California Children's Services, Reseda Medical Therapy Unit, Reseda CA

Adam M. Huber, MSc, MD, Assistant Professor, Division of Pediatric Rheumatology, IWK Health Centre; Associate Professor, Dalhousie University, Halifax NS Canada

Lisa F. Imundo, MD, Assistant Clinical Professor, Pediatrics, Columbia University; Pediatric Rheumatology, Children's Hospital of New York-Presbyterian, New York NY

David A. Isenberg, MD, FRCP, Arthritis Research Campaign Diamond Jubilee Professor of Rheumatology and Academic Director of Rheumatology, Professor of Rheumatology, Centre for Rheumatology, University College London, London UK

Minal S. Jain, MS, PT, PCS, Pediatric Physical Therapist, Rehabilitation Medicine Department, Mark O. Hatfield Clinical Research Center, National Institutes of Health, DHHS, Bethesda MD

Ildy M. Katona, MD, Professor of Pediatrics and Medicine, Department of Pediatrics, Uniformed Services University of the Health Sciences, Bethesda MD

Marisa S. Klein-Gitelman, MD, MPH, Head, Division of Rheumatology, Children's Memorial Hospital; Associate Professor of Pediatrics, Feinberg School of Medicine, Northwestern University, Chicago IL

Ann Kunkel, BS, Education Coordinator, Pediatric Rheumatology, Kansas University Children's Center, University of Kansas Medical Center, Kansas City KS

Bianca A. Lang, MD, FRCPC, Associate Professor, Dalhousie University; Head, Division of Pediatric Rheumatology, IWK Health Centre, Halifax NS Canada

Donna LaRue, RN, BSN, Family Care Consultant, Rheumatology Nurse, Division of Rheumatology, Children's Memorial Hospital, Chicago IL

Arlette Lefebvre, MD, Child Psychiatrist and Director of the Physical Disability Team, The Hospital for Sick Children, Bloorview MacMillan Children's Hospital, Toronto ON Canada

Carol B. Lindsley, MD, Professor of Pediatrics, Department of Pediatrics, Chief, Pediatric Rheumatology, University of Kansas Medical Center, Kansas City KS

Lori A. Love, MD, PhD, Senior Advisor for Clinical Science, Office of Regulatory Affairs, U.S. Food and Drug Administration, DHHS, Rockville MD

Daniel J. Lovell, MD, MPH, Joseph E. Levinson Professor of Pediatrics, University of Cincinnati; Associate Director, William S. Rowe Division of Rheumatology, Cincinnati Children's Hospital Medical Center, Cincinnati OH

Aida N. Lteif, MD, Assistant Professor of Pediatrics, Mayo Clinic College of Medicine; Pediatric and Adolescent Medicine, Mayo Clinic Rochester, Rochester MN

Susan M. Maillard, MSc, SRP, MCSP, Specialist Physiotherapist in Paediatric Rheumatology, Great Ormond Street Hospital, London UK

Peter N. Malleson, MBBS, MRCP(UK), FRCPC, Professor of Pediatrics, Division of Rheumatology, Department of Pediatrics, University of British Columbia, British Columbia's Children's Hospital, Vancouver BC Canada

Margaret A. Marcon, MD, FRCPC, Director, Dysphagia Clinic, Division of Gastroenterology, Hepatology and Nutrition, The Hospital for Sick Children, Toronto; Assistant Professor, Department of Pediatrics, University of Toronto, Toronto ON Canada

Susanna A. McColley, MD, Division Head, Pulmonary Medicine, Children's Memorial Hospital; Associate Professor of Pediatrics, Feinberg School of Medicine, Northwestern University, Chicago IL

Cynthia J. Mears, DO, Assistant Professor of Pediatrics, Feinberg School of Medicine, Northwestern University; Medical Director, Arai Middle School Health Center, Co-Director of Adolescent Medicine Clinics, Chicago IL

Frederick W. Miller, MD, PhD, Chief, Environmental Autoimmunity Group, Office of Clinical Research, National Institute of Environmental Health Sciences, National Institutes of Health, DHHS, Bethesda MD

Laura J. Mirkinson, MD, Associate Professor of Pediatrics, George Washington University School of Medicine; Department of Pediatrics and Medical Education, Holy Cross Hospital, Washington DC

Chester V. Oddis, MD, Professor of Medicine, Division of Rheumatology and Clinical Immunology, University of Pittsburgh School of Medicine, Pittsburgh PA

Nancy Y. Olson, MD, Clinical Associate Professor, Allergy/Immunology and Pediatric Rheumatology, University of Kansas; Chief, Allergy/Immunology, Department of Pediatrics, University of Kansas, Kansas City KS

Elif Arioglu Oral, MD, Assistant Professor of Medicine, Department of Internal Medicine, Division of Endocrinology and Metabolism, University of Michigan, Ann Arbor MI

Barbara E. Ostrov, MD, Professor of Pediatrics and Medicine, Departments of Pediatrics and Medicine, Penn State College of Medicine; Chief, Division of Pediatric Rheumatology, Allergy and Immunology; Division of Rheumatology, The Milton S. Hershey Medical Center, Hershey PA

Lauren M. Pachman, MD, Professor of Pediatrics, Division of Rheumatology, Feinberg School of Medicine, Northwestern University; Director, Molecular and Cellular Pathobiology Program, The Children's Memorial Research Center, Chicago IL

Amy S. Paller, MD, Walter J. Hamlin Professor and Chair of Dermatology, Professor of Pediatrics, Northwestern University's Feinberg School of Medicine, Children's Memorial Medical Center, Chicago IL

Sandra Parker, RN, BScN, MA Ed (Candidate), Rheumatology Clinic Nurse Coordinator, The Hospital for Sick Children, Toronto ON Canada

Murray H. Passo, MD, Director, Fellowship Program, William S. Rowe Division of Rheumatology, Cincinnati Children's Hospital Medical Center; Professor of Pediatrics, University of Cincinnati College of Medicine, Cincinnati OH

Megan Perron, RN, BScN, Ambulatory Care Nurse, Bloorview MacMillan Children's Centre, Toronto ON Canada

Clarissa M. Pilkington, MBBS, Consultant in Paediatric and Adolescent Rheumatology, Great Ormond Street Hospital and Institute of Child Health, London UK

Angelo Ravelli, MD, Dirigente medico I livello, Dipartimento di Pediatria, Università di Genova; Unità Operativa Pediatria II, Istituto di Ricovero a Carattere Scientifico G. Gaslini, Genova Italy

Ann M. Reed, MD, Chair, Pediatric Rheumatology, Mayo Clinic Rochester; Professor, Pediatrics, Mayo Medical School, Rochester MN

Robert M. Rennebohm, MD, Division of Pediatric Rheumatology, Columbus Children's Hospital; Associate Professor of Pediatrics, The Ohio State University College of Medicine and Public Health, Columbus OH

Patricia A. Rettig, RN, MSN, CRNP, Pediatric Nurse Practitioner, The Children's Hospital of Philadelphia, Philadelphia PA

Lisa G. Rider, MD, Deputy Chief, Environmental Autoimmunity Group, Office of Clinical Research, National Institute of Environmental Health Sciences, National Institutes of Health, DHHS, Bethesda MD

Kelly A. Rouster-Stevens, MD, PharmD, Fellow, Division of Rheumatology, Children's Memorial Hospital, Chicago IL

Nicolino Ruperto, MD, MPH, IRCCS G. Gaslini, Pediatria II—Dipartimento di Pediatria Università de Genova, Reumatologia PRINTO, Genova Italy

Jane G. Schaller, MD, Executive Director, International Pediatric Association; Visiting Professor, Pediatrics, University of British Columbia, Vancouver BC Canada

Janine A. Smith, MD, Deputy Clinical Director, National Eye Institute, National Institutes of Health, DHHS, Bethesda MD

Michaele R. Smith, PT, MEd, Education Coordinator, Physical Therapy, Rehabilitation Medicine Department, Mark O. Hatfield Clinical Research Center, National Institutes of Health, DHHS, Bethesda MD

Beth Solomon, MS, CCC-SLP, Chief, Speech and Language Pathology Section, Rehabilitation Medicine Department, Mark O. Hatfield Clinical Research Center, National Institutes of Health, DHHS, Bethesda MD

Barbara C. Sonies, PhD, CCC-SLP, Scientist Emeritus, Department of Rehabilitation Medicine, WG Magnuson Clinical Center, National Institutes of Health, DHHS; Research Professor, University of Maryland, College Park MD

Charles H. Spencer, MD, Chief, Division of Rheumatology, LaRabida Children's Hospital; Professor of Pediatrics, The University of Chicago, Pritzker School of Medicine, Chicago IL

Kathryn A. Spooner, Programs Manager, The Myositis Association, Washington DC

Joyce L. Sundberg, RN, Family Care Coordinator and Pediatric Rheumatology Nurse, Division of Rheumatology, Children's Memorial Hospital, Chicago IL

Robert P. Sundel, MD, Director, Rheumatology Program, Children's Hospital Boston; Associate Professor of Pediatrics, Harvard Medical School, Boston MA

Ilona S. Szer, MD, Director, Pediatric Rheumatology, Rady Children's Hospital and Health Center; Professor of Clinical Pediatrics, University of California San Diego School of Medicine, San Diego CA

Janalee Taylor, RN, MSN, CNS, Clinical Nurse Specialist, Associate Clinical Director, William S. Rowe Division of Rheumatology, Cincinnati Children's Hospital Medical Center, Cincinnati OH

Renee Thomas, Facilitator, Partners in Education; Past Chair, American Juvenile Arthritis Organization, Chagrin Falls OH

Emily von Scheven, MD, Associate Professor of Clinical Pediatrics, Pediatric Rheumatology, University of California, San Francisco CA

Patience H. White, MD, MA, Chief Public Health Officer, Arthritis Foundation; Professor of Medicine and Pediatrics, George Washington University School of Medicine and Health Sciences, Washington DC

Kristi Whitney-Mahoney, MSc, BScPT, Physical Therapist, Department of Rehabilitation Services, Division of Rheumatology, The Hospital for Sick Children, Toronto ON Canada

Lori S. Wiener, DCSW, PhD, Coordinator, Pediatric Psychosocial Support and Research Program, National Cancer Institute, National Institutes of Health, DHHS, Bethesda MD

Patricia Woo, CBE, PhD, FRCP, FRCPCH, FMedSci, Academic Head and Professor of Paediatric Rheumatology, University College London; Consultant, Paediatric Rheumatology, Great Ormond Street Hospital for Sick Children, London UK

Susan J. Wright, OT, Occupational Therapist and Research Assistant, Pediatric Rheumatology, University of Kansas Medical Center, Kansas City KS

Carolyn L. Yancey, MD, Medical Officer, Center for Drug Evaluation and Research, U.S. Food and Drug Administration, DHHS, Rockville MD

Introduction

When a child develops myositis (pronounced "my-oh-SIGH-tis"), the lives of many people in that child's life are affected. Myositis literally means muscle inflammation, and children with myositis experience muscle weakness and often a skin rash. It is considered an autoimmune disease, in which the body's own immune system attacks a child's healthy tissue. (See *Chapter 1, What Is Juvenile Myositis?*, for a more detailed definition of myositis.)

This book was created primarily for the parents and families of children with myositis (which includes juvenile dermatomyositis [JDM], juvenile polymyositis [JPM], and related conditions) to provide information to you about the concerns, uncertainties, frustrations, and fears that often accompany this rare and mysterious group of disorders. This book cannot be used as a substitute for medical advice from your medical professional, but we hope that it will be a valuable resource for families, friends, teachers, other caregivers, and even healthcare professionals as they seek to work together to respond to the challenge presented by myositis. We have generally addressed the book to the parents of children. *Chapter 2, Explaining Juvenile Myositis: A Kid's Guide*, is written for parents to consider using as a script to explain myositis to their child or for older children to read. *Chapter 32, Approaching Adolescence*, has sections for parents and for teens, thereby providing an opportunity for the family to discuss the material together after a reading.

We were compelled to write this book because there are so few resources readily available to families that present useful information about juvenile myositis. Furthermore, the rarity of myositis can make families feel isolated and alone and uncertain about where to turn for medical information and for guidance, compassion, and practical help.

The goals of this book are:

- To discuss what we know and don't know about juvenile myositis in order to foster understanding and relieve unnecessary anxiety. As part of the knowledge gained, you will understand that the pattern of each child's illness is different, requiring virtually individualized decisions based primarily on experience, not always fact. By sharing our knowledge, we hope to empower parents to become more informed and involved in the healthcare decisions for their children.

- To provide support to families by directing them to the resources that can help them adjust to and overcome these illnesses.

- To encourage and inspire everyone who interacts with children with myositis to understand that love, understanding, and hope are as important as medicines and physical therapy in treating myositis.

Our intent is to provide a comprehensive overview of all aspects of juvenile myositis, including perspectives from medical, psychological, legal, and personal viewpoints. To this end, many people have responded to our requests to donate their time in sharing their expertise and wisdom to create this book, and we thank all the contributors for their selflessness and dedication to this effort. The care of a child with myositis involves a complex partnership among the child, parents, family members, friends, healthcare providers, teachers, and others who interact with the child and family. We have reached out to all these groups to obtain their unique perspectives and input into this book.

Use this book as a resource or handbook, a reference book if you will, to include broad information on a wide number of issues pertinent to patients with juvenile myositis. It is not meant to be read cover to cover in one sitting, and in fact you would be overwhelmed if you tried. It is meant to be used chapter by chapter, section by section, as needed throughout your child's illness as you want information on a particular topic. Technical information has been included in the book for your reference. If you are finding portions difficult to read, you may want to skip through those sections and read on.

The first part of the book, written by physicians and researchers, opens with *What Is Juvenile Myositis*, to explain the basic characteristics of the illness, how we think about the different types of myositis, and who becomes ill. The authors discuss the current understanding of the factors that lead to a child becoming ill with juvenile myositis and the pathways in the illness.

At the Beginning is a series of chapters that is particularly helpful to parents of children who have been recently diagnosed with myositis. It reviews the first signs of the illness, how to find appropriate healthcare for your child, and how to sort through the many challenges that you might face. It provides an understanding of the tests that are needed to confirm your child's diagnosis and a discussion of the first medicines that may be given to help your child recover.

Coping with Juvenile Myositis provides helpful suggestions for reorganizing your home and describes adaptive equipment that could be useful to enhance your child's day-to-day functioning. A second chapter helps you keep in touch with your emotions and provides strategies for handling the ups and downs that you, your child with myositis, and your other children may experience.

Following Your Child's Progress consists of two chapters that help you understand how your child's myositis doctor and other healthcare professionals will assess your child's myositis at follow-up visits, including the types of examinations and tests that might be done to see that your child is on the right path for recovery.

Treatment Options provides an in-depth look at many of the medicines frequently used after the initial months of treatment, particularly in the case of children who do not respond to the first round of medicines. This section emphasizes the potential benefits as well as some of the potential side effects, although most children experience few or only mild side effects from the medicines. Another integral part of the recovery process is rehabilitation, which includes a graded exercise program prescribed by a physical therapist or other rehabilitation health professionals. Because some families are interested in complementary and alternative medicines, including more naturalistic approaches, we also inform you about some possibilities as well as their limitations and potential for harm. Also described are exciting new medicines, called biologic therapies, which appear promising.

Important Issues on the Road to Recovery consists of fourteen chapters on specific problems that your child may face. These chapters are intended to be read when you require more information on a particular issue, since no child will face every single problem in this section. Often your child's myositis doctor will engage other healthcare specialists to help with these issues.

Hopes of Recovery describes what the long-term future may hold for your child with myositis. Although the care and treatment of children with myositis is not standardized, we have made tremendous progress in the past several decades toward understanding the variations that can occur in children with myositis. This section also assists with preparing for your child's future and the challenges of adolescence. It also addresses questions parents often face about their child's future ability to have children.

Resources and Opportunities provides practical information on your rights in getting appropriate care for your child and in obtaining reliable medical information. It also covers handling insurance coverage for all of the different costs, working with schools to enable your child to attend school but also meet medical needs, and possibilities for a summer camp experience. In addition, we provide information on the research process and how new information is learned about juvenile myositis. We hope that all of the knowledge you have gained will then empower you to help others with juvenile myositis by raising public awareness and by fundraising.

The book concludes with an appendix of resources, including ways to contact helpful organizations, books, pamphlets, Internet sites, and services that may be helpful for your child with myositis. Some chapters end with additional resources about that topic. A comprehensive index is found at the end of the book, so that you can more easily find information on a particular topic at a later date.

Each chapter begins with a statement about the content of the chapter—what the reader can expect to find. This is followed by a personal statement from a child or parent or friend describing their experience relating to the topic of the chapter, "From the family's point of view...." Chapters are written as a series of questions, inspired by the most common questions we have been asked over the years, followed by answers about issues relating to the topic of the chapter. The text often refers to a girl with juvenile myositis ("she") but is meant to apply to both girls and boys. The decision to use the female gender was based on the fact that girls are affected by juvenile myositis twice as often as boys. Although we would like this book to be useful to international audiences, we have focused on practices and information sources most relevant to children living in the United States. Each chapter concludes with key points, followed by resources on the specific topic that may be helpful to families ("To Learn More"), as well as reports from the medical literature for families or health professionals who seek additional information of a more technical nature.

You will see the term "juvenile myositis" (JM) used throughout the book as a general term for the many forms of myositis that children can develop. When we are referring to a specific form, such as juvenile dermatomyositis (JDM) or juvenile polymyositis (JPM), we will use the appropriate term. We have tried to make this an easy book to read, but some chapters dealing with more complex issues are necessarily more difficult to understand than others. You will find some of the more commonly used and technical terms in the glossary at the end of this book. We encourage you to discuss with your child's doctor any concepts that remain unclear after reading the information.

We have also included references to medical articles or books in the "Reports in the Medical Literature" section at the end of each chapter, although we realize that medical professionals have written these for the medical community rather than for patients and their families. Many of these medical references can be found in electronic form on the Internet using a searchable web site supported by the National Library of Medicine known as PubMed (www.pubmed.gov). A service of the National Institutes of Health, PubMed Central, available at www.pubmed central.nih.gov, provides free, open access to scientific journal articles. Some of the journals at this site provide immediate open access, whereas other published research papers are available here on a delayed basis, after appearing first in their primary journal. Alternatively, these articles can often be found in paper form in a university or medical school library. A few are also available on The Myositis Association's web site, www.myositis.org/jmbookresources.cfm. Again, these may be resources that you can obtain from, or discuss with, your own healthcare professional.

Much of what we understand about juvenile myositis today has been the result of decades of basic and clinical research. Yet, as much as we have learned, we are still in the early stages of our understanding of juvenile myositis. We still do not understand the underlying causes, all of the ways in which the complications may occur or be prevented, and how to develop the best treatments in a rigorous, scientific way with the least number of side effects. We have much to learn. We have only just cracked open the door, and much important research still needs to be done to improve the care and outcome of children with myositis.

This book is not meant to be a substitute for professional care. You should discuss any medical concerns and questions with your child's myositis doctor, who should always be your primary medical resource for your child. We have tried to be as complete, practical, and accurate as possible. But given the incredible breadth and technicality of information that is available, the uncertainties about many aspects of juvenile myositis that still remain, and the rapidly changing approaches to these disorders, information in this book is not necessarily a complete compendium of all available knowledge. It is also reasonable that some of the information in this book will become outdated by new findings. Additionally, different doctors advocate different approaches because they have different knowledge, experiences, and philosophies about the evaluation or treatment of children with myositis. Therefore, it is possible that the information in this book may not be exactly the same as what you hear from your child's doctors—and this may be for good reasons specific to your situation. Finally, juvenile myositis includes a wide range of disorders, which are often expressed very differently and sometimes uniquely in each child, so the general descriptions and guidance offered in some of the chapters might not apply to your child.

Despite these necessary realities and limitations, we hope that *Myositis and You* will have something for everyone who is seeking more information about the problems of and approaches to treating juvenile myositis. We anticipate that it will provide information and resources for learning more about a particular issue, as well as inspiration and hope.

—The Editors
Lisa G. Rider, MD, Lauren M. Pachman, MD,
Frederick W. Miller, MD, PhD, and Harriet Bollar

Disclaimer of Medical Advice and of Liability

This book is provided for informational purposes and is not medical advice. The book is not a complete statement in context of all potentially relevant information related to myositis, nor each reader's situation, and cannot be used as a substitute for a medical review, examination, diagnosis, and informed medical advice and consent in relation to any specific person, condition, or medical and treatment needs.

In addition, the information about medicines and treatments discussed in this book is of a general nature. It does not and cannot cover all possible uses, actions, precautions, side effects, or interactions of the medicines or treatments mentioned, nor is the information intended as medical advice for individual problems or for making an evaluation as to the risks and benefits of taking a particular drug or course of action. The absence of a warning for a given vitamin, mineral, herb, plant, prescription or non-prescription drug, or any combination of these substances or treatments is not intended and shall not be construed to indicate that the substance or course of action is safe, appropriate, or effective for any given person or for any particular situation.

In sum, the information in this book cannot be used as a substitute for or to delay consultation with appropriate, certified medical healthcare provider(s) to obtain proper and complete medical advice for your specific situation or that of your family member.

Also, inclusion of information in this book is not intended to be, and may not be construed as, any endorsement of that information, a certification or warranty of the accuracy of the information, or a recommendation for any treatment or course of action by or for any person. Moreover, information contained in or suggested by this book that otherwise is accurate at the time of publishing can become outdated, invalid, inaccurate, and/or subject to debate given rapid advances in medicine and general knowledge.

The publisher, editors, contributors, and sponsors of this book, as well as The Myositis Association and Cure JM Foundation, and their respective executive directors, board directors, officers, staff, volunteers, members, and donors, are not making any representation or warranty, expressed or implied, regarding the contents of this book. All liability is disclaimed for any direct, indirect, special, incidental, secondary, or consequential damages resulting from any direct or indirect use of the book or the information or ideas in it or suggestions implied by it, whether such use was intended or not. This includes, but is not limited to, references to web sites in this book, which does not imply and does not constitute endorsement of the web sites or the organizations publishing them, which remain solely responsible for their content.

What Is Juvenile Myositis?

CHAPTER 1

What Is Juvenile Myositis?

Lisa G. Rider, MD, and Frederick W. Miller, MD, PhD

In this chapter...

We define juvenile myositis and provide information about who gets sick with juvenile myositis and how your child's doctor can confirm a diagnosis of juvenile myositis. We discuss the different types of juvenile myositis and compare juvenile and adult myositis.

From the family's point of view...

"During the school years, many kids experience growing pains, but be careful—sometimes these pains are not just from growing up. I know this from experience: I was diagnosed with juvenile dermatomyositis recently, but began having the symptoms long before. Dermatomyositis is an autoimmune disorder in which your own immune system attacks your muscles and skin. The first sign is often a skin rash. It usually appears to be a dry red patch but after time becomes a red or purplish rash that can be very itchy. This rash appears on your eyelids, fingers, and can appear other places. Not everyone experiences the rash first, though. Some people feel like they are getting weaker."

What Is Juvenile Myositis?

Myositis (pronounced "my-oh-SIGH-tis") is a group of illnesses that involve muscle inflammation. The word *myositis* comes from the roots *myo,* which means muscle, and *itis,* which means inflammation. Approximately one in five people with myositis have juvenile myositis (JM), which begins in people younger than eighteen years of age. Even adults can have persistent juvenile myositis if they first became sick as a child.

Juvenile myositis is also referred to in medical reports as idiopathic inflammatory myopathies, commonly abbreviated as IIM. Idiopathic means the cause is not known or understood, inflammatory means that swelling or inflammation is present, and myopathy is a sickness of muscle. Juvenile myositis is a broad name for several different illnesses that have slightly different symptoms. All of them involve muscle weakness. Some involve characteristic skin rashes, particularly juvenile dermatomyositis (JDM), and some do not, such as juvenile polymyositis (JPM).

Adult myositis is similar to juvenile myositis with a few critical differences. The different types of juvenile and adult myositis are discussed later in this chapter.

Juvenile and adult forms of myositis are thought to be autoimmune diseases. This means that the immune system, which normally protects the body by attacking infections and other harmful entities, does not work right and attacks part of your own body instead. If you have myositis, your immune system will attack your muscles and some other tissues, causing weakness, swelling, and pain. This results in inflammation (the immune cells entering the affected tissues, resulting in redness, pain, and swelling). Your immune system may be attacking for a good reason, or it may be attacking because it mistakenly sees your muscles as something not belonging to your body. Either of these situations may occur in juvenile myositis; we don't know for sure, but we think autoimmunity, where the immune system attacks your own tissues, is occurring.

We don't know exactly what causes juvenile myositis. But we think that in order to become sick with juvenile myositis, a child needs to come in contact with one or more factors from their surroundings (called environmental exposures), including certain infections, sunlight, life stressors, or other stimulants of the immune system or muscle. A specific combination of genes (probably many genes) is also needed. Genes are the inherited material inside your body's cells (DNA) that make up your body and give directions for your body to work as it should. Probably because a combination of environmental exposures and many genes is necessary for juvenile myositis to develop, it is not very common. It is important to be reassured that juvenile myositis is not contagious, like a cold or the flu. You will learn more about the possible causes of myositis and the role the immune system plays in the illness in *Chapter 3, The Pathways to Juvenile Myositis*.

Who Gets Juvenile Myositis?

Myositis can affect people of any age. Most children who get sick with juvenile myositis are four to fifteen years old. The average age at onset of JDM, the form with characteristic skin rashes, is six to seven years. Children with JPM, the type of JM that does not have certain rashes, or with myositis overlapping with another autoimmune disease (overlap myositis), in which myositis is present along with another autoimmune disease, tend to get sick when they are a few years older.

Most forms of juvenile myositis affect girls twice as often as boys, even before the onset of puberty. Juvenile myositis affects children of all racial and ethnic groups throughout the world.

How Common Is Juvenile Myositis?

We know that juvenile myositis is rare, but we do not know exactly how often it develops. This is because the actual frequency of a rare disease is difficult to measure. Our best guess, based on a recent study, is that at least three children in a million develop JDM each year in the United States. If this estimate is correct, then approximately two hundred to five hundred new cases of JDM will develop each year in the United States. Estimates from other studies conducted around the world suggest that one to five children in a million will get sick with juvenile myositis each year. The total number of children and adults who currently have juvenile myositis is also unknown. We believe it is well under one hundred thousand individuals and perhaps only several thousand individuals. Juvenile myositis occurs about one-fifth as often as adult myositis. Some studies suggest that the frequency of myositis might be increasing.

What Are the Main Symptoms of Juvenile Myositis?

In most children who get sick with juvenile myositis, the illness develops slowly over a period of weeks to months but sometimes can come on suddenly.

Muscle Weakness

Almost all forms of juvenile myositis involve lasting and worsening muscle weakness. Usually, the weakness is proximal, which means that it involves muscles close to the body, such as upper arms or thighs. The axial or trunk muscles can also frequently be involved; they include the neck, abdominal, or back muscles. When these muscles are affected, many kids have trouble doing sit-ups or lifting their head off the bed. Distal muscles (those below the elbow or knees such as in the wrists, hands, and feet) can also be involved, especially in people with JPM and those more severely affected with JDM.

Although nearly all patients have weakness, the first signs of illness can be more subtle. These signs might include tiredness or crankiness after activities, difficulty keeping up in sports or with friends, trouble climbing stairs or getting into a car or school bus, trouble combing or shampooing hair, or trouble getting dressed. Muscle pain and tenderness can also be prominent. If the illness is untreated, patients can eventually become so weak that they have difficulty getting out of bed or even feeding themselves.

Rashes

Children with JDM, the most common form of juvenile myositis, often have rashes instead of muscle weakness as their first problem. In JDM, the skin develops certain rashes, called Gottron's papules and the heliotrope rash. Gottron's papules are red and raised or rough scaly patches over the knuckles, elbows, knees, insides of the ankles, or even over the toe joints (Figure 1.1). The heliotrope rash, named after a lilac-colored flower (Figure 1.2), is a purple or red coloring over the eyelids that can also cause eyelid swelling. The presence of Gottron's papules or the heliotrope rash is needed to confirm a diagnosis of JDM. Children with JDM can have a number of other rashes, including some that may be caused or worsened by sunlight. The various rashes of JDM and ways to treat them will be further discussed in *Chapter 16, Skin Rashes and Sun Protection.*

■ Figure 1.1. (See color plate 1 on page 227.) Gottron's papules.

Gottron's papules are red and raised or rough scaly patches present over the knuckles. They may also be seen over the elbows, knees, insides of the ankles, or even over the toe joints.

■ Figure 1.2. (See color plate 2 on page 227.) Heliotrope rash.

The heliotrope rash is a purple or red coloring over the eyelids that can also cause eyelid swelling. It is named after a lilac-colored flower.

Other Symptoms

Juvenile myositis is a systemic illness and can be associated with inflammation in other parts of the body, such as the joints, intestinal tract, lungs, and heart. Other possible symptoms of juvenile myositis include fever, weight loss, and tenderness or pain in the joints (arthritis). Difficulty swallowing, change in voice quality, trouble breathing especially during exercise, and stomach pain can also be frequent symptoms. Learn more about the early signs and symptoms of juvenile myositis in *Chapter 4, First Signs of Illness.*

Once the diagnosis or presence of juvenile myositis is confirmed, the symptoms can be treated with medicines (see *Chapter 7, Treatment Possibilities in the Beginning* and *Chapter 12, Possible Medicines During the Course*). Most children also require physical therapy (see *Chapter 13, Rehabilitation of the Child with Myositis*). Many symptoms of juvenile myositis often respond to treatment. In some patients, the symptoms go away with treatment and no further medicine is needed, a situation we call "remission." In others, the symptoms may become worse or return despite treatment, which we call an illness "flare." The usual indicators of a flare are worsening symptoms of muscle weakness, tiredness, skin rashes, greater swallowing difficulty or stomach pain, or arthritis. The changes in symptoms and signs of juvenile myositis over time, which we call the disease course, will be discussed further in *Chapter 30, The Clinical Course and Outcome of Juvenile Myositis.*

How Is Juvenile Myositis Identified?

It can often be difficult for your child's doctor to confirm whether your child has juvenile myositis. This is because juvenile myositis can resemble many other illnesses; different children with juvenile myositis can have different symptoms; and many doctors are not familiar with juvenile myositis because it is so rare.

Doctors need to rule out other illnesses before they can confirm that your child has juvenile myositis. They need to consider the symptoms (problems the child experiences), the signs (findings that are recognized by a physical examination), and the results of laboratory tests. For these reasons, your child's doctor might have to perform many tests and see your child several times before confirming the diagnosis of juvenile myositis, or your child's doctor might refer you to a specialist in rheumatology, neurology, or dermatology.

To confirm that your child has juvenile myositis, doctors must examine your child and test the strength of the muscles (see *Chapter 11, Assessing Muscle Strength, Endurance, and Function*). The presence of certain skin rashes, called Gottron's papules or heliotrope, helps a doctor to identify JDM, but these symptoms and signs are not present in JPM.

What Tests Are Used to Confirm That Your Child Has Juvenile Myositis?

Blood tests. Blood testing often shows that children with JM have unusually high activity in one or more muscle enzymes, which are proteins in the muscle that help the muscle make energy or carry out other metabolic processes. These enzymes include creatine kinase (CK), aldolase, lactate dehydrogenase (LD), aspartate aminotransferase (AST), and alanine aminotransferase (ALT). Children with juvenile myositis have high blood levels of one or more of these enzymes because muscle cells leak these enzymes into the blood when they have been injured by inflammation. Enzyme levels tend to increase in the blood when myositis worsens and decrease as it improves.

EMG. Another tool used to help confirm that your child has juvenile myositis is an electromyogram (EMG). An EMG uses a needle inserted into the muscle to measure its electrical activity. An EMG can help determine whether the muscles are abnormal, and whether the muscle injury is due to inflammation. Sometimes muscle weakness can be caused by nerve damage rather than muscle damage. When needed, other electrical tests of the nerves can be done with the EMG, called nerve conduction velocity. These can help determine whether the nerves that stimulate the muscles are functioning properly. The EMG test is not always needed to confirm your child has myositis. Your child's doctor will decide to do this test when it becomes helpful to distinguish myositis from other conditions that mimic myositis.

Muscle biopsy. Your child's doctor might also request that a muscle biopsy be done. This test involves removing a small piece of muscle tissue, either by using a needle or by making a surgical cut, and then examining it under a microscope. If your child has a muscle biopsy, she is either put to sleep or given medicine so that she does not feel any pain during the procedure. The results of the muscle biopsy show your child's doctor whether and how the muscle fibers are damaged and whether other causes of muscle damage are present. It also can help the doctor figure out which type of myositis your child has. A biopsy is the best test to be sure that other causes of muscle weakness are not present and is especially helpful when the rash or other signs of juvenile myositis are not present. Again, many children with myositis will not undergo a muscle biopsy test, particularly if the child's doctor feels more certain that myositis is the diagnosis based on the child's strength, skin rashes, and blood tests or EMG.

Other tests. Some additional tests might be done but are not done by all doctors or in all patients. Another test your child's doctor might order is magnetic resonance imaging (MRI) of the weak muscles, most often the thigh muscles. MRI uses a strong magnet to create a detailed picture of your child's muscles and shows where the inflammation and muscle damage is. This picture of your child's muscles can help your child's doctors decide where to do a muscle biopsy or EMG, or it can help to confirm a diagnosis of myositis.

Doctors might also test your child's blood for autoantibodies, which are proteins made by the immune system that recognize specific parts inside of cells in the body. Different autoantibodies are described later in this chapter. Doctors might also test the blood for infectious illnesses to be sure that your child does not have a virus or other infection that can mimic juvenile myositis. The tests used to assist in confirming that your child has juvenile myositis are discussed in more detail in *Chapter 6, Tests Your Child's Doctor Might Order.*

Guidelines for Identifying Juvenile Myositis

Your child's doctor can identify (or diagnose) juvenile myositis by first ruling out all other possible causes of muscle weakness and then by finding at least three of the following five features:

- Muscle weakness in the shoulders or hips
- Specific skin rashes associated with JDM
- High blood levels of muscle enzymes
- Muscle biopsy changes
- EMG findings

Although these rules for diagnosing myositis were developed almost thirty years ago (Table 1.1), they are still the most useful way to tell myositis from other kinds of muscle disease. Newer rules to diagnose myositis have been suggested and others are being developed, but they have not yet been proven helpful in identifying myositis or deciding what type of myositis is present.

Distinguishing Juvenile Myositis from Other Illnesses

When your child first gets sick, your child's doctors will need to consider the possibility of several other illnesses before they can confirm that your child has juvenile myositis. In children with both muscle weakness and skin rashes, sys-

Table 1.1. How doctors identify a child with juvenile myositis.

First, the doctor will need to be sure the child does not have other sicknesses causing these problems.

The presence of three of the five findings below indicates that myositis is the probable diagnosis, and at least four of five findings indicates definite myositis. Dermatomyositis requires skin changes (#5).

1. Weakness of muscles close to the body (proximal muscles = the shoulders and hips)

2. Elevated blood levels of muscle enzymes

3. Electromyogram (EMG) has abnormal electrical activity in the muscle and findings consistent with muscle inflammation

4. Muscle biopsy (examination of piece of muscle tissue under the microscope) demonstrates characteristic changes with inflammation in the tissue and other findings

5. Skin rashes of dermatomyositis: Gottron's papules (red, scaly rash over joints) or heliotrope rash (purplish to red discoloration over eyelid)

Modified from Bohan A, Peter JB. Polymyositis and dermatomyositis. *New England Journal of Medicine.* 1975 Feb 13;292(7):344–47.

temic autoimmune diseases, such as systemic lupus erythematosus (SLE), systemic sclerosis, and juvenile rheumatoid arthritis, will be considered, because the rashes and widespread complaints are frequently part of these other illnesses. Certain skin conditions, including psoriasis, eczema, and seborrhea, can have rashes that are similar to those characteristic of JDM. Some viral, bacterial, and parasitic infections can mimic JDM and JPM. Certain drugs and toxins can cause rashes similar to those common in JDM or can make the muscles weak, which can mimic JPM (see also *Chapter 4, First Signs of Illness* for more information on other illnesses your doctor will consider before confirming that your child has JDM).

For children who have only muscle weakness without the characteristic JDM rashes, your child's doctor will likely consider several other disorders before being able to confirm that your child has juvenile myositis. These include thyroid disease, diabetes, body salt (electrolyte) imbalances, and muscle diseases, including muscular dystrophies (muscle illnesses in which a gene for a particular part of the muscle is abnormal), metabolic myopathies (muscle illnesses in which the digestion of sugar or fat is disrupted), and mitochondrial myopathies (illnesses in which the cells that supply energy inside of muscle and other tissues do not work correctly). We believe that a muscle biopsy is required if your child has muscle weakness without skin rashes in order to rule out these other conditions that mimic juvenile myositis.

How Many Types of Juvenile Myositis Are There?

There are several types of juvenile myositis. Doctors can tell them apart by what problems your child has, as well as by the muscle biopsy findings (Figure 1.3).

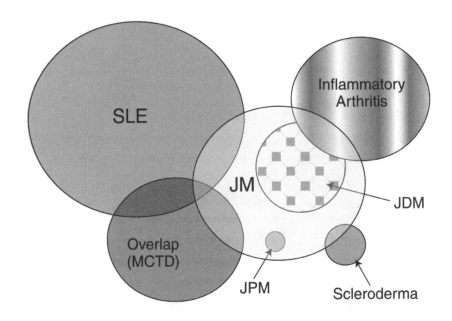

■ **Figure 1.3. Venn diagram of juvenile dermatomyositis and juvenile polymyositis relative to other rheumatic diseases of children.**
Juvenile myositis (JM) is composed of juvenile dermatomyositis (JDM) and juvenile polymyositis (JPM), overlap myositis, and other rarer forms of myositis (not shown), which must be differentiated from each other. Juvenile myositis shares some components with diseases like inflammatory arthritis, systemic lupus erythematosus (SLE), scleroderma, and overlap syndromes, such as mixed connective tissue disease (MCTD), but is quite different from them overall.

Juvenile Dermatomyositis

The main form of juvenile myositis is juvenile dermatomyositis (JDM). Up to 85% of all patients with juvenile myositis have JDM. These children have the characteristic rashes of Gottron's papules or heliotrope rash (Figures 1.1 and 1.2), but they can also have other skin rashes (see *Chapter 16, Skin Rashes and Sun Protection*).

In addition, JDM patients can have other problems that are specific to JDM, such as: calcinosis, in which small lumps or sheets of calcium are deposited in the skin, fat tissue, and muscle (see *Chapter 17, Calcinosis*); ulcerations of the skin or gastrointestinal tract (that is, the stomach and intestines); as well as lipodystrophy, a loss of body fat tissue (see *Chapter 26, Too Much Body Fat Loss*).

These problems do not occur in most children with JDM but are troubling when they do occur.

Less Common Forms of Juvenile Myositis

There are also several other less common forms of juvenile myositis.

Juvenile polymyositis (JPM) causes muscle inflammation and weakness without the characteristic rashes of JDM (*poly* means that many muscles are involved). This form of myositis occurs in 5%–10% of children with juvenile myositis.

In some children, myositis occurs together with or develops into another autoimmune disease. This is called overlap myositis, found in 5%–10% of juvenile myositis patients. Many different autoimmune diseases can be found in the same child who also has myositis, including systemic lupus erythematosus, scleroderma, thyroid disease, diabetes, psoriasis, and celiac disease, among others. The feature of overlap myositis and the associated autoimmune diseases will be discussed further in *Chapter 28, When Your Child Has More Than One Autoimmune Disease.*

Juvenile dermatomyositis sine myositis is also known as amyopathic dermatomyositis (*amyopathic* means the muscles are not involved). Patients with this condition have only the characteristic skin rashes of JDM. All tests for muscle problems, including muscle strength testing, blood tests for enzyme levels, and other specialized tests, indicate that the muscles are not weak or inflamed. This form of myositis accounts for a very small portion of all JM cases.

Rare Forms of Juvenile Myositis

The other types of myositis are quite uncommon in children but not completely unheard of, and some are more frequent in adults. For some of these, there are only rare case reports involving children.

A form of juvenile myositis called focal myositis can occur in a single group of muscles in the body, such as one arm, one leg, or the chest. The affected muscles are weak or painful. Focal myositis can go away without treatment or progress to a more serious form that requires treatment. When the affected muscle is one that moves the eyes, the condition is called orbital myositis or ocular myositis. Orbital myositis can cause eye pain (particularly with movement), double vision, and eyelid swelling.

Macrophagic myositis is another form of focal myositis. It occurs after certain vaccines and involves the muscle group where the vaccine shot was given. It causes pain, swelling, tenderness, and weakness in that muscle only. Macrophagic myositis can be identified clearly through muscle biopsy because macrophages, a type of white blood cell, are very prominent in the tissue.

In eosinophilic myositis, a certain blood cell that has an orange-red color when prepared for viewing under a microscope, called the eosinophil, is present in the muscle tissue and can be seen under the microscope as part of a muscle biopsy. There also might be a higher-than-usual number of eosinophils in the blood. Certain drugs, toxins, and infections cause this type of myositis.

Inclusion body myositis is rare in children, but it is one of the most common forms of myositis in adults over age fifty. It is named for small structures called inclusion bodies, which contain broken-down muscle cell proteins and can be seen under the microscope as part of a muscle biopsy. In this form, muscle weakness worsens slowly over time. The distal muscles (muscles in the hands or feet), as well as thigh muscles are frequently involved. Falling episodes and trouble swallowing are common.

Cancer-associated myositis is also fortunately very rare in children but relatively more common in older adults with myositis. This type of myositis develops within two years after the cancer starts. It may worsen or improve as the cancer worsens or improves.

In this book we will mainly focus on JDM because it is the main form of myositis in children, but we will also provide some information about juvenile polymyositis and overlap myositis. Some of the information in this book can be applied to the other forms of juvenile myositis, although they might not be mentioned specifically.

What Are Autoantibodies?

Another way to figure out what type of juvenile myositis a child has is to test for certain autoantibodies. Autoantibodies are proteins made by the immune system that recognize specific structures on the surface or inside of cells. Many autoantibodies recognize all cells, not just muscle cells, inside their body. Autoantibodies found only in patients with myositis and not in patients with other autoimmune diseases are known as myositis-specific autoantibodies. Those found in patients with myositis as well as in patients with other autoimmune diseases are called myositis-associated autoantibodies. Although autoantibodies cause harm to tissues in some diseases, it is not clear that the myositis-specific autoantibodies harm the muscles or cause myositis. Even so, we use these autoantibodies to help figure out what type of illness your child has.

These autoantibodies tend to bind to things inside of all cells that are involved in putting together proteins, unwinding DNA, or other basic cell functions, and by doing so, stop them from functioning. Because these autoantibodies attack cellular components, they may inhibit the basic functions of those cells. For example, autoantibodies to aminoacyl-tRNA synthetases, or simply synthetases, are directed against enzymes located inside all cells that build proteins by joining amino acids (the basic building blocks of proteins) together. Antibodies to the signal recognition particle (SRP) are directed against a group of proteins that help in moving newly made proteins into a specialized compartment inside cells in order for the protein to be changed further. The Mi-2 autoantibody is directed against an enzyme that unwinds DNA to help it make other molecules called RNA that help make proteins inside of cells. For some autoantibodies we do not yet know their target; this is the case, for example, for anti-p155 autoantibody, which is the most frequent autoantibody identified to date in JDM patients.

Several different myositis-specific and myositis-associated autoantibodies have been identified in approximately 10%–45% of patients with juvenile myositis. Although some children do not have known autoantibodies, this is an active area of research, and new autoantibodies are still being found. Many juvenile myositis patients have autoantibodies that are not yet detected by the usual tests.

It is difficult to test for these autoantibodies, and reliable tests are available only in certain research labs. Such testing may not be necessary or appropriate in all patients. Your child's doctor will decide whether he or she thinks that an autoantibody test will be valuable. Sometimes the results might help your child's doctor to decide which treatment to use or to predict whether your child's illness is likely to progress.

Patients with myositis-specific autoantibodies have certain problems in common. In some cases they may respond in similar ways to treatment, or their illness may progress in similar ways. Following are some examples:

- **Anti-synthetase autoantibodies.** Children with JDM, JPM, or overlap myositis (as well as adults with the corresponding adult form of myositis) can have these myositis-specific antibodies. The most common type of anti-synthetase autoantibody is called anti-Jo-1. Patients with anti-synthetase autoantibodies frequently develop moderate to severe muscle weakness, very high levels of muscle enzymes, fevers, arthritis, and lung problems. They may respond to the usual treatments for myositis, but their illness usually gets worse when medicines are reduced.

- **Anti-SRP autoantibodies.** Patients with antibodies to the signal recognition particle, also called SRP, have polymyositis that often starts quickly in the fall season. They have severe muscle weakness involving many muscle groups and very high levels of creatine kinase and other muscle enzymes in the blood. They also have serious trouble with muscle thinning or atrophy, frequently requiring extensive rehabilitation. They do not respond well to many of the medicines used to treat juvenile myositis. Often they need combinations of medicines to control their illness.

- **Mi-2 autoantibodies.** Patients with these autoantibodies have juvenile or adult dermatomyositis. They tend to have mild to moderate muscle involvement and certain skin rashes, especially rashes made worse by sunlight (photosensitive skin rashes). They respond reasonably well to the usual treatments.

Some of the myositis-associated autoantibodies also have certain clinical patterns of illness, but we won't be able to go into all of them here (see *Chapter 6, Tests Your Child's Doctor Might Order*). For some autoantibodies, the associated clinical features are still being researched. The disease courses for these autoantibody subgroups will be described further in *Chapter 30, The Clinical Course and Outcome of Juvenile Myositis*.

How Is Juvenile Myositis Different from Adult Myositis?

Myositis that develops in people over 18 years of age is adult myositis. Although the types of myositis found in children also occur in adults, their frequency and related complications differ from those in children. Some examples of differences between juvenile and adult myositis include:

- Polymyositis, inclusion body myositis, and cancer-associated myositis are much more common in adults than children.

- Adults are more likely than children to have myositis-specific autoantibodies. However, our understanding of this could change as new autoantibodies are found.

- Children and adults can develop many of the same problems with their illness, including muscle weakness, skin rashes, swallowing and digestive system difficulties, arthritis or less flexibility in their joints, etc. Adults seem to develop heart and lung problems more often than children.

- Children are more likely than adults to have certain problems with their dermatomyositis. Children more frequently develop calcinosis, skin or digestive tract ulcers, or lipodystrophy, a loss of body fat.

- Juvenile myositis or its treatments can affect children's growth and development (discussed further in *Chapter 20, Growth and Development*).

- Although juvenile and adult myositis are treated similarly, patients with juvenile myositis seem to respond better to treatment and may be able to recover more completely (see *Chapter 30, The Clinical Course and Outcome of Juvenile Myositis*).

- Some of the genes that put people at risk of getting sick with myositis appear to be the same in people with juvenile myositis and those with adult myositis. However, there may be differences in some genetic and environmental risk factors between juvenile and adult myositis.

There are probably more similarities and differences between juvenile and adult myositis that we do not yet fully understand.

Key Points

- Juvenile myositis is a group of uncommon childhood diseases involving inflammation of the muscles and muscle weakness (*myo* means "muscle" and *itis* means "inflammation").

- Only about three children per million develop juvenile myositis each year. Girls are affected about twice as often as boys.

- Signs, symptoms, and lab tests to assist your child's doctor in diagnosis include:
  - Muscle weakness (the child is unable to walk, run, or climb normally, and tires with activities)
  - Abnormal blood tests: elevated levels of enzymes such as
    - creatine kinase [CK]
    - aldolase
    - lactate dehydrogenase [LD]
    - aspartate aminotransferase [AST]
    - alanine aminotransferase [ALT]
  - Specific rashes
    - purplish areas on the eyelids or around the eyes, called the heliotrope rash
    - scaly red bumps over the knuckles or elbows or knees, called Gottron's papules
  - Muscle tissue by biopsy shows muscle inflammation, when the tissue is looked at under a microscope
  - Abnormal electrical activity of the muscles (determined by electromyographic [EMG] testing)

- Juvenile dermatomyositis (where characteristic rashes are present) is the most common form of myositis in children. Other forms of myositis exist in children, including one form of muscle weakness of many muscles without the characteristic rashes (juvenile polymyositis), one without significant muscle involvement (amyopathic dermatomyositis), and those where another connective tissue disease like lupus is present (overlap myositis).

- The presence of certain autoantibodies, called myositis-specific and myositis-associated autoantibodies, may help in defining groups of JM patients with similar problems and responses to treatment.

- Juvenile myositis has certain features in common with adult myositis and some differences.

To Learn More

The Myositis Association (TMA).

What is juvenile myositis (JM)? Available from: www.myositis.org/jmbook resources.cfm.

Juvenile myositis [printable brochure]. Available from: www.myositis.org/jmbook resources.cfm or 800-821-7356.

Find more on the juvenile myositis pages of www.myositis.org.

Cure JM Foundation.

What is JM? Available at: www.curejm.com/info/jm.htm or 760-487-1079.

Find more at www.curejm.com.

For more information, see Myositis-Specific Organizations *and* Other Support Organizations *in the Resource Appendix.*

Reports in the Medical Literature

Bohan A, Peter JB. Polymyositis and dermatomyositis. *New England Journal of Medicine.* 1975 Feb 13;292(7):344–47.

Mendez EP, Lipton R, Ramsey-Goldman R, Roettcher P, Bowyer S, Dyer A, Pachman LM; NIAMS Juvenile DM Registry Physician Referral Group. U.S. incidence of juvenile dermatomyositis, 1995–1998: results from the National Institute of Arthritis and Musculoskeletal and Skin Diseases Registry. *Arthritis and Rheumatism (Arthritis Care and Research).* 2003 Jun 15;49(3):300–5.

Rider LG, Miller FW. Idiopathic inflammatory muscle disease: clinical aspects. *Bailliere's Best Practice and Research. Clinical Rheumatology.* 2000 Mar;14(1):37–54.

Rider LG, Miller FW. Classification and treatment of juvenile idiopathic inflammatory myopathies. *Rheumatic Diseases Clinics of North America.* 1997 Aug;23(3):619–55.

Wedderburn LR, Li CK. Paediatric idiopathic inflammatory muscle disease. *Best Practice and Research. Clinical Rheumatology.* 2004 Jun;18(3):345–58.

CHAPTER 2

Explaining Juvenile Myositis: A Kid's Guide

Lauren M. Pachman, MD,
with the help of children with juvenile myositis and their families

In this chapter...

We present a way to help younger children understand what is happening to them. Parents can read along with their child and explain how the general statements in each section may or may not apply to them—such as seeing a doctor in a hospital as opposed to an office nearby.

From the patient's point of view...

"My fighting cells in my body are being tricked. They think my muscles are the virus. The medicine I get in my port is telling my fighting cells to stop going after my muscles, that they are not the virus. Boy, that is tricky."

This chapter is divided into two sections. The first section has suggestions for material that a parent might tell or read to the child. The family might use this section to explain JM to their young child—usually one who is six to eight years old or younger. Some children might also prefer not to read about JDM on their own. The second section is for older children who want to read about juvenile myositis for themselves.

Section 1: For the Young Child

What's Different About Me Now?

It seems that you maybe are not as strong as you used to be. Sometimes it is much harder to run and keep up with your friends or climb stairs or even get out of bed—and that can make you feel cranky or mad or sad. Sometimes your skin may feel hot or itchy—that is part of the problem, and medicines will make it feel better. We understand that sometimes you just don't feel good. Sometimes the medicine you take to help your muscles might make you feel moody, so that one minute you feel like crying, and the next minute you feel just great. Let your family and the doctor know about the stuff that bothers you, so they can help figure out how to make things better!

Did I Do Anything Wrong to Get This Way?

No, there is nothing that you did or didn't do that caused the problem. Myositis just happens to some kids, and even doctors aren't sure why that is—but they are trying to figure it out!

Why Am I Going to See a Doctor?

You see your doctor so that you can feel better. There are a lot of people who will help you get better—your family, your doctors and nurses, and the physical therapists, the people who give you exercises to make you stronger. Your teacher wants to help you, too!

Why Do I Need Blood Tests?

The doctors need to test your blood to figure out how much and what kind of medicine to give you. You can ask for a white cream to put on your arm that takes the "ouch" out of getting the blood, so it does not hurt.

Why Do I Need Medicine?

Medicines can be liquid or they can be pills—some are big and some are little. You can take most of the medicines by mouth. Some of the medicines for the skin can be put on the red places directly. Other medicines must go straight to the muscles through your veins (blue lines on your arm) so that you can get better faster. Once you start taking the medicines, you will begin to feel better and stronger. It may take a long time to feel better all the way and completely strong again, and it may take even longer for the rash, if you have one, to go away.

How Can I Help Myself to Get Better—As Fast As Possible?

- Wear sunscreen and a hat when you go outside. Wear long sleeves when you can, and stay out of the sun as much as possible.
- Drink lots of milk, and eat foods that are good for your body, not the salty or fatty ones.
- Let your body take a nap when it is tired.
- Stretch and do your exercises to make your muscles stronger.
- Take the medicines that are special for you.

You will get better! You will run and play again! Just wait and see!

Section 2: For Older Children

What Is the Name of What's Wrong with Me?

There are several names for slightly different illnesses. First, there's the general label of "juvenile myositis"—which just means that people under eighteen years of age have a special version of myositis. The "myo" part means "muscle," and the "itis" part means that there is inflammation or swelling.

The most common form is juvenile dermatomyositis. The "dermato" part means "skin," and both your muscles and your skin are involved. The other type of myositis in children is called juvenile polymyositis. The "poly" means that there are "many" muscles that are affected, but there is no rash.

What Will Happen to Me?

You may feel more tired when you run, or you might not be able to do a lot of things that you could do well a few weeks or months ago, like keep up with your friends, climb stairs, comb or shampoo your hair, or other things. Some children have red rashes on their face or the knuckles of their hands or other places. These rashes might feel itchy and even sore.

Why Do I Need to See a Doctor?

When your car breaks down, you take it to a mechanic. When your body stops working right, you have to go to someone who knows how the body works to check you out. You may have been to several doctors who have helped to figure out that you have juvenile myositis. There are special doctors who just take care of children with illnesses like yours. You may get to see your doctor several times to find out what exactly is happening in your body. Your doctors, nurses, and their team may become special friends to you, because they understand what you are going through.

How Do They Find Out What's Wrong?

To be really sure about what's going on with your body, they need to check you over and see how strong and flexible you are and how the myositis is affecting your skin and other parts of your body. They need to take blood so they can run tests on it. Your blood can tell the doctor many things about what is happening inside your body; for example, it shows signs of muscles being damaged because damaged muscles leak out enzymes into the blood. Another way they find out what is wrong is by taking special pictures of the muscle (the machines are called MRIs or special X-rays) to get really specific information about the muscle problems that are bothering you. Some other tests may be really important to understand what kind of myositis your body has. Not all the doctors do all the tests on every child who has myositis.

Here are the names of the tests that are used most often to figure out the different types of problems in your muscles. One of these tests involves seeing how much electricity is in your muscles. This test is called an electromyogram, and it is done with special equipment. If a muscle biopsy is needed to help figure the problem out, your doctor will explain that you will have to go to the hospital for a few hours. You will be given a medicine that makes you sleepy. A special doctor, called a surgeon, will take a very small piece of muscle (about the size of several pieces of hair). Other doctors will look at the muscle under a microscope to see why you are weak and to make sure you get enough of the right medicine.

What's Going On in My Body?

When you have an infection like a cold or flu, the germs might cause some of the immune cells in your body to start to fight to protect you. In dermatomyositis and polymyositis, the cells get so excited by the idea of protecting you that they lose track of "the enemy" and start to attack your own muscles and blood vessels instead. Some of the blood tests help track exactly where these excited cells are and if they are causing damage to the muscle. If the muscle is attacked, sometimes it leaks out the stuff inside into the blood (the stuff that leaks out is called "muscle enzymes"). If the blood vessels are attacked, they often change their shape, and some of them shut down. One way some doctors look at these blood vessels is to examine the skin just behind your fingernails by using a special light or camera and comparing photographs taken on the visits from one time to the next.

What Do the Medicines Do to Help Me?

The medicines that you take will help to quiet the battle in your body. Sometimes it's hard to match the amount of medicine with the fierceness of the battle—so you might not feel as good as you would like right away.

Why Are Some Medicines Given by Vein and Some by Mouth?

You will take most of the medicines by mouth—with a big glass of water! If there are a lot of battles going on in the blood vessels (inflammation), then it is harder for the medicine to get from your mouth to the muscle battlefield. To get a more "direct route," the medicines might be injected directly into your veins, so they can get to the muscles more easily. Some other medicines do fine when they are taken by mouth—like vitamin D and calcium—and they help to keep your bones strong. For some medicines, there are blood tests that can determine if the amount of medicine you are taking is "just right" or needs to be changed.

Why Do I Need Blood Tests When I Visit the Doctor, If I Feel Better?

Because the blood tests can give the doctor an idea about what is going on inside of you, they give an early warning if a new attack on your muscles is about to happen. For example, the blood tests can warn of an attack when they show that the contents of the damaged muscles (muscle enzymes) have leaked into the blood or that the number of immune cells (the soldiers in the battles) is higher or lower than normal. These results mean that you should keep taking your medicine, not reduce it or stop it. The blood tests also show when you are getting better. If the results of these tests go along with other improvements that your doctor sees in your skin or muscle strength or other things, then you might be able to take a little less of the medicine and gradually decrease this amount over time.

Will I Ever Get Better?

Most of the children who have myositis are sick at the beginning, take their medicine, and then get better. They can slowly lower the amount of medicine that they need until they don't need any more medicine. About 20%–30% of children have a few "bumps" in the road—sometimes the muscle weakness and rash come back. If so, you need more medicine for a while. Usually, if the myositis returns, you do not feel as sick as you did the first time. If you do notice that you are not feeling as well and that some of the signs of your myositis are returning, you should tell your parents right away, and they will talk to your doctor. Your doctor has many different medicines to help you feel better. Doctors are working to develop new medicines, too.

What Can I Tell My Friends If I Am Too Tired to Play with Them?

Some children tell their friends that their body is working hard to get better, and so there isn't enough energy left to run around. You can invite your friends to do things like watch a movie, play a computer game, or build a model with you. Use your imagination, and keep having fun! Laughter is good medicine!

Why Do I Need to Take Medicines If I Feel Much Better?

Most doctors give medicines to take by mouth that help quiet the immune system. It is very important that you take all of your medicines just the way that your doctor has asked you to take them. If you do not follow your doctor's plan, you cannot get and stay better. You may get partway better, but if you suddenly stopped taking your medicines, then the myositis might return in full force. Some doctors with a special interest in myositis are trying to figure out exactly what and how much medicine is needed for each child, because each child is different. Sometimes the medicines (especially prednisone) can make you feel moody or gain weight. Always let your parents know how you feel. If you are not feeling much better with the medicines that have been ordered for you, your doctor can then try other medicines or add to the medicines that you are taking now.

How Can I Help Take Care of Myself?

- Take your medicines the way the doctor told you and do not miss any doses.

- Take enough calcium to keep your bones strong (at least three servings of milk a day) and enough vitamin D to help the calcium get into your body.

- Pay attention to how much and what you eat: fruits and vegetables are good for you, but salty and fatty foods will contribute to increased weight gain.

- Let your body rest when you feel tired—sleep is the best doctor.

- Use a sunscreen that is 30 SPF or greater to protect your skin, which may help make the immune attack less severe.

- Follow the directions of the people who do exercises with you because the exercises will stretch your muscles and make you strong. Do these exercises at home by yourself when asked to.

- Let your parents know when you feel better and when you don't!

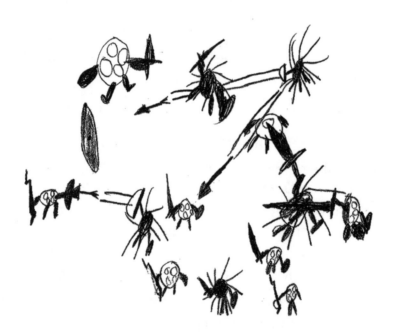

■ **Figure 2.1. A child's view of the immune system.**
This illustration by a seven-year-old boy, Ben W., shows his concept of the battle of the immune system against invaders. He has drawn the immune system to show that the immune cells, which are fighters with circles in them, are trying to protect us against invaders (the stars). The invaders (stars) can sometimes attack their own troops (the immune cells and the muscle, which is the shaded cell with a dot inside).

To Learn More

The Myositis Association (TMA).

Juvenile Myositis. Available from: www.myositis.org/jmbookresources.cfm. Age-specific information for parents, teens, and kids, helpful in dealing with different aspects of myositis, including school issues, coping as a family, and awareness. See these pages for biographies of children who have myositis.

The Myositis Association (TMA). *The JM Companion,* A TMA publication. Quarterly publication written for patients, families, and friends affected by juvenile myositis, with *Just for Me* pages especially for children. Copies available from TMA at 800-821-7356 or tma@myositis.org.

Cure JM Foundation.

Faces of Cure JM; Cure JM Heroes; and *Cure JM's Family Support Network.* Pictures and biographies of JM patients of all ages; stories about JM patients and others who have done something extraordinary to help the JM community; and information about regional family support groups, Bear Hugs program, and helpful tips from families dealing with JM.

Cure JM Foundation. *Cure JM News.* Quarterly publication of the Cure JM Foundation featuring positive stories about patients with JM and their families. Receive a free subscription by filling out the Patient Registration at www.curejm.com and obtain back issues by sending a request to info@curejm.com.

For additional resources, see Resources for Children and Family Support *and* Books and Online Diaries *in the Resource Appendix.*

CHAPTER 3

The Pathways to Juvenile Myositis

Lauren M. Pachman, MD, and Ann M. Reed, MD

In this chapter...

We describe some of the pieces of the puzzle that contribute to juvenile myositis (JM) as one of the autoimmune diseases. We explain some of the specific genetic and immune components that play a role in JM susceptibility and outcome. We then describe the circumstances at the beginning—that is, the environmental conditions and your child's history of infections.

From the family's point of view...

"As a parent, you have to wonder what caused your child's illness. We wish we knew how it all started—how and why the immune system attacks the muscles and the skin. Is there anything we could have done to prevent our child from getting myositis?"

Can You "Catch" JM?

JM is not a communicable disease like measles or chicken pox. You, as parents, or other children who have contact with the child with JM are not responsible for the illness. In fact, it is very rare to have more than one child in the same family with JM. We think that the inflammatory myopathies develop as the result of specific environmental exposures (contact with the surroundings) or immunologic experiences in a child who has a genetic predisposition or "the right combination of genes." Researchers are learning more about the actual pathway that JM follows once it starts. We are just beginning to learn that certain genetic factors influence the length of the inflammatory process (short compared to a long illness). We are learning, too, that the child's environment may play a role at the beginning (starting the process off) as well as in keeping the immune process activated (for example, whether your community gets more or less exposure to ultraviolet light). We are expanding our knowledge about the blood vessels that are one of the major targets of the immune activation.

What Is an Autoimmune Disease?

Autoimmune disease is a term used for a large group of illnesses, which include the inflammatory myopathies (JM, juvenile dermatomyositis [JDM], polymyositis [PM], and related disorders). An illness is called "autoimmune" when the person's immune system mistakes part of the body as being "foreign" and signals for those tissues to be destroyed. These illnesses are not uncommon, for they occur in 5%–8% of the population of the United States. They include conditions such as Crohn's disease, diabetes, rheumatoid arthritis, systemic lupus erythematosus, and multiple sclerosis. Autoimmune diseases are thought to be an overreaction of the body's natural protective immune system. In normal circumstances foreign substances or cells from outside the body (called antigens) are attacked by an immune response cell. In autoimmune diseases, some of the body's own proteins (such as DNA in the nucleus of cells) are seen as "foreign," and the person's immune system overreacts to them (forming anti-DNA, one of the hallmarks of lupus). Some people are prone to autoimmune diseases because they have certain genetic factors (some of which are described later) that allow this self-attack to occur.

Autoimmune diseases are diverse and can target a single organ (called an organ-specific autoimmune disease) or involve many parts of the body (called a systemic autoimmune disease). An example of an organ-specific autoimmune disease is diabetes, in which the person's pancreas is the major site of destruction, even though there may be secondary problems elsewhere. In contrast, JDM is systemic, with inflammation occurring around small and medium-sized blood vessels in many areas of the body, including muscle, skin, and the digestive system. In autoimmune disease, antibodies and cells from the immune system appear to play a role, but the amount that each of them contributes to the trouble varies with the specific type of problem.

What Attacks My Child's Body?

Antibodies are liquid proteins made by the immune system that can attack foreign invaders. They are called *auto*antibodies when they attack part of your own body. In myositis, autoantibodies are commonly seen, but we do not know whether they cause the illness. The type of autoantibody that the person has, however, may be a critical factor in determining their pattern of illness and whether it is likely to be resolved over time (see *Chapter 1, What Is Juvenile Myositis?*). For example, children with myositis might have an autoantibody called anti-Jo-1, which is associated with moderate to severe arthritis and lung disease. In contrast, children with PM who have an autoantibody to a protein called signal recognition particle (SRP) may have a sudden onset of severe muscle weakness, which can be difficult to treat. Other children with myositis and a rash may have an overlap syndrome and an antibody called Ribonuclear Protein (RNP) or have an antibody associated with another variant of the rheumatic diseases, such as polymyositis/scleroderma (PM–Scl) (discussed in *Chapter 28, When Your Child Has More Than One Autoimmune Disease*).

Cells of the immune system that may play a role in the inflammation found in JDM are shown in Figure 3.1. As in Figure 3.1, the *foreign substance* could be a microbe, a virus, or part of the child's own system that has been altered by infection. Several types of immune cells, called antigen presenting cells, are often used to catch the antigen and break it down into little pieces, so that the "would be" self-defense can proceed. The types of cells that patrol the body and recognize something as an invader include macrophages (literally, "large mouths" because they are scavengers that break down the antigen), dendritic cells (cells with long thin projections, which process and recognize special kinds of antigens), and the B lymphocytes (they were first found in the bursa of the chicken) that produce a specific antibody to protect you from a particular antigen. All of these "patrol" cells change the antigen into something with which the "T" lymphocytes can react.

As the cartoon in Figure 3.1 illustrates, we believe that one of the next big steps in the immune response involves "antigen reactive cells." The "T" cells (they are formed in the thymus) come in several varieties, each of which can be in various stages of being "turned on" ("activated") or "turned off" ("suppressed" or "quiet"). Within the T lymphocyte group, there are variations that range from memory cells (they have met that antigen before) to naïve cells (those not previously exposed to an antigen). The main types of T cells are called helper T lymphocytes (CD4), cytotoxic T lymphocytes (CD8), and natural killer (NK) cells, as well as NK cells that are *not* part of the T cell family but recognize invaders, too.

■ **Figure 3.1. (See color plate 3 on page 227.) A possible sequence of events in the immune system of children with juvenile dermatomyositis.**
A substance that is foreign to the body's "antigen" is processed into small pieces by one of the antigen presenting cells (i.e., dendritic cells, macrophages) so that the antigen reactive cells (T cells, NK cells) are "turned on." Sometimes B cells are turned on as well to make antibody. Many of our current medications block the activated immune cells so that target tissue damage is reduced.

There isn't much information about the role of each of these cells in myositis, for their number and state of activation varies with each stage shown in Figure 3.1. In many children with JDM, when a lot of inflammation is present early in the disease course, the absolute numbers of each type of lymphocyte in the blood change from normal. As the inflammation decreases, the distribution of the lymphocytes returns to normal levels for the child's age. When blood from untreated children with active JDM was tested, researchers found that they had low levels of T and NK lymphocytes that carried a specific adhesion marker for the stickiness of the cells (ICAM-1). The investigators suspected that those cells might have left the circulation (in Figure 3.1, these are called capillaries) to migrate to the areas of the body, such as the skin and muscle to become involved in the tissue inflammation. As seen in Figure 3.1, skin and muscle inflammation appears to proceed by different pathways, but both types of inflammation involve the blood vessels. The changes in the number of lymphocytes often parallel the level of activity of the child's myositis symptoms. For some children with JDM, this special blood test of the specific type of lymphocyte numbers can be used to follow the immune activity level as they are treated. The blood vessels are often either "shut down" by the early immune response or may be stimulated to repair as the child's body heals.

How Does Inheritance Play a Role?

Specific genetic factors associated with myositis are under intense study. Researchers are still learning about the genetic characteristics of children with myositis. For example, a set of genes associated with the same proteins that are important in bone marrow transplantation, called the Human Leukocyte Antigens (HLA), appear to be involved in JM. These genes, which help the immune system react, are located on human chromosome 6. In several studies these immune response genes had the strongest association with myositis and other autoimmune diseases. However, these genetic factors do not cause myositis because other family members can have similar markers and be fine. Other non-HLA genes have been reported to be less strongly associated risk factors in myositis. It is an exciting time to study the genetics of myositis because new laboratory methods are becoming available, which may allow us to identify new genes that contribute to the process of JM.

Each gene has a specific location on the chromosome, but the gene might have several different forms or variations, called polymorphism, in different people. There are so many combinations of polymorphisms in HLA genes that it would be unlikely that any two people in a large football stadium would have the same HLA genes unless they are close blood relatives. This great diversity of types or polymorphisms of human genes probably arose many years ago as different groups of people moved around the world and encountered different infections or other stresses from their surroundings.

Based on studies of other autoimmune diseases, it is likely that a large number (several dozen?) of genes need to be present and "turned on" in order for a person to develop myositis. As in other autoimmune diseases, the HLA and non-HLA genes that are associated with myositis are influenced greatly by ethnic background and race, and they may be different in people from different geographic locations or with different environmental exposures. Some of these aspects are being investigated in human studies, as well as in animal models, which help us understand the process of myositis. In the United States, children with many forms of JM seem to have these same HLA genetic markers, suggesting a possible common mechanism for the initiation of muscle inflammation.

Although myositis was first described in the 1800s, only in the past twenty years has laboratory evidence helped us better understand this group of diseases. The HLA genes come in two major forms. These are called Class I and Class II genes (the Class III genes seem to play a lesser role at the moment). They direct the production of protein markers that sit on certain immune cells (B cells, dendritic cells, and macrophages) and serve up the chopped up antigens (either foreign or self) to T lymphocytes, so that they can respond appropriately to defend the body. Of all the possible HLA genes, the HLA-class II genes DRB1*0301 and DQA1*0501 and DQA1*0301 seem to be the strongest genetic factors for the main types of myositis in adults and children. These genes are part of a string of genes that are usually inherited together called "HLA-A1- B8-Cw7- DRB1*0301- DQA1*0501- C4A*Q0" and are found about twice as frequently in children in the United States with myositis compared with healthy children. In the United States children with many forms of JM seem to have these same HLA genetic markers, suggesting a possible common mechanism that is related to the start of muscle inflammation.

Some of the cells in our bodies come from another source—our mother—which might provide further information about disease susceptibility. Chimerism occurs when a small number of cells in a person's blood or tissues comes from someone else, such as a child's mother. The first reports of chimerism in children were in children with JDM. In children with JDM cells from the mother have been found in the child's blood that affect muscle tissue. During normal pregnancies cells from the child and mother cross into each other's bloodstream. These cells have been found years after a child is born in both the child and in the mother. In most individuals, these cells remain quiet and go unnoticed.

However, in cases of autoimmune disease, such as JDM, many of the mother's cells are present in the child, and some investigators suggest that the mother's cells might stimulate the child's immune system to react. These investigators have found that if the mother has the DQA1*0501 genetic marker, more of her lymphocytes are present in the JDM child's blood. Maternal cells have also been detected in the muscle tissue from patients with JM. This area is an active field of research, and there is much more to learn about the differences between a normal protective pathway and one that is associated with autoimmunity.

Tumor necrosis factor alpha–308 (TNF-α–308) is another immune-response HLA gene, which appears to play a role in the more chronic symptoms of JDM and is associated with forming calcium deposits in the soft tissues of the body. One section of the TNF-α gene (in the part that promotes genetic coding) at position –308 has several variants that are distinguished by their different components, called alleles. There are two basic alleles, A and G, which can combine in three different ways, AA, AG, and GG. The most common type (polymorphism) of this gene in normal people is when TNF-α–308 has the "GG" format. In contrast, the "A" form of the TNF-α–308 gene is associated with increased production of

TNF-α, which is a protein that promotes inflammation in your child's body as well as the blood.

A team of investigators found that more children with JDM had either a single or a double A allele—either TNF-α–308 AG or AA—and that this A allele occurs more frequently in children with JDM who have a longer disease course and calcifications compared with children with JDM whose symptoms of JDM clear more quickly (see *Chapter 30, The Clinical Course and Outcome of Juvenile Myositis*). The Class II genes may be related to susceptibility, while the TNF-α genes may be associated with disease severity, but these are still research tests under intense investigation and are not available for general use.

Does Infection Play a Role?

Genes and infection both appear to play a role at the start of the inflammatory process involved in myositis. One of the ways the body fights infection is to "turn on" genes that help produce the immune cells that do the fighting. In a study of many genes expressed in the muscles of children with untreated JDM, the genes related to a microbial response were highly "turned on," or activated. The expression of those same genes *was not increased* in the muscles of normal children or children with Duchenne muscular dystrophy. This is the first clue that the start of the disease process in JDM may involve an immune response similar to what happens when your body is fighting off a microbe.

Infectious agents may play a role in the development of myositis symptoms, but which ones are more likely suspects? Although some studies have suggested the possible role of specific infectious agents (such as bacteria or viruses), several studies tested children for many different infectious agents but could not identify any specific agents in most patients examined. Studies performed on children with myositis (unclassified as to type) more than thirty years ago found that some children with myositis had developed antibodies to group A beta hemolytic *Streptococcus* and influenza A virus. Other viral candidates include a form of enterovirus that causes stomach flu, the Coxsackievirus. Other recent reports have suggested that group A beta hemolytic *Streptococcus* infection could trigger myositis. Furthermore, lymphocytes from children with JDM recognized and responded to a specific part of the streptococcal antigen that is different from the part of the antigen associated with rheumatic fever. This association with group A *Streptococcus* emphasizes the fact that when your child gets a sore throat, a throat culture should be done to see if group A *Streptococcus* is present. If infection is present, it should be treated promptly.

Earlier studies tested for antibodies in the blood to see if the child had recently had a particular kind of infection. More recent studies have used sensitive procedures to amplify, by over a million times, the genes that are "turned on" in response to the agent—whatever that agent is. We now know that the genetic expression profile of the immune response cells in JDM is very similar to the immune response to known viral antigens, but the specific agent has yet to be identified. These fragmentary results from a range of different studies indicate that we simply do not yet know the true answer to the question "What causes JM?"—but many investigators are eager to find out!

One group of investigators found that an immune response to infection might be what pushes the immune system into the JM pathway. They interviewed the parents of eighty children with newly diagnosed JDM in a case control study and compared their answers with responses from parents of their playmates or of children with juvenile rheumatoid arthritis who lived in the same neighborhood. The investigators found that children with JDM had more signs of an infection in the three months before the first definite symptom of JDM (rash or weakness) than children of the same age and from the same region without JDM. They also found that many other factors, such as the child's class size in school, breast versus bottle feeding, life stressors—such as a death in the family, moving, or divorce— were not related to the child getting the symptoms of JM.

In a follow-up study five years later, the parents of 323 children newly diagnosed with JDM were interviewed as part of a JDM Research Registry, funded by the National Institute of Arthritis and Musculoskeletal and Skin Diseases. In this much larger study the infection that the children had before the JDM symptoms involved the upper respiratory tract in 57% of the group as demonstrated by a history of cold, cough, fever, sore throat, or ear infection. Other symptoms were related to stomach and intestines, with a history of vomiting, diarrhea, or stomach aches in 37% of children. In fact, antibiotics were given to over 64% of the whole group of children with signs of infection that preceded JDM. Surprisingly, a subset of these children with infection had a history of exposure to sick animals—but the specific types of animal could not be determined. Once again, there did not appear to be an association between the onset of JDM and specific environmental factors, such as the season of the illness's onset, latex exposure, location or age of the home, exposure to a known toxin, or stressful life events.

What About the Environment in JM?

Environmental factors may, in fact, contribute to the development of myositis in some children. Geography, particularly as it relates to ultraviolet light exposure, is also thought to influence the pattern of illness in myositis. A survey of rheumatology centers in Europe found a difference in the relative frequency of adult dermatomyositis (DM) based on latitude (distance from the equator). A higher frequency of DM relative to all cases of myositis was seen in more southern regions compared with northern centers. This finding has been confirmed in the first worldwide study of myositis and was shown to be associated with the amount of ultraviolet light exposure at each city studied. The Mi-2 autoantibody associated with dermatomyositis also followed this same pattern, and its frequency in these different populations was related to the amount of ultraviolet light exposure. Because most of the subjects in that study were adults with myositis, it is not clear how applicable these results are to JM. Excessive sunlight exposure, however, has been reported in a number of patients (both adults and children) before the onset of dermatomyositis.

Silica has been linked to a variety of connective tissue disorders, including systemic sclerosis, rheumatoid arthritis, and systemic lupus erythematosus. There has not been a careful study of the possible role of silica in children with myositis. However, there are reports of persons developing adult DM and lung involvement after silica exposure.

The characteristics of the individual children play a role in their immune response. For example, the age of the child (young or older), gender, the length of time before diagnosis, and the intensity of therapy all have an impact on studies of immune system function. A national study found that the length of time that the child has been untreated from the first symptom of JDM (rash or weakness) to diagnosis is associated with the level of muscle enzymes: they were often in the normal range in children with a period of untreated active disease that was more than five to six months.

Are Most Children's Symptoms the Same?

It is important to understand which aspects of myositis are similar among children with myositis and which are unique for each child. Children respond to inflammation in an individual manner. For example, your child might become weak, and the muscle enzymes might not be very elevated, but a muscle biopsy could provide evidence of acute and widespread muscle injury, which would benefit from aggressive therapy. The biopsy material from the muscle could also sort out illnesses that appear to be similar but in fact have specific and different hallmarks of muscle pathology. In the same way, a skin biopsy can separate out the rash component into the changes that are typical of JDM from those that are more commonly seen in psoriasis or in scleroderma—each of which has its own distinct appearance.

The pieces of the puzzle are shown in Figure 3.2, and they have yet to be organized into a "big picture" of JDM. In this puzzle are the factors related to when a child becomes ill, genetic endowment, and environment, including the response to a possible viral or microbial agent. Several kinds of cells may chop up the agent and present the specific antigen to the reactive T and NK cells. These immune system cells respond to the challenge and produce interferons (IFN-α/β, IFN-γ), which activate a cascade of immune response genes that can be increased or decreased by cytokines such as TNF-α.

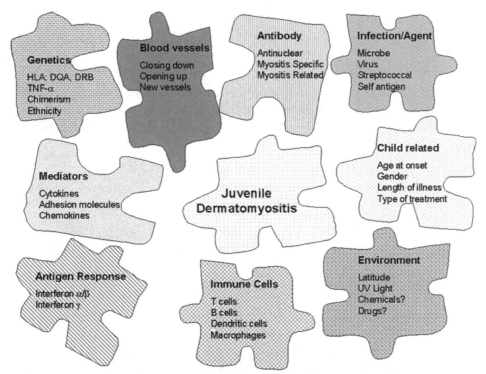

■ Figure 3.2. The pieces of the puzzle that make up the big picture of myositis in children.

We have yet to fit them together.

Key Points

- JM is not a transmissible disease.

- The duration of active inflammation affects the level of muscle enzymes and the cells involved in the immune reaction.

- Certain genetic markers are associated with JDM, but JDM is rare in more than one family member. Those markers, DRB1*0301, DQA1*0501 and DQA1*0301 are part of the human lymphocyte antigens (HLA) on chromosome 6.

- Another immune response gene, which controls the production of tumor necrosis alpha, TNF-α–308, has three forms. The A allele is associated with increased production of TNF-α, a protein important in inflammation of the muscles and other tissues. It is also more common in JDM patients with a prolonged disease course and calcifications.

- Some factors in the environment, such as sun exposure or infections, may contribute to the development of JM.

- More than half the children with JM have a history of symptoms of infection before the diagnosis of JDM, but the specific type of infection is not known.

- Genes that regulate the immune response are "turned on," with a marked change in the specific kinds of immune cells that are in the circulation. Monitoring the gene activation and/or the specific number of immune cells may prove useful for treating the illness.

To Learn More

National Institute of Arthritis and Musculoskeletal and Skin Diseases (NIAMS).

Questions and answers about autoimmunity. Available from: www.niams.nih.gov/hi/topics/autoimmune/autoimmunity.htm or 877-226-4267.

> Answers to frequently asked questions on diagnosis, treatment, and current research related to autoimmune diseases.

American Autoimmune Related Diseases Association (AARDA).

Patient information. Available from: www.aarda.org/patient_information.php or 586-776-3900.

> General information on more than sixty autoimmune diseases.

For more information, see Government Resources *in the Resource Appendix.*

Reports in the Medical Literature

Christopher-Stine L, Plotz PH. Myositis: an update on pathogenesis. *Current Opinion in Rheumatology.* 2004 Nov;16(6):700–6.

Pachman LM, Lipton R, Ramsey-Goldman R, Shamiyeh E, Abbott K, Mendez E, et al. History of infection before the onset of juvenile dermatomyositis: results from the National Institute of Arthritis and Musculoskeletal and Skin Diseases Research Registry. *Arthritis and Rheumatism.* 2005 Apr 15;53(2):166–72.

Pachman LM, Abbott K, Sinecore JM, Amoruso L, Dyer A, Lipton R, et al. Duration of illness is an important variable for untreated children with juvenile dermatomyositis. *Journal of Pediatrics.* 2006;148(2):247-53.

Pachman LM. Juvenile dermatomyositis: immunogenetics, pathophysiology, and disease expression. *Rheumatic Diseases Clinics of North America.* 2002 Aug;28 (3):579–602.

Reed AM. Chimerism in myositis. *Current Rheumatology Reports.* 2003 Dec;5(6):421–24.

Reed AM, Ytterberg SR. Genetic and environmental risk factors for idiopathic inflammatory myopathies. *Rheumatic Diseases Clinics of North America.* 2002 Nov;28(4):891–916.

SECTION TWO

At the Beginning

CHAPTER 4

First Signs of Illness

Lauren M. Pachman, MD, and Carol B. Lindsley, MD

In this chapter...

We describe the first symptoms of myositis—with and without the rash that defines JDM—as well as the possible effect of these symptoms on your child's daily routine.

From the family's point of view...

"We didn't think much about it when she began to say that she was tired— we had just moved, and we had been saying that we were tired, too. Then we noticed that the sunburn on her face had not gone away. We suddenly realized she was now having trouble getting into the car and dressing in the morning—things she had been doing for a long time."

What Are the Main Signs of Myositis?

Children who have myositis with a rash as well as those without a rash might develop muscle complaints. Muscle aches and pains are common problems that usually stem from unaccustomed exertion or minor injury. This sort of muscle damage usually heals quickly and the soreness disappears quickly without treatment. When muscle pain develops without obvious external cause and persists or worsens over weeks to months, it is possible that the pain is related to a generalized muscle illness. Related weakness can develop slowly and not be initially apparent, especially when pain is a prominent feature that limits activity. This combination of muscle pain and weakness is the hallmark of inflammation of muscle, termed "myositis." Other problems affecting muscle can also cause these same symptoms, for example genetic problems with the muscle structure itself (like the muscular dystrophies), specific infection in the muscle, or changes in the metabolism of the muscles related to endocrine and other metabolic disorders.

The word "myositis" means inflammation in the muscle, and when myositis occurs in young people, it is called juvenile myositis or JM. The most common type of myositis in childhood, juvenile dermatomyositis (JDM), causes both muscle weakness and a rash. If the myositis develops as part of another autoimmune problem, in which other illnesses have a role, then we call this "overlap myositis" (see *Chapter 28, When Your Child Has More Than One Autoimmune Disease*).

Your child might not have all the symptoms described in this handbook. Some children are very mildly affected, having only mild rashes and very subtle or minimal muscle weakness. Others cannot make it out of bed and have trouble taking minimal care of themselves. They are homebound and unable to attend school, and may even be hospitalized at the time the diagnosis is established.

Rash and weakness, the hallmarks of JDM, may not be first recognized at the same time. Rash is the first sign of a problem in over 50% of children who are diagnosed with juvenile dermatomyositis (JDM). For the rest of the children, both rash and weakness are recognized together in about 25%, and weakness is the first symptom in the remainder. The characteristic rashes are not a feature of a closely related muscle disease, polymyositis (JPM). The elapsed time between the first symptom of JDM and the time that the illness is diagnosed and medicine is usually started ranges from a few weeks to several years. It is encouraging that this time interval has been getting shorter in the past ten years—it is now about three to five months—as more people learn about the signs of myositis in children.

Your child's rashes may first appear as long-lasting redness and may follow sun exposure. Often, doctors note whether the rash is present in "sun-exposed areas," in contrast to those parts of the body that have not been exposed to sun. The area around the eyes may be violet in color (called heliotrope) with swelling of the eyelids or redness and dilated small blood vessels at the eyelid margins or at the edge of the fingernails (the cuticles), which initially become dry and then itchy. The most common location of the rash is on the back of the hands, across the knuckle joints where the skin can become thickened and red (called Gottron's papules). These raised, reddened, sometimes nodular areas can occur in other parts of the body as well, such as over the knees, elbows, or the insides of the ankles. Table 4.1 shows the frequency of the most common skin findings in children with JDM.

Table 4.1. Frequency of observed skin features in juvenile dermatomyositis patients at diagnosis.

Sign	Percentage
Gottron's papules	91%
Heliotrope rash	83%
Nailfold capillary changes	80%
Malar/facial rash	42%
Gingivitis (inflamed gums)	42%
Mouth sores	15%
Skin ulcers	6%
Calcinosis	3%

Modified from Ramanan AV, Feldman BM. Clinical features and outcomes of juvenile dermatomyositis and other childhood onset myositis syndromes. *Rheumatic Diseases Clinics of North America.* 2002;28:833–57.

On the face, the redness is often palpable and extends over the cheeks and ears and often crosses the bridge of the nose (malar rash). Your child's rashes might include redness and itchiness that extends over the neck and front of the chest (V-sign) or over the shoulders on the back (shawl sign). The inflammation may be limited to the arms and the legs or appear to be a generalized rash that covers the stomach and entire chest. The buttocks and the scalp can be affected as well. Ulcerations or breaks in the skin or gastrointestinal lining often indicate extensive involvement of blood vessels and can be a sign of serious illness that merits intravenous intensive therapy. In general, the children with more skin involvement have more severe nailfold capillary changes, which are different from blood vessel changes seen in children with overlap syndromes. For further information on the skin rashes involved in JDM, see *Chapter 16, Skin Rashes and Sun Protection.*

Many of these rashes or areas of redness are particularly associated with JDM. Children with JPM by itself generally do not have the rashes seen in JDM. Sometimes children with other problems that include myositis, particularly systemic lupus erythematosus (SLE), also have rashes that become worse with sun exposure. Depressions or painful open cracks in the skin at the tips of the fingers are frequent in an overlap syndrome, such as mixed connective tissue disease. Children with myositis might have some elements of scleroderma, and their skin might become stiffer so that it is difficult to bend the fingers. Pits in the fingernails themselves may be seen in children with psoriasis, who often have a scaly dry rash that may be difficult to distinguish from JDM, but improves, not worsens, with sun exposure.

Weakness or loss of strength is most frequently found when your child is not able to perform daily life activities, such as playing, running, dressing (including putting on socks), climbing stairs, or combing or shampooing hair that she could do previously. Tiredness or fatigue is another main sign of muscle weakness, especially when it is a new feature. Weakness might not be as obvious in the very young child, becoming apparent only when age-appropriate behavior (such as dressing oneself) does not progress normally. The weakness usually involves the muscles that are close to the trunk or center of the body—the flexor muscles of the neck (which control holding the head upright) as well as the muscles of the shoulders and hips. The neck flexors are often the first muscles to show weakness and the last to return to normal strength. If your child has neck flexor weakness, she will have trouble holding up her head. Therefore, all situations where head control is important (such as rides in amusement parks, trampolines, or gymnastics) should be strictly avoided until your child regains normal strength. Table 4.2 lists tasks that may be difficult for a child with myositis. If your child has JPM, these signs of weakness are often the first and major signs of illness. For children with overlap myositis, weakness is present, but it can be milder, and the significant features of the overlapping illness may be more troubling, such as arthritis or heart and kidney problems.

> ## Table 4.2. Levels of symptoms of weakness in children with myositis.
>
> ### Mild
> • Can't run as fast as friends in play and sports activities
> • Tires more easily
> • Prefers quieter activities, such as coloring, TV, and crafts
>
> ### Moderate
> • Difficulty combing or shampooing hair
> • Loss of ability to dress self, put on socks
> • Trouble getting in and out of car, bed ("Lift me up")
> • Needs to hold on to banister to be able to climb stairs
> • Trouble with gym—running, "monkey bars" (upper arm strength)
> • Complains of pain or "aches" in muscles after walking
>
> ### Severe
> • Wants to be carried everywhere
> • Has trouble with swallowing—water goes "down the wrong pipe"
> • Has to be helped to go from lying down to sitting up position
> • Trouble walking—walks with a wide-based shuffling gait

Specific tests of muscle strength and function are very important in documenting and measuring the extent of the muscle weakness. These would be performed when your child first comes to the doctor and then repeated over time to monitor your child's progress (see *Chapter 11, Assessing Muscle Strength, Endurance, and Function*).

What Are Some of the Other Symptoms of JM?

The most common symptoms reported by doctors at diagnosis are shown in Table 4.3. All the children had the definite rash and weakness associated with JDM. There are other symptoms that require prompt attention in children with myositis, some of which are a direct consequence of weak muscles (swallowing, breathing, occasionally heart, lung, and voice problems). Some of the other issues relate to the involvement of blood vessels or chronic inflammation in the skin. The most frequent muscle-related problems encountered in children with myositis are discussed next.

Swallowing difficulties arise when the muscles in the esophagus are weak, which results in food getting "stuck." This symptom is among the most serious signs of JM. This weakness could be life threatening when severe, for it means that food

Table 4.3. Symptoms present in 79 children with newly diagnosed juvenile dermatomyositis.

Symptom	Percentage of children with this problem
Rash	100%
Weakness	100%
Muscle pain	73%
Fever	65%
Trouble swallowing	44%
Hoarseness	43%
Stomach pain	37%
Arthritis	35%
Calcifications	23%
Blood in stool	13%

Used with permission of *The Journal of Rheumatology*. Modified from Pachman LM, et al. Juvenile dermatomyositis at diagnosis: clinical characteristics of 79 children. *Journal of Rheumatology*. 1998;25:1198–1204.

particles or liquid can enter the child's breathing passages and lungs during the act of eating or swallowing liquids (which can go down the wrong tube). If this happens, lung infections, such as pneumonia, may occur. Severe difficulty in swallowing is often associated with extreme neck flexor weakness, so that your child may not be able to lift her head from the bed.

X-ray tests such as the "cookie swallow" (modified barium swallow exam), in which the child drinks thin barium, can be used to show that the muscles of the mouth and swallowing tube are not functioning in a normal fashion and can help determine that the child's airway is unprotected. Because difficulty swallowing is one of the most serious signs of JM, it should be treated promptly and aggressively, often requiring hospitalization for both medicines given by vein (intravenous or IV) as well as for precautions related to eating. For further information on swallowing difficulties, see *Chapter 18, Swallowing and Other Digestive Problems*. Other complaints, such as constipation or diarrhea, are often associated with weakness in the muscle function of the digestive system (gastrointestinal [GI] tract). In children with JM, if the inner lining of the GI tract is irritated, then sometimes blood can be found in the stool (which appears black and tarry). If there is severe stomach pain, your child should get prompt medical attention. A less dramatic problem occurs when there is slow bleeding from the intestinal tract. The child's level of red blood cells (hemoglobin) should be checked on a regular basis, and a replacement blood transfusion may be needed on a rare occasion if the level of the red blood cell count is too low (see *Chapter 18, Swallowing and Other Digestive Problems*). The function as well as the structure of the digestive tract can also be involved in JM, so that the nutrition from the food does not get absorbed. Despite eating adequate amounts of food, your child may not be gaining weight or growing as fast as the rest of her friends (see *Chapter 19, Nutrition and Your Child's Weight*).

Arthritis involving the small joints of the hands and feet or the large joints—hips, knees, and elbows—is a common finding in children with JM before they begin medicines. There may be pain and swelling of the small joints, as well as loss of range of motion of the joints (contractures). The result is that your child may not be able to curl her fingers to touch the palm of the hand or fully extend the elbows. The joint symptoms often respond to the first medicines but may reappear at the end of the treatment and require the use of arthritis-specific medicines. Arthritis may also develop in children whose initial JDM evolves into an "overlap" syndrome, as well as in children with JPM. For further information on joint related issues, see *Chapter 21, Maintaining Flexibility: Joints and Other Considerations*.

Fever, particularly a low-grade temperature around 101 or 102 degrees Fahrenheit that persists throughout the day, may be present when the symptoms of myositis begin. Over half the children with JDM will have fever at diagnosis. A national study provided data indicating that older children are more prone to elevated temperatures than are children younger than six years of age. Fevers are also common in untreated children with JPM and overlap myositis.

Other symptoms include a change in the quality of the child's voice, which occurs when there is weakness involving the soft palate at the roof of the mouth. Her voice may have a more nasal tone (as when congested) when she pronounces the letter "e" (see *Chapter 23, Tune to Your Voice*). On the other hand, your child's voice may become very soft, for weakness in the chest muscles is common in myositis and makes it hard to take a deep breath. As a result, nodules may form on your child's vocal cords from overwork, as a result of trying to "speak loudly enough." Shortness of breath is a symptom that may be related to both weakness in the chest muscles as well as to inflammation in the lung tissue itself (see *Chapter 24, When Children Have Difficulty Breathing*).

Calcifications have been reported in as many as 25% of children at diagnosis in the past (see *Chapter 17, Calcinosis*). This appears to be less frequent now, down to 5% in some areas, as children are diagnosed earlier and aggressive medical therapy becomes more effective.

Death occurs very rarely in children with JM—currently, only about 1% of the time in newly diagnosed cases of JDM. The most frequent associations are with lung disease, infection, or severe gastrointestinal involvement.

What Else Could My Child Have?

Under current guidelines a firm diagnosis of JDM requires the presence of the characteristic rash as well as at least two other diagnostic criteria for JM. These almost always include muscle weakness and tests for elevated blood levels of the muscle enzymes. However, if the myositis symptoms have been present for a long time (months or years) or the rash is the major symptom, the concentrations of muscle-derived enzymes in the blood may be in the normal range. Electromyography and/or muscle structure abnormalities, seen on images from magnetic resonance imaging (MRI) or the microscopic study of a muscle biopsy, may also be present. See *Chapter 6, Tests Your Child's Doctor Might Order* for further information on how you can be more certain that your child really has juvenile myositis. If your child does not have the rashes of dermatomyositis but does have at least three of the other signs of myositis named above, then your child could have JPM.

Your child's doctor will consider other illnesses before deciding that your child has JM. Other considerations in a child with weakness include myositis following an infection and primary problems with the structure of the muscle itself. Early in the disease course, before all the symptoms and signs have appeared, figuring out the exact diagnosis can be difficult (Table 4.4).

Table 4.4. What else could this problem be?*

A. Myositis with a prominent rash

1. Other connective tissue disorders (systemic lupus erythematosus [SLE] or scleroderma)
2. Rash more prominent feature than weakness (psoriasis, eczema)
3. Myositis associated with infections (viral, such as influenza or coxsackievirus or bacterial infections)

B. Myositis without a rash

4. Infectious myopathies (viral or bacterial)
5. Endocrine diseases (thyroid problems, diabetes)
6. Muscular dystrophies (Duchenne)
7. Metabolic and mitochondrial myopathies (potassium—too high or too low, sugar metabolism problems)
8. Drug and toxin-induced myopathies

* These are just some of the possibilities.

Infections with common bacteria, such as streptococcus, can be associated with the symptoms of myositis, but muscle pain and weakness are particularly associated with certain viruses. Patients with infections often have severe muscle pain but relatively little inflammation. The calf muscles of the lower leg are prominently involved, not the muscles close to the trunk. The illness typically runs its course in several weeks, after which time the child recovers fully. Other rare causes include parasitic and staphylococcal infections.

Dystrophies and metabolic problems are also major considerations in a young child with weakness. These types of problems stem from the way that the muscles were formed. Especially when the characteristic rashes of JDM are not present, your child's doctor may consider whether your child has one of the muscular dystrophies or trouble with parts of the cells that make up the muscle, such as mitochondrial and other metabolic myopathies. A diagnosis of one of the muscular dystrophies, in which one of several genes that makes the muscles work properly is not functioning, may be suggested by someone else in the family having a muscle disorder, as well as by a very slow onset, with an absence of rash, or other symptoms such as fever and arthritis.

In metabolic myopathies the weakness often comes and goes and may be related to food intake (or fasting), exercise, or illnesses with fevers. There can be cramping in the muscles. Finally, mitochondrial myopathies often have associated symptoms, such as weakness of the eye muscles or strokes. These can be distinguished from myositis based on the findings of exam, blood testing, and the muscle biopsy. Hormonal disorders, including thyroid disease, diabetes, and others, can all cause muscle weakness. Blood testing for the hormone levels will help to distinguish them from myositis.

Key Points

- *The symptoms of the inflammatory myopathies are diverse and of a wide range of severity.*
- Rash is the first symptom in over 50% of children with definite JDM.
- Weakness is the first symptom in approximately 25% of children with JDM, and both rash and weakness are first noted at the same time in another 25%.
- In children with JDM, the most serious symptoms are trouble with swallowing and inflammation of blood vessels in the bowel associated with bleeding into the stools and severe stomach pain.
- In children with JPM, the most serious symptoms relate to weakness, including swallowing and trouble breathing, which may reflect lung involvement.
- It is important that your child receive medical attention as soon as possible after the rash or weakness is recognized.
- *It is important that your child's doctor consider many other conditions before concluding that your child has juvenile myositis.* Careful diagnostic testing can help define the particular type of myositis.

To Learn More

Paediatric Rheumatology International Trials Organisation (PRINTO).

Juvenile dermatomyositis. Available from: www.printo.it/pediatric-rheumatology/information/UK/3.htm.

Drug therapy. Available from: www.printo.it/pediatric-rheumatology/information/UK/15.htm.

General information about juvenile dermatomyositis, symptoms, tests, and treatments, as well as different medicines used to treat myositis and possible side effects. Information provided in different languages from the PRINTO homepage (www.printo.it/pediatric-rheumatology).

For additional resources, see the Resource Appendix.

Reports in the Medical Literature

Compeyrot-Lacassagne S, Feldman BM. Inflammatory myopathies in children. *Pediatric Clinics of North America.* 2005 April;52(2):493–520, vi-vii.

Rennebohm R. Juvenile dermatomyositis. *Pediatric Annals.* 2002 Jul;31(7):426–33.

Pachman LM, Hayford JR, Chung A, Daugherty CA, Pallansch MA, Fink CW et al. Juvenile dermatomyositis at diagnosis: Clinical characteristics of 79 children. *Journal of Rheumatology.* 1998 Jun;25(6):1198–1204.

Ramanan AV, Feldman BM, Clinical features and outcomes of juvenile dermatomyositis and other childhood onset myositis syndromes. *Rheumatic Diseases Clinics of North America.* 2002 Nov;28(4):833–57.

Wedderburn LR, Li CK. Paediatric idiopathic inflammatory muscle disease. *Best Practice and Research Clinical Rheumatology.* 2004 Jun;18(3):345–58. [Complete article also available on The Myositis Association's web site at www.myositis.org in the juvenile myositis section.]

CHAPTER 5

Finding Help

Janalee Taylor, RN, MSN, CNS; Sandra Parker, RN, BScN, MA Ed (Candidate); Miriam S. Granger, MSW, RSW; and Murray H. Passo, MD

In this chapter...

We describe how you can help provide care for your child with juvenile myositis as a parent, caretaker, and advocate. Some of the suggestions focus on finding medical help and preparing for the medical visits to make the most of the available help.

From the family's point of view...

"We were overwhelmed! We knew something was wrong with our five-year-old—she had gotten so clingy, asking to be carried all the time! We didn't know where to begin to find help for her."

What Can I, As a Parent, Do to Help My Child?

If your child is diagnosed with a potentially long-lasting illness, such as juvenile myositis (JM) or juvenile dermatomyositis (JDM), that can create many feelings and concerns. You will probably have a lot of questions about the diagnosis, illness, and treatments for your child. Questions will come up regarding day-to-day activities: school, insurance, and how to help your child and family adjust to these changes. As a parent, much of the responsibility for implementing your child's care and treatment will fall on you. Sometimes, parents feel somewhat helpless when their child is first diagnosed with an illness such as JM. Although you might feel that you alone are responsible for your child's health, know that your child's care will be a team effort. The most important members of your child's healthcare team are *you and your child!* Parents know their children the best. *You* are your child's best advocate.

Your child's medical team may consist of several health professionals, including doctors (both a pediatrician and a "myositis doctor" who is trained in pediatric rheumatology or neurology), nurses (including home health nurses or nurse practitioners), physical and occupational therapists, speech language pathologists, nutritionists, social workers or mental health specialists, and pharmacists. Other experts may be part of the team, depending on your child's specific needs, such as a dermatologist for skin or a gastroenterologist for intestinal issues. Many children do not have all or even most of these health professionals involved in their care.

It is important for all members of the healthcare team to be familiar with your child's progress and treatment plans. Communication is an important part of working as a team, and you are often the essential link in a team that provides a wide range of services. Think of yourself as a hub of a wheel and each doctor as the end of a spoke (Figure 5.1).

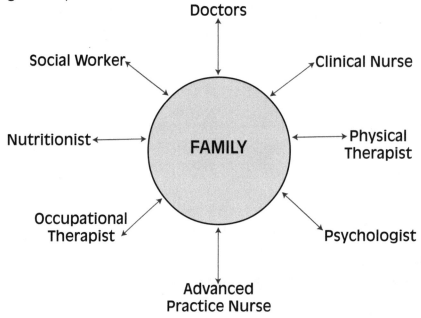

Figure 5.1. Your child's healthcare team.

Finding the Right Doctor to Take Care of Your Child's Myositis

This is one of the most important steps in the care of your child. Because myositis is quite uncommon in children, your primary care physician may have never treated a child with JM. In fact, many primary physicians (pediatricians or those in family care practice) have not had extensive training in muscle, joint, and bone diseases affecting children. If your pediatrician or family doctor does not have experience treating children with myositis, do not hesitate to get a second opinion. Generally, your child's myositis doctor (discussed more thoroughly later in this chapter) will be the primary person managing your child's myositis, but in some situations your pediatrician or family doctor may work closely with the myositis doctor to carry out some of the plan established by the myositis doctor.

Many insurance companies, such as health maintenance organizations (HMOs) require a referral from your primary care provider in order to see a specialist. Be sure to check with your insurance about "in" or "out" of network referrals. If your doctor does not know a myositis doctor or there is none in your HMO network, then see *To Learn More* at the end of this chapter to get help finding a specialist.

Questions to Ask the Myositis Specialist

These questions are designed to help you choose an experienced doctor. It is probably a good idea to ask these questions before you make an appointment. It may be helpful to talk with the nurse, nurse practitioner, or social worker before the appointment.

It may be helpful to discuss the following items:

- Is the doctor a specialist in caring for children with myositis? (Is he or she a pediatric rheumatologist or a pediatric neurologist?)

- Is the doctor board certified in his or her specialty? If not, ask for a referral to a doctor who is certified. In some areas, an adult rheumatologist or neurologist may be available but not a pediatric subspecialist.

- Pediatric subspecialists are preferred whenever possible, as they are aware of the special issues important in growing children. An adult rheumatologist or neurologist could be helpful when a pediatric subspecialist is not available in your area, particularly if your child is older.

- How many children with myositis has the doctor treated within the last several years? How many children whose conditions are similar to your own child's illness has the doctor treated? Remember, JM is a rare disease, so the numbers may not be large. If the answer is "none" or "very few," ask the doctor for the name of another doctor who has cared for more children with myositis.

- If things are not going as expected with your child's illness, is the doctor willing to consult with a juvenile myositis expert about your child's care, even by telephone? Does the doctor seek out the latest information on myositis research?

Once I Get an Appointment with My Child's Myositis Doctor, How Will I Know Whether That Doctor Is the Best One Available for My Child?

First of all, you should feel comfortable talking with your doctor and be able to ask questions and get satisfactory answers. You want to find a doctor who takes time to explain what is happening. A translator should be available if needed. It is often helpful to talk with other families dealing with the same disease. Ask the myositis doctor whether he or she can connect you with other families with a child who has myositis. There are many approaches to the treatment of myositis. Your child's myositis doctor will be one who will make the most informed and best choices for your child's illness and clinical care. You may want to learn more about myositis yourself, so that you can make informed choices. We urge you to read all you can about the type of myositis that has affected your child. You can check out some of the new information about your child's myositis on the Internet and in this book (see *Resource Appendix*). Finally, if things are not going well for your child and your resources permit, consider seeking a second opinion, particularly one from a doctor with a special interest in juvenile myositis.

Expectations of Your Child's Medical Visits

Once your child has been diagnosed with JDM or JM, it is important to understand the treatment goals. Your child's healthcare team will have several treatment goals. The main ones are to:

- Understand the extent and severity of the illness
- Design a treatment plan for your child
- Decrease pain
- Control inflammation with the treatment
- Minimize side effects of treatments
- Prevent complications of the illness
- Improve muscle weakness and function
- Help families learn how to manage at home
- Encourage your child to take part in some of her normal activities as tolerated

You and your child will be seeing members of your healthcare team often. They will also rely on you and your child (depending on her age) to share any progress and observations that you have noticed. It is also important to share your own goals with the healthcare team. It is often helpful to try to plan what needs to be discussed and what questions you would like answered at each visit. Below is a list of ideas that have been helpful for families when visiting the doctor or healthcare team member.

Checklist for Before, During, and After the Doctor Visit

Before the Visit

- Make appointments ahead of time, preferably when it is not an emergency.
- Write down your questions before your appointment.
- Encourage your child (if she is old enough) to write down her own questions.
- Make a list of all the medications and doses your child is taking. It is also important to include any over-the-counter medications, health food supplements, or medications prescribed by another doctor.
- Make a list of any refills or prescriptions you need.
- Make some brief notes or a progress report to let the doctor know how your child is doing. It might be helpful to start a journal. It will help you to keep track of changes. Include things such as how she is responding to the treatment, how she is tolerating her medications, whether you notice any side effects from the medications, what problems you might have, and how you and your child are coping with all the changes.

- Schedule appointments with other team members, such as occupational or physical therapists, nutritionists, etc. If possible, it is helpful to schedule these *before* your doctor appointments so that your child's doctor will have as much information as possible to make informed decisions about your child's treatment.

- Consider getting some of the more routine laboratory blood tests *before* your child's visit so that you can discuss the results. However, the doctor may want to get some additional tests at the time of the visit, which might increase the number of times that your child has blood drawn. The doctor might also request some blood tests at regular intervals to check progress.

During the Visit

- Encourage your child (if she is old enough) to ask and answer questions. This promotes involvement, self-management, and communication skills.

- Encourage older children (twelve and up) to spend some time (even five to ten minutes) alone with healthcare providers. Gradually increase the time as they get older. This will also promote independence, skill building, and trust.

- Take notes during the visit, especially on any changes in medication or treatment.

- Ask your most important concerns first (your time and your doctor's may be limited).

- Ask about what to expect from a recommended treatment, including adverse reactions (side effects).

- If you don't understand something, ask to have it explained.

- Ask for written patient education materials or have the nurse or other healthcare team member explain something you do not understand.

- If it is a follow-up visit, ask for any needed prescription refills at the start of the visit.

- If you are concerned, ask about the cost of medications, alternatives, or treatment plans.

- Sign a "Release of Information" form if you need members of your healthcare team to talk with people outside the hospital, such as the teacher, coach, etc., about your child's condition.

After the Visit

- Make sure you and your child follow the recommended treatment program.

- If the treatment, medical or physical, appears not to be tolerated or causes a problem for your child, let your doctor or healthcare team know right away.

- Don't change your child's medications or treatment program on your own; always check with the doctor or healthcare team first.

- Don't try any new treatments, including complementary and alternative therapies, without checking with your healthcare team first.
- If you have questions, call the doctor's office; if necessary, leave several phone numbers where you can be reached at various times during the day.
- Monitor your child's progress, and report any changes.
- Schedule the next appointment.
- Schedule any referrals to other specialists or healthcare providers.
- If you want a second opinion, ask your child's doctor to suggest a consulting physician.
- Discuss with your doctor the findings of other specialists.

What Shall We Tell the Doctor About Our Child?

1. Note any changes in behavior—both emotional and physical—for either better or worse.
2. Are there signs of fever or infection?
3. Have the rashes gotten worse or more apparent?
4. Has my child lost the ability to cope with frustration?
5. Has there been a change in the child's ability to do things that she could do before without help?
6. If your child is taking medicines, has the schedule and dosage been followed as directed?

What Questions Should We Ask the Myositis Doctor?

1. What type of myositis does my child have?
2. What is the effect of the myositis on her body? And how long will it last?
3. What is the purpose of the treatment for the myositis? What are the choices that are available for this treatment?
4. How will the treatment make my child feel better?
5. When can I expect my child to feel better?
6. Should I expect some negative effects from the treatment? How often do they occur? What should we do about them?
7. For which symptoms should I call the doctor's office?
8. What other health professionals are available to see my child?
9. What lifestyle changes will we have to make? What kind of assistive devices (orthotics, reacher, walker) might be helpful?
10. How often will we need to visit the doctor?

How Can We Organize All This Information?

1. Some families with myositis find it useful to keep a notebook or journal for themselves to keep track of things that are helpful or troublesome. Your doctor may suggest that your child have a special book to write things down about how they feel or to keep a record of small victories that add up to recovery.

2. Write down your questions and ask your child's nurse or doctor to explain any information that isn't clear.

3. You can ask your child's doctor or nurse for an appointment outside of regular clinic hours, which will give you a chance to speak with the doctor without your child present.

4. There are some good Internet sites that can give you accurate information (see *To Learn More* at the end of this chapter and *Resource Appendix*), but be careful of sites that ask for your money. Any information you read that you have questions about you should bring to your child's doctor for discussion (see *Chapter 34, Protecting Your Child's Rights*).

5. Develop a system to keep information organized. Some parents keep a journal or loose-leaf notebook where they record their questions and any medical information they are given. Some parents file doctor's notes, laboratory reports, and X-ray reports in a file cabinet. Others keep it all on a computer, in a program such as Microsoft Office. Keeping track of appointments and medical information can be challenging, so try different ways of organizing this information until you find something that works for you. If you are feeling stuck, ask other parents for ideas. There are chat rooms on the web sites of Cure JM and The Myositis Association, for example, where you can ask what has worked for other parents.

Who Will Examine My Child, and What Are They Looking For?

Your child's doctor or members of the healthcare team will evaluate the following areas: 1) general growth and development; 2) important body indicators such as blood pressure and pulse; 3) changes in activities or daily tasks; 4) skin changes (rash, areas of skin breakdown, or "knots or bumps" under the skin called calcinosis); 5) nail changes, scaly rash on knuckles (Gottron's papules), and redness around the fingernails; 6) changes in strength or weakness; 7) difficulty swallowing or problems with "gagging" or choking while eating; 8) difficulty breathing; 9) stomach pain or bowel problems; 10) joint pain, swelling, or loss of motion; and 11) difficulty speaking or voice changes (for further information, see *Chapter 4, First Signs of Illness*).

What Kind of Tests Can I Expect My Child to Have?

You can expect that your child will have blood tests, X-rays, and other kinds of tests at the beginning in order for your doctor to establish the specific type and activity of the myositis. For information about these tests and what they may show, see *Chapter 6, Tests Your Child's Doctor Might Order.*

There are also several methods to check your child's strength. Many physicians or practitioners can do this, but it is sometimes done by a physical therapist or an occupational therapist. For a complete description of tests that evaluate muscle strength and function, see *Chapter 11, Assessing Muscle Strength, Endurance, and Function.*

What Can I Expect in Terms of the Course of This Disease?

The outcome is not predictable at the beginning of this disease. Even having severe symptoms at the beginning of the illness does not predict a severe course. Children with JM generally fall into three groups.

- Group one will have the disease from several months to one or two years and will recover with treatment.

- Group two will have periods of improvement but with relapses (setbacks). Typically, these children recover from relapses by having their treatment changed; however, children in this group can have symptoms that last for several years with up-and-down cycles.

- Group three has a very difficult condition to suppress and consequently will have active illness for extended periods of time. In most cases, the sickness will finally go away, although it might persist into adulthood, with weakness or rashes and some complications of therapy.

For further information, see *Chapter 30, The Clinical Course and Outcome of Juvenile Myositis.*

How Do We Address Issues About Sports, School Attendance, Discipline, and Restrictions?

Always try to treat your child as normally as possible. Participation in sports is not restricted forever. During times of significant weakness and high doses of corticosteroids it is probably not possible for children to participate in contact sports such as football or in gymnastics or other programs that require strength. *In addition, play activities, such as riding roller coasters, bouncing on trampolines, and so forth, should be strictly avoided even when your child has fully recovered from neck flexor weakness.* It is important, however, that children remain active and have some limited degree of muscle strengthening and stretching while recovering from JM so that the muscles do not deteriorate. Recent studies have shown that minimal muscle use does not deter healing of the muscles. Your doctor and physical therapists will help you make decisions regarding participation and restriction of sports (for further information, see *Chapter 13, Rehabilitation of the Child with Myositis*).

Appropriate play and learning activities are important. If applicable, your child should attend school, once the acute phase of the illness has passed. School attendance is important, and that is your child's responsibility. Social and academic skills are best learned through play and the school environment. If other restrictions are necessary, because of weakness or immunosuppressants, this will be decided by your healthcare providers (see *Chapter 36, School Issues*).

Key Points

- Learn and understand as much as you can about your child's illness.
- Take an active role in your child's care. Speak up, and ask questions.
- Keep a notebook of the material you have been given (names and telephone numbers of healthcare team, appointments, medicine charts, list of medicines, test results, etc.).
- Understand the goals of treatment, the medications, and their side effects.
- Follow your healthcare team's recommended treatment plan.
- Be familiar with the signs of JM, and report flares of symptoms promptly.

To Learn More

To find a physician, see *Finding a Doctor or Specialist* in the *Resource Appendix*, specifically:

American College of Rheumatology (ACR)
American Academy of Neurology (AAN)
American Academy of Dermatology (AAD)
American Academy of Pediatrics (AAP)
American Academy of Family Physicians (AAFP)
American Medical Association (AMA)
Canadian Rheumatology Association (CRA)
National Health Service (NHS)
Paediatric Rheumatology European Society (PRES)

CHAPTER 6

Tests Your Child's Doctor Might Order

Richard S. Finkel, MD; Kevin E. Bove, MD; and Lauren M. Pachman, MD

In this chapter...

You will learn which special tests your child's doctor might use to help determine whether your child has juvenile myositis (JM). We describe some of the blood, radiologic, and muscle tests that are commonly requested. We explain why they are needed as well as the information that they provide. Some of these tests may be repeated to monitor your child's progress.

From the family's point of view...

"When we noticed that our child had trouble getting into bed, our pediatrician took some blood tests, which showed that the problem was in the muscle—but they couldn't sort out what kind of muscle problem it was. So we saw a specialist, who asked for an MRI of her legs and a battery of other tests to check for and possibly rule out certain conditions. We hadn't realized that there were a lot of different things that could be wrong."

What Are the Diagnostic Criteria for JM?

As discussed in *Chapter 1, What Is Juvenile Myositis?*, the diagnostic criteria for juvenile dermatomyositis (JDM) include two clinical findings (the characteristic rash and symmetric proximal muscle weakness) and three laboratory tests (blood tests, electromyogram, and a muscle biopsy). To diagnose juvenile polymyositis (JPM), the rash is omitted, but the rest of the criteria are used. Radiographic imaging is also being used more frequently to find the areas of patchy inflammation to decide where to place the muscle biopsy and to map out the extent of the inflammation.

Why Are These Tests Needed?

When myositis is suspected, it is important for your child's myositis doctor to determine which body regions are affected, such as skin and the digestive system, and to figure out the specific type of muscle problem (myositis or another cause).

The goal of this medical evaluation is to determine the exact label or diagnosis so that appropriate treatment may be given. Not all physicians use the same methods to assess the extent of the inflammation: for example, rheumatologists who are also trained in immunology might use blood tests that indicate immune activation, but neurologists rely more on electromyography (EMG) data that indicate whether the nerves or the muscles are working normally.

Are My Child's Complaints a Single Problem or Part of a Larger Problem?

The doctor's goal is to determine whether the problems that caused your child to seek medical care are part of a larger set of concerns. For example, as seen in Figure 1.3 of *Chapter 1, What Is Juvenile Myositis?*, myositis can be part of many pediatric rheumatic diseases, and it is important to determine right away whether your child's myositis is connected with another condition. Your child's doctor needs to confirm the specific type of problem or diagnosis and at the same time to exclude other possible illnesses from consideration. To do this, a number of different types of tests are often necessary. Many useful tests can be performed on blood and body fluids to help identify the nature of an illness that affects muscle alone in addition to changes in other body systems, such as the blood vessels. (Some of the tests are listed in Table 6.1.) It is particularly helpful to obtain a small sample of involved tissue, such as skin or muscle, for detailed examination under the microscope. This procedure is called a biopsy, which literally means "to look at life." This section will try to answer some frequent questions about JM, such as:

- Can the diagnosis be made on clinical signs and symptoms alone?
- How is the test done, and is there any related discomfort or risk to my child?
- What does the testing measure?
- How are the test results used to make the diagnosis and to treat my child?
- Which tests are done to confirm the diagnosis of JM versus excluding other possible "mimics"?
- Are the tests done because the doctor routinely does this testing in all patients with suspected JM?

Which Tests Are Necessary for Diagnosis of JM?

In this section we first discuss the tests used to fulfill the diagnostic criteria for the inflammatory myopathies, then in the next section we describe the tests that are often used to exclude other diseases in which myositis can be present as well. Table 6.1 shows some of the tests used to evaluate children with symptoms of myositis.

Blood Tests

Blood tests are the most frequent tests that are ordered by most doctors. Blood samples are obtained by sticking a small needle into a patient's vein and withdrawing a few teaspoons of blood. A small amount of discomfort and sometimes a

Table 6.1. Tests for pediatric inflammatory myopathy.

This table generally shows how experts in myositis approach the clinical evaluation and testing in a child with suspected myositis.

Common diagnostic tests

Basic blood tests

- Muscle enzymes

    Creatine phosphokinase (CK)

    Aldolase

    Lactic acid dehydrogenase (LDH)

    Serum aspartate aminotransferase (SGOT/AST)

Other tests

- Magnetic resonance imaging (MRI)
- Electromyogram (EMG)
- Muscle biopsy

Optional diagnostic tests

Blood tests

- Complete blood count: hemoglobin, white blood count, platelet count
- Antinuclear antibody (ANA)
- Myositis-specific antibodies (MSA) to:

    SRP

    Jo-1

    Mi-2

- Myositis-associated antibodies (MAA) to:

    PM-Scl

    Scl-70

    SSA/SSB

- Flow cytometry
- Neopterin

Vascular studies

- von Willebrand factor antigen (blood)
- Nailfold capillary studies
- Heart: echocardiogram, chest X-ray, EKG

Urine

    Routine urine: protein, hemoglobin, cells, calcium/creatinine ratio

Other organ involvement

- *Bone:* DXA, blood tests for bone loss
- *Digestive system:* swallowing studies; hemocult stools for blood
- *Lungs:* pulmonary function; chest X-ray; high resolution CT scan
- *Eye:* funduscopic examination; red/green color blindness

The Diagnosis of JM is generally made by abnormality seen in at least two of the items under *Common diagnostic tests*. Tests under *Optional diagnostic tests* are done at the doctor's discretion depending upon individual circumstances.

small bruise can temporarily result, although an anesthetic cream (EMLA) that numbs the skin is available so that your child will not feel the poke. These blood tests are important for the initial diagnosis, and most likely many of them will be repeated at each office visit to monitor your child's progress (see *Chapter 10, Charting Your Child's Progress*) or to check for possible side effects of the medicines.

Muscle Enzyme Tests

Most doctors agree that muscle enzyme tests are a necessary part of the diagnostic evaluation. Elevated blood levels of the muscle enzymes occur in several muscle illnesses, not just myositis, when the muscle is injured or missing an essential factor, as well as when inflammation is located in the muscle. Muscle injury causes enzymes to leak from inside the muscle cell into the bloodstream.

The most commonly measured muscle enzymes are creatine phosphokinase (CK, also known as CPK), serum aspartate aminotransferase (AST/SGOT), and lactic acid dehydrogenase (LDH). These tests are usually performed in your hospital's central laboratory, and the results are available the same day. Another basic test of muscle enzymes, the aldolase test, is often sent to a specialized laboratory. The result takes several days and may be elevated when all the other tests are in the normal range. The CK level in blood is typically less than 180 units, but the normal values in children vary somewhat among labs. Teenage boys may normally have a higher CK value, about 750, which may be related to intensive exercise; girls who exercise or play sports may also have an elevated CK level.

The blood level of CK can also be elevated, not just from muscle illnesses, but also in problems that affect the heart, liver, and brain. An elevation in CK, therefore, is not diagnostic of JM, but is supportive of a diagnosis if other symptoms are also present. Furthermore, in one study, only 64% of children with juvenile dermatomyositis (JDM) who had both rash and weakness had an elevated CK level at the time of diagnosis, so it is even more important that blood tests for *all* the muscle enzymes are obtained at diagnosis. This is also true after diagnosis, because the CK level may decrease rapidly, whereas other muscle enzymes, especially aldolase, are slower to respond. Another fact to remember is that the longer the disease is untreated, the more frequently the concentration of enzymes is within the normal range in the child's blood, even though the inflammation in the skin can be quite severe. Finally, the results from some or all of these tests may be elevated for other reasons, including other disorders.

Muscle Imaging Tests

Muscle imaging tests take pictures of the muscle and identify features of inflammation; they include magnetic resonance imagining (MRI), scan ultrasound, and computed tomography (CT) scan. Although the results of each test are not specifically diagnostic of JM, they can help confirm the diagnosis. Certain patterns in these studies can be highly suggestive of JM. Identifying the precise location of muscle inflammation is very helpful for selecting the place for a muscle biopsy or an EMG, as well as in defining the extent of inflammation.

MRI scan is very sensitive to changes in muscle caused by inflammation. It can be used to assess the activity of the disease process; for example, the severity and extent of the inflammation in the muscle and the damage or scarring that has resulted from this inflammation.

MRI takes a picture of the muscles using a very strong magnet, not X-rays. This test requires sedation of younger children, because they must lie very still for thirty minutes to an hour while the pictures are being taken. On one type of MRI picture, brightness in the muscles corresponds to the areas of inflammation (Figure 6.1a). MRI shows which muscle group is affected, and so it can be used to locate the place for the muscle biopsy. On a different type of MRI picture, the muscle can be evaluated for thinning or atrophy and any scarring or fibrosis (shown as white patches inside the muscle tissue, see Figure 6.1b).

■ Figure 6.1a. (See color plate 4 on page 227.) A T-2 weighted MRI scan of the thighs.
This is a T-2 weighted scan with fat suppression. Note that the black arrows indicate symmetrical white areas of affected muscle; the dark muscles are less affected. There is increased fascia (membrane) surrounding the muscle (white arrow).

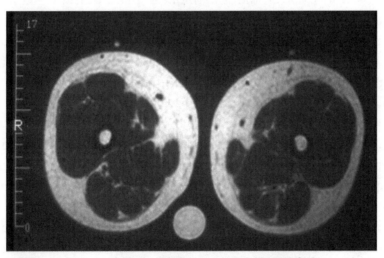

■ Figure 6.1b. A T-1 weighted MRI scan of the thighs.
This scan shows that some of the muscle groups are atrophied (thin or shrunken), and scarring or fibrosis can be seen as white patches within the muscle mass. (Note: The central white circles are bone.)

If an EMG or muscle biopsy test was done before the MRI, it can leave some bruising in the muscle for a few days to a few weeks, and this can show up as areas of abnormality on the MRI, so it is usually more efficient to perform the MRI first.

A muscle ultrasound test uses sound waves to show inflammatory changes in muscle. It is not painful but does require significant experience by the person performing the test, and the child is required to remain as still as possible. Because the inflammatory changes in muscle caused by JM are usually patchy, the ultrasound test is another way to identify a possible site for biopsy.

A CT scan of muscle can identify both inflammation and areas of calcification (calcinosis). This test also requires your child to hold still for a period of time. The test involves a small amount of radiation and sometimes the injection of iodine dye in the vein. These are small risks, but they need to be kept in mind because this test should not be repeated frequently. The study should be performed where your child can be sedated safely, if needed.

Electromyography (EMG) and Nerve Conduction Testing

These tests are part of the diagnostic criteria but might not be performed when your child has several other classic signs of myositis and when your child's doctor feels certain of the diagnosis without undertaking further tests.

EMG testing involves placing a thin wire (needle) through the skin into the muscle. The tip of this wire serves as a microphone, picking up the electrical signals from the muscle. These signals can be heard and watched on a computer screen. The doctor gently tests a few muscles in the arm and leg with the muscle fully relaxed and then during varying degrees of muscle contraction. This requires some cooperation and effort by your child. It is uncomfortable, but with the new, smaller wires used in children there is minimal pain. Some EMG labs will sedate children for this testing or apply a numbing cream where the needle enters the muscles. The test can cause some brief discomfort or bruising, but infection or significant bleeding is rare. One kind of an EMG pattern is seen in inflammation, and other kinds of patterns are seen when there is nerve damage or a primary muscle problem, such as muscular dystrophy.

Nerve conduction testing is not always performed with the EMG study, but if the doctor suspects that the nerves are damaged, your child's doctor will also order this component of the test. This test involves stimulating nerves in the arm and leg by applying very brief electrical shocks to the skin overlying the nerve. The response is then measured further up or down the nerve path. The size and speed of the nerve's response is then calculated. This testing is mildly uncomfortable but not dangerous. In myositis, the response measured when a muscle contracts after the muscle has been stimulated can be either reduced or normal. This shows that there is inflammation in the muscle, which results in the failure of that muscle tissue to contract properly. The nerves controlling sensation are not usually affected in JM.

Muscle Biopsy

This is a minor surgical procedure performed to obtain a small sample of skeletal muscle to be examined closely under a microscope. There are certain real and potential benefits of having your child undergo the muscle biopsy. For children who do not have the characteristic rashes of JDM, it is our experience that a muscle biopsy is highly recommended and almost always required to help determine exactly which muscle illness your child has. The muscle biopsy is virtually diagnostic in such situations. The muscle biopsy:

1. Helps to confirm the initial diagnosis of an inflammatory illness of muscle. This is especially helpful in children who do not have typical signs or symptoms of myositis or typical results of lab tests (again, especially with children who do not have the characteristic rashes of JDM).

2. Identifies other, less expected or even unsuspected non-inflammatory muscle diseases that produce weakness or muscle pain.

3. Can be used to assess the activity of the disease process; for example, the severity and extent of the inflammation in the muscle and the damage or scarring that has resulted from that inflammation.

4. Gives information about the extent of blood vessel involvement, which may be quite different from the involvement seen in the nailfold capillaries or skin inflammation.

5. Can be used to evaluate the extent of immune-associated inflammation and possible tissue damage (infarcts).

Who needs a muscle biopsy?

Many doctors will not require a biopsy if the diagnosis appears certain, based on clinical and routine laboratory testing. However, other doctors use the data obtained from the muscle biopsy to design a specific plan of therapy for each child. The choice of diagnostic testing, as with the type of therapy that is given, is determined by the physician's mode of practice and the wishes of the family.

How is a muscle biopsy performed?

The procedure is usually performed with the help of mild anesthesia When your child has this test, a piece of muscle tissue should be saved (frozen at -80°C), so that if any further tests are needed or special research tests need to be performed to help with the diagnosis, then the frozen muscle tissue can be used. If your doctor is not able to perform the muscle biopsy and save the frozen piece of tissue, some other pathways for diagnosis could be considered (see the following section, *What Other Tests Might Be Needed to Exclude Other Diseases?*).

Once your child is sedated, a short strip of muscle, no more than half an inch long, is removed from the muscle that tests positive on MRI, usually the outside of the thigh. Major blood vessels and nerves are avoided, and bleeding is usually minimal. The biopsy site heals quickly with a small scar, similar to a small cut in the skin. The muscle sample is sent immediately to the pathology lab where it is prepared for examination with a microscope by using special techniques that are usually available only at hospitals equipped to examine muscle for diagnostic purposes. Features of normal and abnormal muscle biopsies are shown in Figure 6.2. Inflammation is present in both JDM and JPM, but frequently the types of cells that participate in the inflammation are not the same and the location of these cells in the muscle may be different.

What are some of the features of JDM on muscle biopsy?

In JDM, the usual features are noticeable closing or even the loss of the smallest blood vessels, the capillaries, which are surrounded by inflammatory cells. The muscle itself may have smaller fibers at the edge of the group of fibers that make up the muscle mass (see Figure 6.2). Scarring can occur in between the muscle fibers. In JPM the damage may be produced by a different type of inflammatory cell. In some children with JPM an acute reaction can be seen in which polymorphonuclear cells more directly attack the muscle fibers, and the blood vessels appear to be less damaged. In overlap syndromes, such as JM-lupus, different parts of the immune system interact with some of the liquids in the blood that both protect us and can cause damage, such as the complement system. The small blood vessels are not as directly involved.

■ **Figure 6.2. (See color plate 5 on page 228.) Normal muscle biopsy features (panels A, C, E) compared to common abnormalities seen in JDM (panels B, D, F).**
In all panels, muscle fibers (m) are displayed in cross section; a, small arteries; v, small veins. Muscle fiber diameter is normally uniform (panel A) but is very nonuniform in JDM (panel B) because of shrinkage of injured muscle fibers (arrowheads). Collections of small, round, dark inflammatory cells (arrow, panel B) are abnormal lymphocytes, which cause muscle damage in JDM. The tiny, dark-staining dots between muscle fibers (panels C and D, arrows) are capillaries, the smallest blood vessels. Capillaries are reduced in number (panel D, arrowheads) in the zone of muscle fiber shrinkage as a result of the vascular injury that commonly accompanies muscle fiber injury in JDM. Arteries also may be injured and obstructed in JDM (panel F) causing more serious reduction in blood flow.

What Other Tests Might Be Needed to Exclude Other Diseases?
Complete Blood Cell Count

A complete blood count is a test that identifies a possible low red blood cell count (anemia) or low white blood cell count or low platelet count—which could be associated with other illnesses in which muscle problems also occur. These are sometimes present, especially in myositis overlap syndromes. Children with JDM occasionally have a slightly low red blood cell count or anemia, and the percentage of a type of white blood cell called lymphocyte is often decreased. Other tests for inflammation (the erythrocyte sedimentation rate [ESR] and the C-reactive protein [CRP]) are often in the normal range but might also be elevated in some of the other conditions in which myositis may be present.

Urine Analysis

Urine analysis often is used to help assess kidney function. In myositis, when muscle breakdown is severe, the kidneys must work very hard to clear waste material from the damaged muscle; consequently, they may become less effective. In the acute phase of myositis, the doctors will carefully watch kidney function and often they will try to dilute the waste in the urine by administering more fluids. In lupus-myositis overlap syndromes, the urinalysis may show red blood cells, protein, and decreased renal function.

Antinuclear Antibody Test

The results of the antinuclear antibody (ANA) test are positive in over 80% of untreated children with JM. The ANA is the most common autoantibody (a type of antibody made by your child's own immune system that recognizes specific parts on the surface or inside of cells in your child's body as compared with invading proteins from the outside that can harm your child's body). Children with muscle weakness from causes other than JM may also have positive results on an ANA test.

In children with JDM the ANA test has a speckled pattern (Figure 6.3) when the serum from your child with myositis is placed over the test cells. If the pattern is not speckled, then other types of connective tissue disease, such as lupus, must also be considered. If lupus is suspected, other blood and urine tests may be obtained, and a kidney biopsy may be requested.

■ **Figure 6.3. (See color plate 6 on page 228.) Typical ANA in children with JDM.**
Typical antinuclear antibody (ANA) pattern in an untreated child with JDM, showing coarse speckled pattern of staining in the nucleus of the indicator cells.

Nailfold Capillary Studies

The major problem in JDM is that the small blood vessels (capillaries) are the main targets of damage. One of the best places in the body to look at small blood vessels is the base of the fingernail. These capillaries show changes that may be seen in the rest of the tissues, particularly the skin, in children with JDM and overlap myositis, and are associated with the severity of the illness and rash. These capillaries can be evaluated with a hand-held ophthalmoscope. Some centers have the ability to photograph the nailfold changes and compare them over time. Figure 6.4 shows normal nailfold capillaries (panel A) compared with those from a child with active JDM (panel B). These studies provide another available way to document your child's response to therapy.

■ **Figure 6.4. (See color plate 7 on page 228.) Nailfold capillary studies.**
Studies of the nailfold capillaries from a normal child show an even spacing of
hairpin turn capillaries that go down to the edge of the nail (A). In contrast, a child
with active juvenile dermatomyositis not only has a smaller number of nailfold capillaries (dropout), but those that are there are abnormal in shape—dilated and bushy
in formation (B).

Optional Tests of Immune Function

Once the ANA results have been identified as positive, some doctors may test
for less-common autoantibodies by requesting tests for myositis-specific (MSA)
and myositis-associated antibodies (MAA). The myositis-specific autoantibodies,
discussed in *Chapter 1, What Is Juvenile Myositis?*, are present in only 10% of
children with myositis and are not found in children with other connective tissue
diseases. These myositis-associated antibodies develop in children and adults who
have symptoms of myositis, but they may have other connective tissue illnesses,
including lupus and scleroderma, a systemic connective tissue condition that affects the skin and internal organs. The search for new antibodies is actively being
pursued. However, only a few laboratories have the difficult and sophisticated techniques that can accurately detect these different antibodies, although new techniques
will be developed in the near future.

In the early active stages of myositis (as well as after a long period of untreated
illness), the serum levels of muscle enzymes often return to the normal range.
However, other tests may remain abnormal and are often helpful to evaluate the
severity of the disease. Flow cytometry identifies a group of white blood cells,
called lymphocytes, that are in the blood. Untreated children with active symptoms of JDM often show an abnormality in the proportions of the different types of
lymphocytes in their blood. This test can help establish both that there is a change
in the number of immune cells and whether they are activated. Other tests of the
members of the immune system may be helpful as clues to the severity of the
immune activation. For example, a macrophage factor called neopterin is elevated
in children with persistent muscle damage. Finally, tests that reflect damage to the
lining of the vascular system, such as von Willebrand factor antigen (vWF: Ag),
may be useful to indicate the extent of the problem in about two-thirds of the
children and may help guide therapy.

Tests of Other Body Systems

Each of the following areas will be reviewed in a separate chapter in *Section 6,
Important Issues on the Road to Recovery*, but it is also important to consider them
at the time of initial diagnostic testing. The evaluation of muscle function (strength
and performance) is discussed in *Chapter 11, Assessing Muscle Strength, Endurance, and Function*.

Here are some other things that your doctor may consider testing in your child, depending on your child's signs and symptoms. The most worrisome problems are associated with swallowing and digestive symptoms, as well as the less frequent problems in which there is involvement of the child's heart or lungs or both.

Tests for Swallowing and Digestive Symptoms

Children who have trouble with swallowing the saliva that is normally produced (drooling) or swallowing other liquids (choking on the fluid) are at risk of getting fluid and food into their lungs. This symptom should be tested with a thin preparation of barium, called a "cookie swallow" or modified barium swallow, to see whether there is loss of function of the muscles in the mouth, including the tongue and esophagus. If liquid barium goes into the breathing passages during the tests, then your child must have a special diet and learn special positioning while eating (see *Chapter 18, Swallowing and Other Digestive Problems*).

Other frequent complaints include constipation (difficulty passing bowels) or diarrhea (loose or frequent stools). Sometimes there is bloating or stomach pain, particularly after meals, because of changes in the function of the smooth muscles that propel food through the intestines (see *Chapter 18, Swallowing and Other Digestive Problems*).

If the child with JDM has actively inflamed blood vessels, called vasculitis, then the lining of the small intestine may become fragile and bruise easily, and blood may appear in the stool. If blood occurs at the beginning of the digestive tract, the blood will turn black, and stools will appear "tarry" and will be positive for blood on testing (hemocult test). If the part of the intestine that is affected is lower down, then red blood may be seen—although this is less likely. Stomach and abdominal pain can also occur and may worsen over time. These are important symptoms to tell your myositis doctor as soon as possible, so that appropriate diagnostic blood and radiologic tests can be scheduled.

Heart and Lung Tests

If your child complains of a rapid or irregular heart rate, it should be checked out with a heart rhythm test (electrocardiogram, EKG) and possibly with a heart function test (echocardiogram). Many children have an abnormal heart rhythm, in which the rhythm and heart look fine, but the heart is simply beating too fast (often because of the muscle weakness). Occasionally, there are problems with the heart rhythm, in which the conduction pathways are short-circuited. This generally corrects back to normal as the myositis is treated and comes under control. In a test of heart function (echocardiogram), the heart might not contract normally, because the heart muscle is inflamed, or because there is fluid around the heart. If this happens, your child's doctor might order other specialized tests, including a chest X-ray, an echocardiogram, and/or MRI, to further evaluate this condition, and a blood test, called a troponin level, to measure heart involvement. Your child's doctor might also ask a heart specialist to help care for your child.

Sometimes shortness of breath can be associated with heart problems (see *Chapter 24, When Children Have Difficulty Breathing*) and tests of lung function, pulmonary function tests, are needed as well as X-rays that have high resolution (CT scan). Children with myositis might have shortness of breath after doing some exercise or exertion. There may be additional symptoms of breathing troubles, including coughing or shortness of breath when your child is resting. This is frequently related to weakness in the breathing muscles. For children over six years of age, pulmonary function tests may be done to determine how well your child's chest wall muscles work when your child is asked to take a deep breath in and out. Special pulmonary functions tests provide information on diffusion of oxygen across the lung membranes, and X-ray studies may be ordered to take a picture of the lungs. (For further discussion, see *Chapter 24, When Children Have Difficulty Breathing.*)

Tests for Arthritis and Bone Loss

Joint symptoms can occur in over 60% of children at the beginning of myositis. Other forms of connective tissue disease are also associated with swelling of the fingers and with loss of range of motion. An X-ray of the hand shows whether the developing bones of the child's hand appear closer together, which is what happens when there is joint inflammation (arthritis) in a child who has not reached puberty. The X-ray may also show the arthritis, thinning of the bones surrounding the joints, or rarely, punched-out holes in the bone (erosions). The loss of bone in the spine is measured by DXA and should be compared with age-matched pediatric standards (see *Chapter 22, Taking Care of the Bones*). The presence of a rheumatoid factor is determined by a blood test, which can be performed to see whether the joint symptoms could be part of a common related problem, juvenile rheumatoid arthritis.

Eye Exams

Rarely, myositis can affect the eyes, so that an eye examination is usually requested at the time that your child is diagnosed with myositis (see *Chapter 27, Eye Health*).

Key Points

- Because many different illnesses can cause inflammation in the muscle, careful testing is needed to find out which illness your child has and how extensive it is.

- Most doctors use some basic blood tests to measure the levels of muscle enzymes in your child's blood, including creatine phosphokinase (CK), aldolase, lactic acid dehydrogenase (LDH), and aspartate aminotransferase (AST).

- In children with juvenile myositis, the levels of muscle enzymes are often elevated in the blood, but this may also be seen in other muscle conditions. In children with JDM, the muscle enzymes might not indicate the extent of overall disease activity, especially if the inflammation has been going on for a long time.

- A muscle biopsy helps to establish the correct diagnosis. When the muscle tissue is examined under the microscope, it shows immune cells and associated damage to the muscle tissue or blood vessels in children with myositis.

- Imaging studies (MRI and ultrasound) can identify the area of muscle that is inflamed and help determine the site of muscle biopsy.

- An electromyogram (EMG) can be used to determine whether there is nerve damage as well as muscle inflammation.

- To determine whether other organs are involved, your child's doctor might test for bone density loss (DXA, bone mineral blood tests), heart involvement (echocardiogram, ECG, troponin level), lung changes, or swallowing problems (cookie swallow).

- Nailfold capillary abnormalities, reflecting vascular changes in the body, are linked to the rash of JDM and may confirm the diagnosis of JDM.

- Most children with myositis have antinuclear antibodies (ANA). In children with JM myositis-related antibodies are not uncommon. About 10% of children are positive for myositis-specific antibodies, and 25% are positive for myositis-associated antibodies. These antibodies help to identify the child's pattern of illness.

Reports in the Medical Literature

Understanding laboratory and diagnostic tests. In: Lehman TJA, ed. *It's Not Just Growing Pains: A Guide to Childhood Muscle, Bone and Joint Pain, Rheumatic Diseases, and the Latest Treatments.* New York: Oxford University Press; 2004.

Dalakas MC. Muscle biopsy findings in inflammatory myopathies. *Rheumatic Diseases Clinics of North America.* 2002 Nov;28(4):779–98, vi. Review.

Mastaglia FL, Garlepp MJ, Phillips BA, Zilko PJ. Inflammatory myopathies: clinical, diagnostic and therapeutic aspects. *Muscle Nerve.* 2003 Apr;27(4):407–25.

Park JH, Olsen NJ. Utility of magnetic resonance imaging in the evaluation of patients with inflammatory myopathies. *Current Rheumatology Reports.* 2001 Aug;3(4):334–45.

Rider LG, Miller FW. Laboratory evaluation of the inflammatory myopathies. *Clinical and Diagnostic Laboratory Immunology*. 1995 Jan;2(1):1–9.

Smith RL, Sundberg J, Shamiyah E, Dyer A, Pachman LM. Skin involvement in juvenile dermatomyositis is associated with loss of end row nailfold capillary loops. *Journal of Rheumatology*. 2004 Aug;31(8):1644–49.

CHAPTER 7

Treatment Possibilities in the Beginning

Bianca A. Lang, MD, FRCPC; Ann M. Reed, MD;
Peter N. Malleson, MBBS, MRCP(UK), FRCPC; and Lauren M. Pachman, MD

In this chapter...

We describe some of the medications that are used to treat myositis in the first few months after diagnosis, as well as their side effects.

From the family's point of view...

"We were told that several medicines would be needed to control the myositis symptoms at the beginning. Treatment began with three days of intravenous steroids, along with medicine to protect the stomach, adding oral prednisone after four days. We continued IV infusions over the next several weeks. Ten days into treatment, we added methotrexate and folic acid. Somewhere along the way we added Motrin, which made a big difference in managing the soreness."

There is no standardized way to treat children with juvenile myositis (JM). The most current thinking about therapy at diagnosis is that early aggressive therapy will be more effective in improving the long-term outcome of our children. More research is needed to help guide the choice of the most appropriate single drug or combination of drugs to use at diagnosis. The range in treatment options is based on which symptoms your child has and how severe they are, as well as the background and experience of your child's doctors. Their viewpoints concerning the illness process and the effects of specific treatments will determine the type of therapy that is selected. The medicines used at the beginning might also be used later on. However, if they don't work by themselves, then other medicines or combinations of treatments might be used. Information about the long-term use of medicines is discussed in *Chapter 12, Possible Medicines During the Course.*

What Can We Expect for Our Child's Treatment?

Most physicians will start your child with juvenile dermatomyositis (JDM) or polymyositis (JPM) on medication as soon as they have sufficient information about the specific kind of myositis that your child has and the extent of the inflammation. The type and amount of medicines selected for your child's care when JM is finally diagnosed depend on the following factors: 1) the acuteness and severity of the inflammation and the amount of the tissue damage; 2) your child's myositis doctor's training and experiences; and 3) your participation, as a family, in the plan of care. We do not know whether myositis can be cured, but most physicians agree that many children with JM have a treatable illness that is responsive to appropriate medication and that most children with JM will have a good outcome.

To get a picture of how the medicines can work, imagine that the myositis symptoms (inflammation and rash) are like having a fire that has the potential to become a very large problem. The best way to put out this fire is to use as much water (in this case, corticosteroids and other medications) as needed to douse the flames. However, if smoldering embers remain, reflecting persistent disease inflammation, then additional help is needed, and this approach is discussed in *Chapter 12, Possible Medicines During the Course.*

> Corticosteroids: Despite potential side effects, early treatment with adequate doses of corticosteroids is probably the single most important factor that has led to the overall improvement in prognosis of children with JM.

What Are Corticosteriods?

After the diagnosis of JM is confirmed, almost all children are given corticosteroids, also known as glucocorticoids. They are strong anti-inflammatory medications that reduce the inflammation in the muscles, skin, blood vessels, and other organs, and they also inhibit the immune cells that attack the muscle and other body systems (immunosuppressants) (see *Chapter 3, The Pathways to Juvenile Myositis*). The term "corticosteroids" is sometimes shortened to "steroids," which are different from steroids used illegally by some athletes (those are called androgenic steroids). Corticosteroids are used to treat almost every aspect of JM, including muscle inflammation, skin rashes, arthritis, swallowing difficulty, hoarseness, and many other signs and symptoms. Exactly how much steroid your child will need cannot be known in advance because some children have a milder illness or respond better to treatment than other children.

How Long Have Steroids Been Used to Treat JM?

Corticosteroids have been used to treat JM for more than fifty years, and intravenous (IV) corticosteroids have been used to treat children with JDM for more than twenty-five years. The use of the IV route at diagnosis in most JDM patients has gained increasing acceptance in the past ten years. In the 1960s approximately one-third of the children with JM died, another one-third survived but had serious long-term disability from their illness, and the final third survived without any recognized long-term disability. The poor outcome seen in most children before the optimal use of corticosteroids were available to treat JM emphasizes how serious this illness can be.

In the 1970s fewer children with JM (less than 10%) died when corticosteroids were used to treat the illness. Today, with even earlier recognition of JDM, earlier implementation of treatment, and more frequent use of high doses of corticosteroids, along with other medicines that suppress the immune system, the outcomes of JDM seem to be improving, and the death rate has decreased dramatically to 1% (see *Chapter 30, The Clinical Course and Outcome of Juvenile Myositis*).

How Are Steroids Administered?

Steroids are given either by mouth (orally) or by vein (intravenously, IV). The main types of steroids used to treat JM are prednisolone or prednisone. In a child who is not severely ill, daily corticosteroids might be started by mouth (orally), usually in the pill form as prednisone (Deltasone) or the liquid form as prednisolone (Pediapred, Prelone, or Orapred). Many young children like the taste of Orapred. If your child's symptoms indicate the need for more intensive therapy, methylprednisolone (Solumedrol) is often given, which is injected directly into the bloodstream by an intravenous infusion, often called an "IV pulse" when the dosage of steroids is high (thirty milligrams per kilogram per day, or mg/kg/day, with one gram maximal dose per day). Many factors determine whether your child's conditions require steroids given at a low or high dose and which route should be used. The selection of medicines will depend on the severity of the illness at diagnosis and on the usual practice of your child's myositis doctor.

When Is Oral Steroid Therapy Used at the Beginning?

At the beginning of treatment, oral steroids are used in one of two ways—either as the main form of steroid treatment, if your child's myositis symptoms are mild, or at a lower dose in between the IV treatments. Some centers use a starting dose of 2 mg/kg/day divided into one, two, or three doses given daily for the first four to eight weeks. However, some places use lower doses of steroids.

How Frequently Is Oral Steroid Treatment Administered at the Beginning?

Altogether, most children receive eighteen months to three years of daily oral corticosteroid therapy. Once the serum level of muscle enzymes decreases to the normal range or when there is an improvement in other critical laboratory tests, as well as clinical improvement in muscle strength and other signs of illness, the daily dose of corticosteroids can be slowly reduced. The doses may then be consolidated, first to twice a day and then, if all is stable, to once a day. A few doctors prefer using steroids as a single dose once a day, either from the beginning or certainly later in the course of treatment. In our experience, steroids given every other day (missing a day of steroids) do not effectively control the symptoms of JM, and they have no role in the initial treatment of JM. As your child improves, the amount as well as the frequency of the prednisone will be decreased. Initially, small decreases in the dose may be made monthly, although this may vary with each child's response. As the total dose of medicine is decreased, however, the amount the dose is reduced each time will be smaller, and the time between each change in dose will become longer. This process of reducing the dosage is called tapering. Tapering is necessary because once your child starts taking corticosteroids, her body stops making them naturally. By tapering them, it gives the body a chance to start making them again. The body needs steroids to function, so if the body is not making them and you stop taking them before your body has readjusted and started making them again, you can make yourself very sick.

> Warning: Steroids should never be stopped abruptly. Your child can become very ill if they are stopped suddenly.

Unfortunately, on this regimen of oral steroids alone, a significant proportion of children with JM experience a worsening of their symptoms (called a flare) after their illness initially comes under control. In this situation, the steroid dose often has to be increased again. Your child will be monitored closely for changes in muscle strength, skin rashes, and other evidence of disease activity, including laboratory tests.

If your child has not responded as well as you and your child's myositis doctor would like, other medicines may be started along with the steroids to try to gain better control of the inflammation in the muscle, skin, or other body systems. These are called second-line medicines (see *What Other Medications May Be Given at the Diagnosis of JM?* in this chapter).

> The early initiation of treatment with high doses of daily corticosteroids, followed by a slow taper over many months to years, has dramatically improved the long-term outcome of children with this disease.

When Is Intravenous Therapy Used?

Corticosteroids will usually be given intravenously to a child with JM who has evidence of moderate to significant inflammation and immune activation at the diagnosis of the disease, particularly if there is marked inflammation of the blood vessels (known as vasculopathy). Other indications for IV injection are severe edema (swelling of the arms or lower extremities) or involvement of the heart and lungs, as well as the presence of other types of rheumatic diseases (see *Chapter 28, When Your Child Has More Than One Autoimmune Disease*). The intravenous route may also be preferred initially if a child has difficulty swallowing or has signs that her vascular system or gastrointestinal tract is affected so that medicine may not be absorbed properly.

Intravenous steroids are used because they are delivered directly to the blood-stream and can get to target tissue faster than oral steroids (which must go through the digestive system first). Because the major problem in JDM is a systemic vasculopathy, which means that small blood vessels (capillaries, arterioles) are damaged, the absorption of nutrients and medicines from the gastrointestinal tract into your child's bloodstream may be impaired. Intravenous steroids can also be given when the illness is severe or if there are other myositis problems that need to be controlled more immediately. IV steroids provide higher doses of steroids than can be given by mouth. In fact, preliminary data have shown that children with JDM and active inflammation of blood vessels have less absorption of corticoster-oids when given by mouth as opposed to intravenously. If your child receives frequent pulses of high-dose IV steroids, she'll be able to take lower doses of daily oral steroids. This could result in fewer overall side effects from steroids.

There are several reasons why the IV route, rather than the oral route, might be more effective, especially early in the disease course. The much higher dose that is achieved in the bloodstream might be necessary to turn off the immune system that is involved in the inflammation. It is well known that very high dosages of corticosteroids are more effective in shutting down certain pathways involved with inflammation. There are several reports that children with JM who were given several high doses of IV steroids until their inflammation was controlled developed less calcification than children who were given lower doses of oral corticosteroids. However, other physicians maintain that the need for intravenous treatment has not been fully proven. The critical questions are: 1) Who will benefit most from high-dose IV corticosteroid therapy? and 2) What are the best indicators of contin-ued disease activity? Once the answers are provided by careful research, then better guidelines for IV steroid therapy will be possible, both at diagnosis and later in the course of illness.

How Frequently Are Intravenous Steroids Administered?

In many centers, the initial treatment consists of one or more doses of IV meth-ylprednisolone. Some physicians give a starting dose of IV methylprednisolone that ranges from 1–2 mg/kg/day given daily, divided into three or four doses. Other physicians (including the authors) have a strong preference for higher doses of 30 mg/kg/day (1 gram/day maximal dose) because that dosage appears to control the inflammation more rapidly. If the child is in critical condition, the steroids can be given at 30 mg/kg/dose (1 gram/day maximal dose) on a daily basis for a long time. Other medicines may be started along with the intravenous methylprednisolone to try to gain better control of the inflammation in the muscles, skin, or other body systems. These are called second-line medications. The additional medication, such as methotrexate or intravenous immune globulin (IVIG), may be started along with corticosteroids at diagnosis. These second-line medications may enable the dose of steroids to be reduced so that the steroid side effects are diminished. They will be discussed briefly in this chapter and in more detail in *Chapter 12, Possible Medicines During the Course.* Finally, if your child is critically ill at diagnosis, other extreme measures might be considered, such as plasma exchange, ECMO (extra corporeal membrane oxygenation), other medications that are less frequently used, or medications that have just been approved for use in children or are part of a special trial of therapy.

How Are Intravenous Steroids Administered?

The first dose of intravenous steroids must be given at the hospital, so that the medical staff can monitor your child's reaction to the medication. A medicine that numbs the skin consisting of a mixture of topical lidocaine and prilocaine (Elamax or EMLA cream) can be used before the IV is started. For children who have trouble holding still, for small children, or for those who have an aversion to needles, a semipermanent catheter, called a "port," can be put in place (see *Frequently Asked Questions*). Additional doses of intravenous steroids can be administered by nurses and sometimes by home health nurses in your own home. Despite the initial set-up costs, one economic-based study provided data that the initial cost of the intravenous route was offset by the shorter duration of disease activity, which decreased the parent's lost time from work as well as the need for prolonged medical and laboratory observation of the child.

How Quickly Will My Child Start to Feel Better?

The response to treatment varies in children with JM. If fever is one of the symptoms, it can usually be resolved within a few days after beginning corticosteroid treatment. Likewise, muscle enzyme levels usually fall within one to several weeks after starting treatment, but improved strength might take several months of corticosteroid treatment. In addition, in some children who have relatively normal muscle enzymes, the immune indicators of disease activity could remain abnormal for longer periods of time, indicating a persistent condition. The skin rash of JDM often improves dramatically with the initial high-dose corticosteroids but could worsen as the corticosteroid dose is decreased. Your child may require other medications to clear the skin entirely (see *Chapter 16, Skin Rashes and Sun Protection*).

After treatment has been started in a child with JM—especially in a child with significant muscle weakness—it is important to notify your child's doctor if there are problems with swallowing, breathing, stomach pain, blood in the stools, or skin ulceration. Any of these symptoms requires urgent reevaluation (Table 7.1).

Table 7.1. Once my child has started treatment for JM, when should I call the doctor?

You should contact your doctor if any of the following develop or get worse:

- Difficulty swallowing or food getting stuck
- Choking on solid food
- Liquids coming out through the nose when swallowing
- Coughing after eating
- Difficulty breathing
- Heart skips beats or beats irregularly
- Voice sounding more nasal
- Obvious increased weakness
- Abdominal (stomach) pain that is severe or increasing
- Vomiting blood
- Passing blood in bowel movements
- Having black bowel movements
- Fever or signs of infection develop
- More severe muscle weakness develops (e.g., difficulty getting out of bed, doing normal activities)
- Deep rashes in the skin that appear punched out or as breaks in the skin (ulcers)
- Another new problem develops that you are worried about
- Vomiting and unable to take corticosteroid medicine

What Are Some of the Early Side Effects of Steroids, Especially in the First Few Months of Treatment?

As with all medications, the risks must be weighed against potential benefits. Although corticosteroids have many side effects, it is important to focus on the fact that *they are often life saving for children with JM.* Furthermore, many of the serious problems with corticosteroids can be avoided if they are recognized early and dealt with appropriately. Some of the adverse effects of corticosteroids that occur early in the treatment of JM are discussed later in this chapter and summarized in Table 7.2. Some side effects, such as marked mood swings within twenty-four hours after the drug is given, might not be present initially but could be noted after the first few weeks of therapy (see following sections). When corticosteroids are given by the intravenous route, some children notice a metallic taste in their mouth, which can be lessened by the use of lemon-flavored hard candy. Other side effects include elevated blood pressure and fluid retention, both of which respond rapidly to medicines. Your child's healthcare team may suggest ways to modify your child's diet (low salt, fewer calories), and they might check for electrolyte imbalance, which can be reduced by adequate intake of potassium, found, for instance, in bananas. Some doctors recommend that your child wear a medical alert tag or bracelet to indicate that she is taking corticosteroids.

Table 7.2. Possible side effects of corticosteroids at any time in the course of therapy for JM.

Area of body affected	Possible effect
Adrenal glands	Unable to make enough natural cortisone in times of stress
Immune system	More susceptible to infections
Bones	Weakened bones (osteoporosis) Damaged bones due to poor blood supply (osteonecrosis)
Muscles	Weakness
Stomach	Stomach upset, heartburn, ulcer
Eyes	Cataracts (later in disease course) Increased pressure (glaucoma)
Skin	Acne Thin skin with poor healing Stretch marks (striae)
Hair	Thinning of hair on head New growth of fine hair on the face/body
Face	Puffy rounded face
Body in general	Increased appetite and weight gain Stunted growth High blood pressure High blood sugars (diabetes) Mood swings, depression, euphoria, disturbed thoughts

Decreased Protection from Infection

One of the functions of corticosteroids is to suppress your body's immune system. In part, this is a desired effect because the immune system is causing the inflammation in the muscles and skin. However, corticosteroids also suppress the normal function of the immune system, which protects us from infection. Because your child's body may not be able to fight infection as well when taking corticosteroids, it is very important that you contact your child's doctor if fever or an illness develops, because it might be necessary to change the way the medication is administered. This becomes even more important if your child is taking another medicine that affects the immune system in addition to corticosteroids (see *Chapter 29, Vaccines and Infection Protection*).

Infection around the toenails (paronychia) is more frequent in children with severe skin involvement and decreased capillary flow. These infections usually respond to soaking and topical antibiotic ointment but may require oral antibiotics. These small infections, if untreated, could cause a flare of the myositis.

Weight Gain

Children with untreated JM are often underweight and less tall than their friends because they may not absorb the nutrition in their food. However, once steroids are started, almost all children will have a better appetite, gain weight, and notice a redistribution of body fat. If your child takes large doses of oral prednisone (more than about 10–20 mg per day), it is likely that she will put on weight, which will usually go away as the dose is reduced. The larger the dose and the longer she continues to take prednisone, the more obvious this weight gain will be. This side effect is known as becoming cushingoid (because it has features similar to Cushing's disease, namely weight gain). The weight gain can be dramatic: many pounds or kilograms can be put on in only a few weeks. The distribution of fat differs somewhat from obesity due to overeating (which also may occur); steroid-induced fat collects in the central part of the body (face, torso, and abdomen) while the arms and legs tend to stay thin. The cause of the increased fat results from a greatly increased appetite and an altered metabolism—which means that the body uses the energy from food to create fat rather than muscle. There is relatively less weight gain from high-dose IV steroids than from relatively lower doses (2 mg/kg/day) by mouth.

Weight gain and water retention, or swelling, caused by steroids can be controlled by keeping the same calorie intake as before the steroids were started, eating low-calorie snacks (vegetables and fruits instead of sweets and salty "junk food"), and reducing salt in the diet (see *Chapter 19, Nutrition and Your Child's Weight*). However, most children find it difficult to control their calorie intake because they feel hungrier. Fortunately, most children start to lose weight as the amount of steroid taken becomes less, and they eventually return to a normal weight when the steroids have been stopped, although this may take a year or two. The puffy, rounded cheeks from taking corticosteroids will resolve completely when the dose is reduced but can be upsetting to adolescents or to the child who is teased by his friends at school.

Steroids and the Skin

Although the rash will often improve with steroids, your child may gain weight and develop stretch marks (known as striae) on the body, arms, and legs, which can be upsetting. The development of stretch marks and thinning of the skin with easy bruising can be minimized but almost never completely prevented. Acne is often exacerbated and should be treated by your doctor, who may suggest a topical antibiotic, as well as good skin care.

Gastrointestinal Effects

Stomach upset, nausea and heartburn, and irritation of the lining of the stomach (gastritis) may occur with corticosteroids. Rarely, bleeding from an ulcer can occur. Prednisone should be taken after eating, not on an empty stomach. These stomach symptoms can usually be controlled with an additional medication to protect the stomach, such as omepraozole (Prilosec), ranitidine (Zantac), or other medications. Sometimes JM itself affects the bowels, so if there is stomach pain, constipation, or diarrhea, letting your doctor know about these symptoms is very important (see *Chapter 18, Swallowing and Other Digestive Problems*).

Mood Swings

Corticosteroids can also cause mood swings (depressed moods and euphoria and, yes, even temper tantrums) as well as disturbed thoughts. Mood changes are quite common. You may find that your child is more emotionally "up-and-down" than before, with bouts of irritability, tantrums, and not getting along well with family members. Some children, especially those receiving divided daily doses, may have difficulty sleeping (insomnia). Some children become truly depressed or develop personality changes or strange, uncontrolled thoughts (psychosis). These emotional changes are probably mainly due to the steroids themselves but are often made worse by the fact that your child has a serious illness that interferes with her ability to do many normal childhood activities, as well as by the obvious change in appearance. These mood alterations go away as the dose is reduced. These effects vary from child to child but will usually subside on a reduced dosage of medication. They can be quite unsettling if they start to become apparent when the medication is begun.

What Other Things Do We Need to Think About When Treatment with Steroids Begins?

Side effects of high-dose intravenous pulse steroids are similar to those described for daily oral steroids. In addition, high or low blood pressure, high blood sugar, headaches, flushing of the skin, dizziness, vomiting, and a metallic taste may be specifically associated with the infusions.

When giving corticosteroids, physicians often provide other medications that protect the stomach. Children receiving steroids should get vitamin D supplements and sufficient calcium to maintain or repair their bone density (see *Chapter 22, Taking Care of the Bones*). Children with JDM need protection from the sun's ultraviolet (UVA and UVB) radiation (see *Chapter 16, Skin Rashes and Sun Protection*), which in turn, decreases the body's ability to produce its own vitamin D. In addition, an eye examination at baseline and every six months is helpful to monitor for cataracts or glaucoma.

Are There Other Choices?

The long list of possible adverse effects of corticosteroids often leads to the question of whether there are alternative therapies, which will be discussed further in *Chapter 14, Complementary and Alternative Approaches to Juvenile Myositis*. One of the most significant risks of alternative medicine as an initial treatment is that they are usually not effective, resulting in a delay in starting medicines that will quiet the immune system. Be sure to tell your doctor about any other treatments you are using, from herbal or nutritional supplements to acupuncture.

> Despite the potential side effects, early treatment with adequate doses of corticosteroids is probably the single most important factor that has led to the overall improvement in prognosis of JM.

What Other Medications May Be Given at the Diagnosis of JM?

Sometimes your child's doctor will start treatment not only with corticosteroids but also with one of the following second-line medicines: methotrexate, hydroxychloroquine, or intravenous immune globulin. These additional drugs usually further enhance the steroid's quieting effect on the immune system.

Methotrexate

Methotrexate is an anti-inflammatory drug that probably inhibits several pathways in immune cells, so it decreases the function of the inflammatory cells that are invading the muscle and other affected tissues in JM patients. Although it originally was used in very high doses to treat cancer, methotrexate (Rheumatrex; Trexall) has been licensed to treat adult and juvenile rheumatoid arthritis for many years. We believe that it is effective in treating JM because several medical reports found that children receiving methotrexate had better controlled JM activity. Starting methotrexate at the very beginning of the illness, at the same time as starting steroids, appears to help reduce some side effects from steroids and the total amount of steroids that need to be given. A few medical reports suggest—but do not prove—that early use of methotrexate, combined with repeated intravenous pulses of steroids, increases the chance of achieving remission of JM and may decrease the rate of calcinosis. Because of these potential benefits of methotrexate, many doctors are using methotrexate in combination with steroids as part of the initial treatment for all JM patients.

How is methotrexate administered? The preferred way to administer methotrexate to patients with JM is by injecting it just under the skin through a small needle, like an insulin shot. This method ensures that the medicine gets into the tissues and is well absorbed. Intravenous infusion is another way to give methotrexate, especially if a port is available. For patients receiving injectable methotrexate, local numbing (anesthetic) creams (Elamax; EMLA) applied to the skin can help reduce the pain associated with the injection. Some patients wonder whether calcinosis might be induced while receiving subcutaneous injections, but this has generally not been a problem in our experience.

Many patients, however, prefer taking methotrexate as pills. In our experience, methotrexate taken by mouth is associated with an increased occurrence of stomach upset. It may not be well absorbed, so the amount reaching the body tissues varies. Preferred dosages range from 0.3–1.0 mg/kg (up to 45 mg per week) administered once weekly. Many patients prefer to receive their methotrexate during a weekend to ensure that they will feel better in time for school. Methotrexate is available in tablet form and in some countries as syrup. The injectable liquid can also be taken by mouth and may be a less expensive alternative to the pills. Methotrexate taken by mouth is best administered on an empty stomach, although taking a light soda or fizzy drink is acceptable. Children metabolize methotrexate faster than adults, so that higher doses can be well tolerated by those with JM as well as other groups of children who have juvenile rheumatoid arthritis. If folic acid (1–2 mg/day) is taken daily or folinic acid (Leucovorin) is given the day after the methotrexate, some of the side effects, such as nausea and hair loss, may be reduced.

What are some of the side effects of methotrexate? The most frequent and annoying side effects are nausea, vomiting, stomach pain, diarrhea, and reduced appetite. Some children report tiredness or not feeling well after they take methotrexate. This feeling usually lasts for a day or two and then goes away. Children taking methotrexate can also develop mouth sores, especially when it is taken orally as a pill or liquid. Hair loss can occur but is nearly always mild and almost never associated with actual bald patches. Getting an injection rather than pills can also help decrease these problems. Liver side effects are uncommon. Short-term liver problems can be detected through repeated blood tests for liver enzymes. This type of problem goes away when methotrexate is stopped. Treatment with methotrexate frequently increases sensitivity to sunlight, so it is important to wear a good sunscreen and to avoid prolonged direct sun exposure (see *Chapter 16, Skin Rashes and Sun Protection*). For further information on methotrexate and its side effects, see *Chapter 12, Possible Medicines During the Course*.

Hydroxychloroquine

Hydroxychloroquine (Plaquenil) was originally used to treat malaria. It has been used for many years to treat skin manifestations of autoimmune disease, including rheumatoid arthritis and lupus, in both adults and children. Many children with JM are given this medicine at a dose of 4–6 mg/kg/day administered by mouth once or twice daily. If your family has a history of red-green color blindness, your child must be tested for color blindness before the drug is started (see *Chapter 27, Eye Health*). If your family has a history of anemia, your doctor might consider a blood test for a G6PD level before hydroxychloroquine is started.

Hydroxychloroquine is used in JM because it does not appear to suppress the immune system as much as the other medications discussed so far. It takes several months to have any noticeable benefit and probably helps the skin rash more than the muscle weakness. It may have a role in preventing or minimizing flares of JM, as it seems to work this way in another autoimmune disease called systemic lupus erythematosus.

What are the side effects of hydroxychloroquine? Hydroxychloroquine seems to be a relatively safe medication. Its most troubling side effect is that, in large doses, it can cause loss of color vision, decreased field of vision, as well as permanent damage to the retina of the eye. Corneal deposits may result in blurry vision or sensitivity to bright light. The effect on the eyes seems to be rare, especially in the doses used for treating JM (less than 6 mg/kg/day). It is strongly recommended that children on hydroxychloroquine be examined at least once a year by an ophthalmologist for evidence of eye damage (see *Chapter 27, Eye Health*).

A fairly common side effect of hydroxychloroquine is stomach pain and nausea. This is usually mild and can often be helped by taking the medicine just before bedtime. If it becomes more severe, the medicine may need to be stopped. Another adverse reaction to hydroxychloroquine is a skin rash that can mimic the JDM rash (but spares the palms) and is scalier. A perceptive child may notice some lightening of hair color.

Some dermatologists prefer to use other antimalarial drugs, called chloroquine, quinacrine, or mepacrine, for treating the rashes of JDM. These might be used if your child does not appear to respond to hydroxychloroquine. With some of those medicines, a yellow tinge to the skin and the eyes can occur, which disappears when the drug is stopped.

Intravenous Immune Globulin

Intravenous immune globulin (IVIG) is frequently given to children who have one of several autoimmune disorders or whose immune system fails to make antibodies. In children with JM, IVIG has been used as part of the initial treatment of JM for children with severe or life-threatening complications, such as severe swallowing difficulties. Several small studies of children with JM suggest that IVIG may be beneficial in those circumstances. The usual dosage is 2 grams (g) per kg given over one to two days monthly for at least three to six months. Sometimes the first five doses are given once every two weeks, and then the doses are given once a month. IVIG starts working rapidly (within hours to days). One frequent observation is that children appear to feel better, even if there is no objective change in laboratory or clinical findings. IVIG is discussed further in *Chapter 12, Possible Medicines During the Course*.

Frequently Asked Questions

Does my child need a PICC (percutaneous intravenous central catheter) or Port-a-Catheter to receive repeated intravenous treatments with IVIG or methylprednisolone? (See also *Chapter 12, Possible Medicines During the Course*.)

Some doctors recommend placement of a more permanent intravenous catheter, particularly when they see the need for repeated blood tests and repeated intravenous medicines (like IVIG and methylprednisolone, or other medicines administered by vein). A semipermanent catheter may be recommended for patients in whom finding a vein is difficult (because the child is very young or because the veins have been scarred by repeated blood pokes and placement of IV catheters). Another reason is needle phobia, especially in the young child, to reduce the stress of the frequent treatments and blood draws. Placement of a semipermanent catheter can usually be accomplished through an outpatient one-day surgical procedure. A Port-a-Catheter is placed when the child is under anesthesia, and it looks like a bump under the skin. The PICC lines are at risk of becoming infected, so always use sterile procedures to access the line and keep the line away from water (from bathtubs or swimming pools). With a Port-a-Catheter children can go swimming, but they should try to avoid being hit on the placed catheter. In both cases, the access line is usually removed after the need for frequent, repeated intravenous drug treatment has resolved.

What other medications can we use for the rash?

Topical therapy is beneficial in conjunction with medication taken by mouth or by vein (see *Chapter 16, Skin Rashes and Sun Protection*). Preparations that help prevent dryness of the skin at the elbows and knees, such as moisturizing creams or lotions, may be helpful. Topical corticosteroids can be used one to four times a day to bring intense local inflammation under control. Topical tacrolimus has been useful in some patients; for others, it acts as an irritant, leaving the skin with more redness. For further information on topical and other therapies to treat skin, see *Chapter 16, Skin Rashes and Sun Protection*.

What are other supportive measures?

As in any long-lasting illness, supportive measures, such as adequate rest and adequate nutrition, are important. We encourage your child to work with physical therapists as soon as the muscle weakness is detected. In active myositis, exercises that help with stretching and improving range of motion, rather than work—such as running—allow the inflammation to calm down (see *Chapter 13, Rehabilitation of the Child with Myositis*).

How important is it to take the medicine in the way recommended by the doctor or pharmacist?

> **Do not change the dose by yourself or suddenly stop the medicine by yourself without directions from your child's myositis doctor.**

It is important to adhere to the medication schedule and dose prescribed by your child's doctor. Take the medicines according to the instructions, including taking them with food or on an empty stomach.

If your child is older, work with her to develop more responsibility to take the medicines on her own. Younger children can practice swallowing pills by using M&Ms, tic tacs, or other small candies.

If your child develops an illness with fever or vomiting, contact your child's doctor while your child is sick. In the case of steroids, it is important to continue administering the medicine, even if your child vomits within a few hours of a dose. If your child continues to vomit, she may need to continue to get her medicine intravenously, and the dose may need to be increased. Most pills (except methotrexate) can be crushed and put in food or something sweet to help make them more acceptable.

Key Points

- There is no standardized approach to treating the child with JM, although corticosteroids are most often used as the first treatment and have saved many patients' lives.

- Corticosteroids are the mainstay of treatment for JM patients and can be given by mouth in moderate to high daily oral doses or higher doses may be given by vein.

- Children with more active JM may heal more quickly if corticosteroids and another agent, such as methotrexate, are both started at the beginning of treatment.

- Children with active inflammation may need high doses of corticosteroid (given by vein at the start of therapy to "turn off" the inflammation effectively).

- Skin disease in JDM is associated with inflammation of blood vessels and should be treated as aggressively as muscle weakness with both systemic medication and topical agents.

- Medicines to protect the stomach and to help the absorption of calcium and vitamin D should also be used in conjunction with extra calcium to protect your child's bones.

To Learn More

The Myositis Association (TMA).

Treatment options for juvenile myositis; Your thoughts and ideas on JM; Juvenile myositis and prednisone: battling side effects; Strategies to help along the journey (Gay R); Emergency alert systems and other aids. Available from: www.myositis.org/jmbookresources.cfm.

The Myositis Association.

Medical alert resources. Available from: www.myositis.org/jmbookresources.cfm or contact The Myositis Association (see *Resource Appendix*).

Zukerman E, Ingelfinger J. ***Coping With Prednisone and Other Cortisone-Related Medicines.*** NY: St. Martin's Griffin; 1997.

Arthritis Foundation.

Medications. In: *Raising a Child With Arthritis: A Parent's Guide.* Atlanta (GA): Arthritis Foundation; 1998. p. 29–36.

2006 Drug Guide. Arthritis Today. 2006 Jan-Feb:p. 73–90. Available from: www.arthritis.org/conditions/DrugGuide or www.arthritis.org/AFstore/CategoryHome.asp?idCat=8 [to order free brochure].

Paediatric Rheumatology International Trials Organisation (PRINTO).

Juvenile dermatomyositis. Available from: www.printo.it/pediatric-rheumatology/information/UK/3.htm.

Drug therapy. Available from: www.printo.it/pediatric-rheumatology/information/UK/15.htm.

General information about juvenile dermatomyositis, symptoms, tests, and treatments, as well as about different medicines used to treat myositis, including possible side effects. Information provided in different languages from the PRINTO homepage (www.printo.it/pediatric-rheumatology).

Reports in the Medical Literature

Fisler RE, Liang MG, Fuhlbrigge RC, Yalcindag A, Sundel RP. Aggressive management of juvenile dermatomyositis results in improved outcome and decreased incidence of calcinosis. *Journal of the American Academy of Dermatology.* 2002 Oct;47(4):505–11.

Klein-Gitelman MS, Waters T, Pachman LM. The economic impact of intermittent high-dose intravenous versus oral corticosteroid treatment of juvenile dermatomyositis. *Arthritis Care and Research.* 2000 Dec;13(6):360–8.

Klein-Gitelman MS, Pachman LM. Intravenous corticosteroids: adverse reactions are more variable than expected in children. *Journal of Rheumatology.* 1998 Oct;25(10):1995–2002.

Lang BA, Laxer RM, Murphy G, Silverman ED, Roifman CM. Treatment of dermatomyositis with intravenous gammaglobulin. *American Journal of Medicine.* 1991 Aug;91(2):169–72.

Coping with Juvenile Myositis

CHAPTER 8

Adapting to Physical Limitations

Kristi Whitney-Mahoney, MSc, BScPT; Dorothy P. I. Ho, PT;
and Susan M. Maillard, MSc, SRP, MCSP

In this chapter...

We describe aides to children's function and mobility. The types of helping agents needed will vary with the child's degree of disability at different times during the illness.

From the family's point of view...

"At certain times during the illness, walking distances became more difficult for her. We found a heavy-duty stroller to use only for those times when she needed a little extra help. Throughout this ordeal with juvenile myositis, we've found smaller, but just as useful, items to use every day, from larger grips on her pencils, forks, and spoons to an electric toothbrush for making brushing easier. All of these helped her keep her independence as much as possible."

Most children with juvenile myositis (JM) experience changes in their ability to function physically. Whereas some children have difficulty competing in sports at their usual level, others may have difficulty getting out of bed, dressing, or walking. Such functional changes vary among children with JM. Physical adaptations are changes in the way your child performs physical activities. They may be needed to ensure safety, optimize independence, and foster recovery. These adaptations are usually temporary, but in some cases long-term adaptations may be required. The specific physical adaptations that are required will change throughout the course of the illness and with possible relapses, remissions, and/or recovery. Each child with JM is unique and has individual needs that vary according to age, family situation, and stage and severity of illness.

The healthcare team, including your child's physical therapist and occupational therapist, will help you to determine and meet those needs. Your child's myositis doctor or the physical and occupational therapy associations (listed at the end of this chapter) may be able to refer you to a pediatric rehabilitation therapist experienced with childhood rheumatic diseases. If you do not have a pediatric physical or occupational therapist near your home, you can contact therapy organizations (listed at the end of this chapter and in the *Resource Appendix*) to help you locate one. You may also want to contact other families of children with myositis in your area who may be able to provide resources that have been beneficial. Adult physical and occupational therapists with rheumatologic experience can provide therapy care; however, pediatric therapists are most able to understand a child's developmental needs. In areas where you do not have access to therapists with specific expertise either in pediatrics or myositis care, your child can still receive appropriate care. You can suggest that your therapist contact another therapist who has the desired expertise to assist in the planning of your child's care. If your therapist is unsure how to find a therapist with this expertise, he or she could start by searching for children's hospitals or rehabilitation centers, or hospitals with a rheumatic disease unit.

Although each child's experience with JM is unique, we address the common physical problems faced by many families and suggest adaptations to resolve these issues. This chapter follows "Evan," a hypothetical child with severe juvenile dermatomyositis (JDM) and his experience as he goes through the stages of his illness. The stages of illness and course of JDM differ among children. Likewise, a child's needs may change at any time. The physical adaptations mentioned for each stage can be applied at any point of the illness depending on the specific needs of your child at a given time. Some of the suggestions or issues may not apply to your child. In addition, excessive and unnecessary adaptations may have a negative effect and inhibit normal function and independence. As with all aspects of managing JM, the final aim is for your child to have a normal and independent life.

Typical questions asked by families, along with suggested strategies to manage these situations are also presented here. If your child has specific needs that are not covered in these sections, please ask a member of your healthcare team (such as your physiotherapist or occupational therapist) for suggestions.

Evan, a six-year-old boy with JDM, At presentation

Evan is a six-year-old boy who has been more moody, less energetic, and has asked to be carried for the past few weeks. He moves more slowly than usual (especially when getting up and down from the ground) and cannot keep up with his friends. Evan has a funny rash on his knuckles and around his eyes.

Over the next month, Evan has more difficulty with his usual activities. He needs to be carried up and down stairs and requires help with dressing and toileting. His rash has worsened, and he is more irritable. After seeing a pediatric rheumatologist and undergoing laboratory tests, Evan is diagnosed with JDM. Evan is now admitted to the hospital for tests and to start treatment. After finally learning what Evan's condition is called, the family is relieved yet scared at the same time.

Common Questions Asked at This Stage

My child is too weak to sit or hold her head up for long. My child also cannot roll over without help and often chooses to lie on her back. What should I do?

It is important for your child to spend some time sitting up to help with her breathing and digestion. Children should sit propped up with lots of surrounding support. You can use high-backed chairs and pillows to support the whole body. At this time, it is especially important that your child's head be supported at all times while sitting (in a chair or in bed).

When in bed, it is also important for your child's position to be changed regularly and carefully. Staying in one position for more than two hours can cause the skin to hurt, break down, and even develop pressure sores. These can be prevented by changing your child's position every two hours and by using special pressure-care mattresses supplied by the hospital.

A chair with an elongated back, a headrest, and pillows or cushions can provide great support when your child is ready to sit in a chair or wheelchair. If chairs, headrests, or cushions are not available, a neck collar can help support your child's head during prolonged sitting.

My child is too weak to get out of bed without my help. What can we do to assist?

When children are this weak, it is important to consider both their safety and your safety in moving them about. When moving or transferring your child, remember that her joints are not protected well by muscles. You should minimize pulling movements and activities. Remember that your child will also have difficulty controlling her neck, which needs to be supported at all times. The other important consideration is your own health, especially that of your back. If possible, get a bed that can be raised and lowered to ensure safety for your back. A social worker or case manager can determine whether your child is eligible for an adjustable height bed for home use (although such beds often are not covered by insurance companies in the United States). You may also want to visit your neighborhood medical supply store as an alternative, which can be found in most telephone directories under "medical supplies" or "therapy supplies."

The safest way to move your child is to encourage her to help you as much as possible. For example, as your child rolls onto her side in bed (keeping head, shoulders, and hips in line with each other), encourage her to sit up over the edge of the bed using her hands for support (Figure 8.1).

If your child is very weak and is six years or older, the safest way to move her is with a hoist (a mechanical device your child can sit in to be safely moved from one place to another, e.g., from bed to chair). Adjustable beds and hoists most often are used temporarily during an acute phase of your child's illness. In this case, you can rent the equipment. This can be done through your local hospital or a medical supplier. If your child has a more severe and chronic course, such equipment may

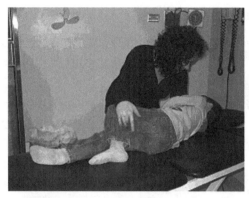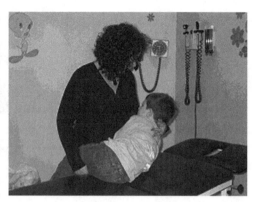

■ **Figure 8.1. Log roll.**
Left, Log roll to help a child sit up. Here, the mother bends the child's top knee and rolls the child as a log onto his side. Right, she provides support under his knees and behind his head and shoulders. *Photos reprinted with permission from N. Mattia and The Hospital for Sick Children, Toronto.*

be required for a longer time, so you might want to purchase the equipment. In most cases, a physician's prescription is required for insurance coverage.

My child has difficulty using the toilet and shower alone. What can I do to help?

Younger children are usually happy to have you help them with bathing and getting on and off the toilet. Older children may want more privacy and independence. When children are weak and tire easily, a raised toilet seat with side handles is helpful (this provides support and allows some independence). In addition, a special bath seat can be used temporarily to ensure safe bathing or showering. If your child needs help with balance while standing in the shower, consider installing a grab bar in the shower for security and support. You may also want to use a non-slip shower mat to minimize slips or falls in the shower. A long-handled sponge is a device that a child can use to reach spots that are difficult to wash. An electric toothbrush and long-handled hair brush can make hair and dental care less tiring.

My child is still very unsteady while walking. Do you have any suggestions?

When children are unsteady on their feet and have active JM, they will also have other difficulties from the muscle weakness. It is very important to explain to your child that she is in danger of falling and hurting herself and therefore needs some help for a while. Physical therapists can teach families how to help their child with walking safely. Walking aids, such as properly fitted walkers or canes, can help children who have limited stability, decreased endurance, or difficulty bearing weight through their legs (especially if arthritis is present). At the same time, these walking aids may be difficult for children with JM to use because of the weakness in their arms and body, which limits proper use and control of such devices. In all cases you should be advised by a professional about the level of support that is appropriate for your child.

My child gets tired quickly, even after taking a few steps. What about a wheelchair?

Children under the age of five can continue to use the stroller they had as a toddler. Special needs strollers, which hold older children of heavier weight, have large tires that allow you to move easily and accessories, such as sunshades and padding.

For older children, however, it is advisable to consider a wheelchair if assistance with mobility is required. Although some children may not want to use a wheelchair for social reasons, it may be needed temporarily to help children get around when the myositis is severe. Keep in mind that wheelchairs can be used intermittently and may be helpful in the beginning for long-distance transport and for energy conservation, but take care to avoid long periods of sitting or immobility. Using a wheelchair for special outings or even going to school can help conserve energy for later activities such as schoolwork.

In most cases wheelchair use is temporary and a standard wheelchair is sufficient. You may be able to borrow a chair from your hospital or rehabilitation center. Rental wheelchairs are available at medical suppliers, typically on a monthly basis. The staff members of medical supply stores can assist you with appropriate chair sizing for your child, should you not have access to a physical or occupational therapist. You may want to consider removable arm rests and adjustable or removable leg rests to facilitate transfers and to provide additional comfort for your child. You may also desire a wheelchair with a reclining back and/or headrest if keeping the head upright is tiring.

If cost is an issue, be sure to explore local charitable organizations, such as the Muscular Dystrophy Association, Easter Seals, and Shriners Hospitals (listed at the end of this chapter and in the *Resource Appendix*). Other local philanthropic organizations might help; often, therapists can direct you to these organizations. Shriners may provide devices including wheelchairs, reviewed case by case.

If a customized wheelchair is needed (although this is rare), consider one that is adjustable (expandable) as your child grows. Many chairs have adjustable seat heights and widths, which would be very helpful in a young growing child. In some instances, older individuals with long-term mobility issues may benefit from the use of a motorized device, such as a scooter. A seat cushion (filled with air, gel, or foam) can help prolong wheelchair sit time while minimizing the development of pressure sores. Wheelchair frames come in different weights (from heavy-duty to ultra-light weight) as well as in collapsible or fixed frames. If your child's environment requires a more durable wheelchair (e.g., to travel non-paved roads) and your child will likely be transported in the wheelchair a lot, you may want to consider a portable active-duty wheelchair frame. Your child's activity level and environment are important factors when deciding the type of wheelchair to get.

Customized wheelchairs, when medically necessary, are best ordered through the collaboration of a rehabilitation therapist and an equipment-supply company because of the therapist's knowledge of the body and the supplier's knowledge of current equipment. In the United States physical and occupational therapists work together with particular equipment-supply companies to determine the best wheelchair for your child.

How do we get the equipment we need?

If equipment, such as a hoist or a wheelchair, is needed for the home, consult your therapists, case mangers, and insurance company to assist with the process. In the United States and Canada a letter of medical necessity (signed by a physician) is usually needed when applying for Medicaid or other insurance funding to cover the cost of specialized equipment. A documented assessment performed by an authorized physical therapist or occupational therapist is often required in Canada and the United States. The resource list at the end of the chapter may provide additional funding sources. In the United Kingdom an assessment by the Social Services Occupational Therapist is needed before financial and practical assistance can be given. Your hospital team can refer you to the appropriate social services team for your area. In the United States your therapist works directly with equipment supply companies to select appropriate equipment.

Therapists recommend equipment based on your child's body type, posture, and overall needs, and the equipment supplier recommends the type or brand of equipment and takes any measurements needed. If you are unable to consult a therapist when selecting equipment, consider looking at catalogues (available through online searches or by contacting your therapy associations) and call the companies directly with any questions you may have regarding their products. A telephone directory or the Internet will list suppliers under "therapy supplies" or "medical supplies," or you can use keywords such as "rehabilitation," "medical" or "therapy equipment."

My child is too tired and weak to keep up with other children. What play activities could interest my child when she is not feeling well?

Play time is vital for children, because they learn important skills while playing. However, children with JM frequently cannot play as much as before they became ill. Early in the illness or during a flare, children can focus on other less tiring activities until they are stronger and fitter. Focus on your child's strengths. Suggest activities such as drawing, painting, working on puzzles, reading, arts, crafts, and board or computer games. Encourage your child to play games with other people to avoid feeling lonely. To prevent your child from getting too tired, set aside small amounts of play and rest time. The length of play time and intensity and difficulty of the activity can be increased gradually.

What things will we need to think about to make our home safe after our child is discharged from the hospital?

If the medical team has cleared your child to go home, you will need to think about how you are going to get your child home (such as by car or public transportation). You may need to use a wheelchair to get to and from or in and out of the vehicle. Remember not to push or pull your child; instead, support her. Once in the car she will need to be strapped in and supported with additional cushions. If you need to take the wheelchair home, think of ways to ensure adequate space in your car. In some circumstances, if your child's neck muscles are very weak, a neck collar may be used for support while riding in the car.

If your child cannot climb stairs safely, you will need to consider the access into your house and bathroom. In multi-level homes, consider temporarily putting your child's bed on the floor with the bathroom, especially if your child cannot safely go up and down stairs without help. Do not carry an older or heavier child up the stairs because of the risk of injuries to you and your child. Children may be able to go up and down stairs on their bottoms with some help, after being taught by a physical therapist. When a child cannot safely travel to the bathroom upstairs, you may want to obtain a bedside commode and sponge bathe her temporarily until her physical function improves.

Extra smooth floors may by too slippery if no shoes are worn, whereas thick carpets can make walking more difficult. For children with small joint arthritis or weakness in the hands, install large or horizontal door handles to make them easier to open.

Evan's Story: In the Hospital, on the Road to Recovery

Evan has been in the hospital for three weeks and is improving. His rash and strength are improving. He still has trouble lifting his head to get up from lying down. He still needs to use a chair or other support to get up from the ground. He can walk with supervision but gets tired quickly and occasionally loses his balance. He has trouble putting on shoes and socks. Sometimes his arms become tired while brushing his teeth or hair for too long.

Evan is attending full-time rehabilitation, which includes time in the gym and hydrotherapy pool (warm water pool). Rehabilitation helps Evan improve muscle flexibility, strength, endurance, and fitness. Evan is especially working toward being ready to get back to school soon.

Evan spent four weeks in total as a patient in the hospital and came home only on the third weekend for a visit. He received daily treatment for an additional two weeks but can now stay home at night. After this period of rehabilitation, Evan gradually returned to school. At first he started with half days for two weeks but is now attending school full-time. Evan's back pain is much better, and now he can walk with his heels flat. He continues to have some mild muscle weakness and some minor tightness in his legs. The biggest difficulty now is tiredness, especially at the end of the school day. Evan also does not feel as physically fit as he was before becoming ill.

My child has improved with the medicines and rehabilitation therapy; however, she is still having difficulty cutting her food. What can we do to help her be more independent?

There are several types of adapted cutlery that your child can use to become more independent. The wider the handle, the easier it is to cut food. Some cutlery is also shaped to make eating easier. It is also a good idea to place a non-slip mat under the plate to ensure that the plate does not move as the food is cut.

My child has difficulty putting on her clothes, especially her shoes and socks. How can we help?

There are many devices to help children dress; for example, there are reach-aids to help with putting on socks and shoes and button-aids to help with closing buttons. A shoehorn can help a child put on shoes more easily. The occupational therapist can work with your child to find easier ways to get dressed. You may also want to have you child wear looser clothing to make dressing easier. Clothes and shoes with elastic or Velcro fasteners make life easier.

My child can walk now and get up from a chair alone, but she still needs help getting up from the ground. How closely do I need to watch her?

Although your child's muscles have recovered considerably, they are still weak, and this may become more evident when she gets tired or is challenged quickly by a bump on the street. Your child is still at risk of falling and being injured; therefore, it is important to explain to her that extra care is needed for a little longer. She still has increased risk of breaking bones caused by the medicines used to treat the myositis, as well as from the myositis itself. Her balance has also been reduced during the time that she was unwell, and this will increase the likelihood of a fall. When standing or walking, have your child stay close to something steady (such as a rail) to hold onto for balance as needed. When more difficult walking surfaces (such as inclines, sand, or rough streets) are anticipated, alert your child or consider alternative routes. Early on, your child may need supervision when attempting a new and more difficult physical task.

Why does my child have pain in the back of her calf when trying to walk and prefer to walk on her toes?

When muscles are inflamed and not moving regularly, they tend to rest in a position of comfort (generally a bent position). The calf muscles and Achilles tendon (the tendon at the back of the heel) can become tight from this positioning. When standing flat, the calf muscle and tendon are stretched, which might cause some pain. The best way to improve this condition is for your child to stretch those muscles and tendons. Your physical therapist can teach her those exercises. The use of night splints (or other interventions such as serial casting) can keep the ankle in a better position, improve flexibility, and prevent more tightening.

My child has a compression fracture in the spine. What can I do to help now and to prevent this in the future?

Compression fractures (a loss of bone height in the spine) happen when the bones become weak (from steroids or inactivity). These fractures are painful but not usually dangerous to your child. We recommend temporarily avoiding body contact activities, sports, or torque motions, such as football, rugby, roller coaster rides, skating, and skiing, where falls and injuries from lack of muscle support are likely (see *Chapter 22, Taking Care of the Bones*). Once the healthcare team assures you that your child's bones and muscles are strong and your child is taking a low dose of prednisone, it is safe to return to these activities. If fractures have occurred, your child's physical therapist can show her mobility and muscle strengthening exercises (when medically cleared) to help ease the pain. Avoid extreme movements, like bending over, twisting, arching the back, and sit-ups, which place stress on the spine; also avoid staying in one position for a long time while the fractures heal. Your child should do exercises to strengthen the back and abdominal muscles to help keep good posture (this includes tightening the stomach muscles for fifteen seconds at a time). Bones become stronger when stress is applied to them. Weight-bearing activities (such as walking on a treadmill) help build bone density and provide other benefits, such as increasing strength and general fitness. It is also important to avoid situations where your child must sit for a long time. Encourage your child to roll like a log to get out of or into bed.

Should I push her to do her exercises now?

It is important to keep up with the exercises to be sure that muscle strength is optimal and that overall fitness improves. Muscle strength improves with the medicines because they reduce the inflammation. However, some muscle strength can only be improved with progressive exercises. At this stage it is important for your child to get as fit as possible because she will then be able to perform daily tasks with fewer adaptations and aids. She might be able to start other activities, such as stationary cycling or modified yoga. However, always check with your healthcare team before trying a new activity. See *Chapter 13, Rehabilitation of the Child with Myositis*, for more information on specific exercises.

My child still seems to tire easily. We are thinking of planning family outings that will require a lot of walking. What should we do?

For younger children, take a wagon or stroller to provide rests. Some older children choose to have a wheelchair handy, whereas other families simply plan short outings with frequent rests. As your child's strength and endurance improve, this will no longer be an issue. Before the trip, work on stretches, muscle strengthening, and overall fitness. Gradually increase the amount of walking your child does at one time. If your child cannot walk for ten minutes without pain, encourage her to walk until she develops pain and then encourage her to walk for an additional two or three minutes longer before taking a rest. Gradually, the distance walked without pain will increase. Occasionally, a wheelchair may be necessary for long distances. It is extremely important that your child only use the chair periodically and spend time both walking and resting. If walking is painful and difficult because of poor positioning of your child's feet, your therapist can suggest a stretching and strengthening program and may recommend orthotics (such as shoe inserts) as needed.

Some additional helpful hints include:

- Obtain a temporary handicapped permit for your car so you can park close to your destination.

- Make reservations in advance (such as for restaurants and movies) to minimize the waiting period.

- Before deciding on a destination, call ahead or check the Internet for handicap accessibility.

- Fun activities specifically designed for children with physical disabilities may be available through your local rehabilitation center or local rotary centers.

- Sensible footwear may also help with some pain and discomfort. Check to make sure your child's shoes have good shock-absorbency and that the shoes are fastened properly. Ankle boots with low heels are often very suitable as they provide good support and are often comfortable.

Evan's Story:
Back to School, but with Some Limitations

Evan has now had JDM for just over two years. He is back at school full-time and manages well; however, he still has some difficulty with participation in sports. He can't run as fast or for as long as his friends. Although he manages well with his schoolwork, he sometimes has difficulty concentrating for long periods of time. He is often a little uncomfortable by the end of the day and is too tired to attend after-school activities. Evan is still taking some medication but is off prednisone. He regularly does the exercises his physical and occupational therapists have taught him.

My child is still on prednisone, but she is reducing her dose and doing well. What activities are safe for her to do?

Until your child's myositis doctors and therapists decide that it is appropriate, activities with risks of falls and body contact should be limited or avoided. Bone density, degree of myositis activity, muscle strength and stamina, and level of steroids are the usual factors considered in this decision. There are many sports, though, that are allowed, such as swimming and walking (on floors, treadmills, and inclines). Once recovery has occurred and your child's muscles become capable again of safely supporting her body, activities such as stationary cycling and modified tae kwon do or yoga are acceptable. However, always check with your healthcare team before trying a new activity.

As a divorced mother, I have a hard time making sure my child is exercising at her father's home. Do you have any advice?

You may want to give your child's father a copy of your child's exercises along with a checklist for your child to fill in when she has completed her exercises. Encourage your child to be responsible for doing her exercises. If your child is also undergoing physical or occupational therapy, encourage dad to attend some of these sessions, so that he can ask questions and feel included in the therapy. If the child lives in two separate homes, many of the devices and home accommodations may need to be set up in both homes.

Table 8.1. Summary of common physical adaptations.

Common problem	Suggested adaptation	Other considerations
My child is too weak to sit or hold her head up and cannot roll over in bed without assistance.	Sit in an adjustable bed with cushions to assist with positioning or a high-back chair with head and neck support and seat belt for safety. A neck collar may be helpful in providing support for prolonged sitting or during transport.	Sitting and changing positions are important to promote proper breathing patterns, aid in digestion, prevent muscle tightness/contracture, as well as to allow for pressure relief and prevent bed sores.
My child is too weak to get out of bed independently.	Help your child to log roll to the edge of the bed and then to a sitting position while supporting the head and neck area. Adjust the height of the bed to your comfort and have your child help as much as possible.	Ensure your child's safety, especially by protecting the neck. Your safety is also a concern; therefore, proper lifting/transferring body mechanics are essential.
My child has difficulty using the toilet/shower.	Adaptive equipment, such as a raised toilet seat, grab bars, and shower bench, can be useful. Nonslip mats are essential.	Equipment may be rented or purchased, depending on the estimated time that it will be required.
My child tires quickly and becomes unsteady walking.	A wheelchair is very useful, in particular, for long-distance use. For younger children, a stroller or wagon may be appropriate.	Many children are reluctant to use a wheelchair due to the social stigma. Reassurance that this is usually a temporary measure may help.
My child wants to play with friends but is too tired and weak.	Focus on your child's current abilities and suggest activities such as puzzles, art, and computer games.	Social interaction with peers is important to children's self-esteem, and age-appropriate play assists with this.
Our child is coming home from the hospital and is still quite weak. How can we make our home more accessible without expensive renovations?	Try to arrange for your child to sleep on the same level as the bathroom. Perhaps a main floor room can serve as a temporary bedroom until stairs are more feasible.	Your child's returning home is an exciting and important step; however, safety must be the primary consideration.
My child has some difficulty with cutting food, opening jars, etc.	Many small devices can be used to assist your child, such as large-handled cutlery, non-slip pads under the plate, and jar openers. These are available at medical specialty shops.	These devices are often covered by government and privately-funded insurance programs with a physician's prescription.

(continued)

Table 8.1. (continued)

Common problem	Suggested adaptation	Other considerations
My child has difficulty getting ready in the morning, especially putting on shoes and socks and brushing teeth and hair.	Shoehorns and sock-aids are simple devices that provide help with dressing. Electric toothbrushes and long-handled extensions for hair brushes are also available.	An occupational therapist can do an "Activities of Daily Living" assessment to identify areas of weakness in these tasks and recommend useful equipment.
My child has tight calf muscles and often walks on her toes.	A stretching regimen performed daily may be helpful. Sometimes the use of night splints can provide a more prolonged stretch. Shoe inserts or day-use braces are occasionally used in conjunction with exercise.	This is a common problem. Stretching programs initiated early on may prevent or minimize this complication. Physical therapists can provide exercise recommendations.
My child has a crush (compression) fracture in the spine. What should we do?	An exercise program that focuses on strengthening the trunk is vital. Early on, a hydrotherapy program will allow for exercise while minimizing pain. Later on, weight-bearing exercise is important to build back bone density.	While such fractures are often painful, they are not usually dangerous. Avoiding sports with body contact or high risk of falls can help to prevent them. Exercise is an important part of recovery.
What activities are safe while my child is still on steroids?	Walking, swimming, and later, stationary biking and yoga or tae kwon do would be acceptable. Participation in other sports depends on the general strength and stamina of your child.	Activity is important for improving muscle flexibility, strength, and improving general fitness. Children on steroids can safely exercise with appropriate supervision.
What are common adaptations made in the school setting?	A graduated return to school starting with half-days may be required. Use of an elevator at school, using lockers or an extra set of textbooks to leave at home may be helpful. A special backpack, such as those on wheels, is a good idea. Adjustable chairs with back support and sloped desks will help facilitate appropriate posture.	Energy should be focused on schoolwork and peer interactions. Energy conservation may be achieved by getting a ride to school rather than walking, and by using photocopied class notes rather than writing them or using a laptop computer.

Key Points

- In the acute phase of JM, always use care when moving your child, to avoid damaging her or yourself.

- Saving energy and planning tasks are vital for ensuring everyone's safety.

- Many of the necessary adaptations are temporary. For some children, these changes may be required at different times throughout their course of illness to encourage independence. Adaptive equipment needs may also change over time and are crucial for providing a safe environment for you and your child.

To Learn More

To find a therapist, see *Finding a Rehabilitation Specialist* in the *Finding a Doctor or Specialist* section of the *Resource Appendix*, specifically:

American Physical Therapy Association (APTA)

American Occupational Therapy Association, Inc. (AOTA)

Canadian Physiotherapy Association (CPA)

Canadian Association of Occupational Therapists (CAOT)

United Kingdom Chartered Society of Physiotherapy (CSP)

Products and Equipment:

These organizations offer mobility equipment for adults and older children, but they may offer alternatives for your younger child. Consult your healthcare team (including a pediatric physical or occupational therapist) when considering mobility equipment. This list is not meant to be all-inclusive but merely a representation of some companies offering mobility products and equipment.

The Myositis Association (TMA).

General aids; *Juvenile myositis-specific products*. Available from: www.myositis.org/jmbookresources.cfm.

Lists of companies and organizations offering aids for daily living and other adaptive products. TMA offers an *OutLook Extra Products Issue*, focusing on products and strategies for daily living.

Allabilities. Zundor Interactive, 831 Burley Avenue, Buhl ID 83316; Internet: www.allabilities.com.

Maxi Aids. 42 Executive Blvd, Farmingdale NY 11735 USA; Phone: 631-752-0521 (for information) or 800-522-6294 (to order); Internet: www.maxiaids.com.

Sammons Preston Rolyan, an AbilityOne Company. 270 Remington Blvd, Suite C, Bolingbrook IL 60440-3593; Phone: 800-323-5547; Internet: www.sammonspreston.com; Email: SPR@abilityone.com.

Wisdom King. 4015 Avenida de la Plata, Unit 401, Oceanside CA 92056; Phone: 877-931-9693 or 760-450-0671 (outside U.S.); Internet: www.wisdomking.com.

Possible organizations to assist in funding of equipment needs (see Other Support Organizations in the Resource Appendix):

Easter Seals

Muscular Dystrophy Association (MDA)

The Shriners Hospitals for Children

Additional Information:

Tucker LB, DeNardo BA, Stebulis JA, Schaller JG. *Physical and Occupational Therapy: Splints, Crutches, and Other Devices.* In: **Your Child with Arthritis: A Family Guide for Caregiving.** Baltimore: Johns Hopkins University Press; 1996. p. 97–101.

Reports in the Medical Literature

Campbell SK, Palsano RJ, Vander Linden DW. *Physical therapy for children.* 3rd ed. Philadelphia: WB Saunders Company; 2005.

CHAPTER 9

Coping with Myositis As a Family

Miriam S. Granger, MSW, RSW; Ilona S. Szer, MD;
and Arlette Lefebvre, MD

In this chapter...

We describe the feelings that children with juvenile myositis (JM), their siblings, and parents might have as they try to cope with the illness. We also provide suggestions for decreasing the stress and other common problems. At the end of the chapter we share some positive experiences of parents and young people who live with juvenile myositis.

From the family's point of view...

"There have been moments when we felt completely overwhelmed. Sometimes we got together with good friends; other times we sought the help of a therapist. And through it all, we educated ourselves about every aspect of juvenile myositis. We found it was important to let our daughter play a part in her care, to encourage honest but constructive expression of her feelings, and to communicate openly with every member of the family. We've decided to take the strengths we built up through this experience and use them in our favor."

Most childhood illnesses develop suddenly and eventually go away with little or no treatment. Families are used to going to the pediatrician and leaving with a clear diagnosis of an ear infection or strep throat and a medication that will cure the problem quickly. A rheumatic disease such as juvenile myositis (JM), which could last several years and has an unpredictable course, is a difficult concept for most families to understand. When an illness such as JM is diagnosed, the initial reaction is usually shock and grief. The grieving process involves various stages of denial, anger, sadness, and finally acceptance. Families move through these stages at their own pace, often visiting one stage longer than another.

Many factors affect how well a family and a child cope with this new challenge. Research suggests that the family environment affects how well children and families cope with the stress of an illness such as JM and that the parents' ability to deal with stress directly affects how well their children deal with stress. Children begin to learn at a very early age how to deal with challenges in life by watching how their parents deal with these challenges. For this reason, this chapter focuses mainly on parents and on what they can do to help themselves and their children.

The Parent's Perspective

When a child is diagnosed with JM, the adults in that child's life often experience a wide variety of emotions, including the following:

- Relief. "I knew something was wrong. Now my child can get the right treatment."

- Fear. "Juvenile *what*? Will my child be all right?"

- Guilt. "Could I have prevented this? Is this genetic? Why didn't I insist that my child see a specialist sooner?"

After the child has been diagnosed and treatment has begun, other feelings may arise.

- Grief. "My child won't have the kind of childhood I wanted for her. My dreams for her will have to change."

- Hopelessness or depression. "This is too much. I just can't live like this!"

- Frustration. "How long will this last? I'm tired of going to the doctor!"

- Hope. "We're through the worst. Things are getting back to normal."

Parents often have more difficulty emotionally and find it even harder to cope than the child with the illness. Why is this?

- Seeing your child unhappy or in pain and not being able to take that pain away is one of the most stressful and painful experiences for a parent.

- Depending on their age, most children have a limited understanding of the potential longer-term impact of this disease. They are not concerned as much about their future and are usually focused on the present. As a parent, you might be wondering whether the disease will limit your child's ability to become an independent teenager or adult, whereas your child's focus is on what she can or cannot do today or next week.

- Parents have the responsibility not only of understanding the illness and treatment but of educating others in the child's life. Trying to explain complicated information to family members, teachers, and friends and trying to answer their questions can be exhausting.

- Parents also have the duty to ensure that their child receives appropriate treatment. This means attending many medical appointments and buying medications that can be costly.

- The financial costs associated with chronic illness can be frightening. Obvious costs for families without health coverage and drug coverage include treatment and medication costs, as well as transportation to and from medical appointments, which could be far away if you do not have a pediatric rheumatologist, pediatric neurologist, or other appropriate subspecialist in your local community. Hidden costs might include time away from work and using up all your vacation time taking your child to medical appointments, so there is no time left for your family to enjoy a break together. Continuous financial and emotional stress can contribute to depression and other mental health problems among parents.

- Caring for a sick child usually results in having less time for other children, for partners, and for oneself. This can lead to frustration, guilt, anger, resentment, and depression.

- Parents understand how complicated and fragile a child's self-esteem can be. You want your children to be confident and to have the skills needed to deal with any problems they will face as they continue to grow older. Parents worry about the possibility that a longstanding illness could affect how their children feel about themselves.

Despite these challenges, you will do all you can to help your child get better. Finding the right myositis doctor for your child is the first important step (see *Chapter 5, Finding Help*). Although it feels like your child is the first child ever to be diagnosed with this illness, she is not, and others have learned before you. Here are some steps you can take to lessen or perhaps even prevent some inevitable difficulties that lie ahead. These suggestions were gathered from parents of children such as yours.

- Educate yourself about JM, but don't expect to remember everything you are told during the first few appointments. Write down your questions and ask your child's nurse or doctor to explain any information that isn't clear. You can ask your child's doctor or nurse for an appointment outside of regular clinic hours, which will give you a chance to speak with the doctor without your child present. There are some good web sites that can give you accurate information, but be wary of sites that ask for your money or that mention cures. Any information you read that seems terrible or wonderful may not be true, so bring the information to your child's doctor for discussion (see *Chapter 5, Finding Help* and *Chapter 38, Searching the Internet for Reliable Information*).

- Develop a system to keep information organized. Some parents keep a journal or loose-leaf notebook where they record their questions and any medical information they are given. Keeping track of appointments and medical information can be challenging, so try different ways of keeping track of this information until you find something that works for you. If you are feeling stuck, ask other parents for ideas.

- Enlist support. This can be difficult, especially if you don't usually need help. There are many different kinds of support, and it is important to be open to receiving it. For example, you might arrange to call or see a friend every week so you can talk about how you are coping with the challenges that accompany the disease. You can accept a family member's offer to babysit your children, so that you can have some time alone with your spouse/partner. If your child is very sick, consider asking a neighbor or friend to help with some of the household chores. If you are getting too many telephone calls from concerned friends and relatives, ask one person to be the main contact for these people. If you feel overwhelmed with others' questions, one coping strategy is to say that you appreciate the concern but cannot go into details until the situation settles down and regular routines are back in place. Most people will understand and respect this. If you are finding it difficult to accept others' offers to help you, ask yourself what you would do if the situation were reversed. Would you want to help a friend whose child was sick? If the answer is yes, then accept that person's offers of help. We all give and receive help at different points in our lives, and in your life, you will have many opportunities to help others. One of the most important things you can do is hook up with other families who also have children with JM. The Myositis Association and Cure JM Foundation have bulletin boards, support groups, and conferences that many families find helpful. Remember that each child's illness and situation is different.

- If your child sees healthcare professionals other than your child's myositis doctor, then meet the people on your child's healthcare team and ask them what they do. Get their names and telephone numbers in case you decide to contact them later. At any point after your child's diagnosis, you may have questions or concerns, or you may experience an unanticipated situation that you do not know how to handle. Sometimes your questions may not seem like the kinds you would ask a doctor. However, the nurses, social workers, physical and occupational therapists, recreational therapist or child life staff, psychiatrists, and psychologists may be able to help you deal with these situations. For example, to handle the financial costs associated with any long-term illness, meet with your child's social worker at the beginning of treatment. This can help you save thousands of dollars in medical bills if you do not have health coverage or a drug plan. You may be eligible for financial assistance from the government, and your child's social worker will be able to give you information about these programs.

- Consider how your faith can give you the courage and strength to help you through the time ahead. Having a seriously ill child can help you reconsider and strengthen your faith in many ways. Speak to someone you trust, and take full advantage of your spiritual or religious supports.

- Consider your parenting style and how and when you discipline your child. Offer lots of choices to your child to give her a sense of control over her life. Remember that your child with JM has just lost the ability to do things that used to come easily. Many parents find it difficult to set limits and to say no to a child who is sick. This can result in difficult situations because children quickly learn how to get what they want from their parents and may take advantage of a situation. Wanting to compensate a child for being sick is normal, but it can be taken too far and can cause big problems for the child and for the family. Consider what is in your child's best long-term interests and what kind of adult you want her to become. Most parents believe that teaching all children to follow rules and helping all children learn how to deal with limitations and disappointments is very important. "Firm but fair" is a common and usually helpful way to approach setting limits on a child's behavior. At every opportunity offer a choice and let the child choose what happens. Reward good choices with the best of special rewards.

- Try not to overprotect your child, even though protecting your child is a normal response to a threatening situation. If a parent is too overprotective, by not allowing the child to experiment or by always being there to catch her before she falls, this can cause long-term emotional harm to the child. Children need to experience childhood, a time of falling and getting up again, before they can enter adulthood. A common example of this is when a parent keeps a child out of school for fear of exposing her to colds and flus, despite being told by the doctor that the child should attend school. If you catch yourself becoming overprotective, ask to meet with a social worker or psychiatrist.

- Take things one day at a time. When your child is very sick, you might feel overwhelmed and find even simple tasks difficult to do. Try to focus on accomplishing one small thing each day, and avoid making big plans. Also, try to be flexible because even the small things you plan might not get done. As your child's health improves, you will be able to return to your usual way of planning and completing tasks.

- When your child is ill, everyone in the family will experience stress. Tempers might flare, and people might raise their voices more than they mean to. Try to stay calm, and try to do things that help you deal with stress or that help you take a small break from the stress, such as going for a quick walk around the block, taking a hot bath, or calling a friend. Encourage everyone in your family to do something that helps them cope with stress. Asking family members what they have found helpful in past stressful situations can be a good place to start.

- Consider the effect of your overall attitude on how you cope, on how your sick child feels, and on how your family copes. Children are incredibly adaptable and will follow your lead. If you are really anxious, your child will probably be anxious, too. If you are calm and have a positive outlook, your child will probably follow your lead and feel the same way. Focus on the positive as much as possible. This does not mean that you shouldn't be aware of the challenges your family is facing or the realities of living with a chronic illness; however, a positive attitude will help you and your family in the long run much more than a pessimistic attitude. For example, try to focus on your child's abilities rather than disabilities, and remember that with treatment, the symptoms of this disease decrease dramatically. Positive changes in your child may occur slowly, so watch carefully for these changes and celebrate them as they happen. Keeping a positive attitude as much as possible will give your child and other family members hope and encouragement.

- Make time for your relationship with your spouse/partner. Most parents focus most of their time and energy on their children, with a bit of time left over for each other and for themselves. When a child is sick, there is usually a lot less time and a lot more stress, and the parents' relationship can suffer drastically as a result. Also, there are many different ways to deal with stress and grief, and if these differences aren't appreciated, they can push parents apart rather than bring them together. Communication and time together are very important for parents of children with health problems. Try to set time aside every week just for the two of you to talk about what's going on and how you both are coping. Also, try to spend time together each week doing something you enjoy. Get a babysitter if you can, or if your child is in the hospital, ask for a volunteer to come at the same time every week so that you and your partner can spend some uninterrupted time together. A good relationship between parents is like any other relationship—it takes time and effort.

- Very importantly, take care of yourself. Remember that if you don't take care of yourself and you become exhausted or sick, you won't be able to care for your child properly. Remember that you are the most important role model in your child's life. Do you want your children to grow up thinking it's okay for adults to get so run down that they get sick? Of course not! You want your children to become adolescents and then adults who take good care of themselves. They learn that best by seeing their parents take care of themselves. Make sure you eat well, exercise regularly, and get enough rest. Meet with your own physician if you start to notice changes that could be due to depression. Your own mental health will significantly affect your child's ability to cope with JM, so take care of yourself, and do not hesitate to ask for help.

Remember that life is filled with challenges and that you have dealt with and survived difficult situations before. You will survive this! Most parents find that the first year is the most challenging; after that, life gets back to normal. It won't be the same as before, but it will be normal nonetheless and probably will be as good as or even better than it was before. For many families, living with a chronic illness forces people to re-evaluate what is important, resulting in changes that benefit the entire family.

The Perspective of the Child with JM

Children's responses to a diagnosis of JM can vary greatly, depending on their age, the degree to which they are affected, their own personal coping style, and their family's ability to cope with challenges. Children diagnosed with JM may experience the following emotions:

- Guilt. "Did this happen because I did something bad?"

- Fear. "What's going to happen to me? Am I going to die?"

- Anxiety. "My arm hurts. Is it from the JM? Is every pain I feel from the disease?"

- Anger. "Why is this happening to me? This isn't fair! How come the bully at my school isn't sick and I am?"

- Depression. "I look ugly because of prednisone. I can't play with my friends because I'm too weak."

- Impatience. "When can I eat my favorite food again? Why do I have to keep taking these pills and getting all these shots?"

These experiences are normal. You can help your child deal with them by discussing them and by giving your child information she can understand. If you are concerned about your child's feelings or if you think your child is depressed, speak with a social worker or psychiatrist.

The Perspective of Other Children in the Family

Brothers and sisters of the child with JM might feel the following emotions:

- Guilt. "Did my brother become sick because I hit him? Is this my fault?"

- Fear. "Will my sister always be sick? Will I get sick too?"

- Jealousy. "Why does my sister get to spend so much time with my mom while I have to go to the babysitter's? How come my brother gets toys and stickers every time he goes to the clinic and I don't get anything? How come my brother doesn't have to do as many chores as I do?"

- Impatience. "When will my dad spend time with me instead of always being with my sister? When will things get back to normal in my home?"

These feelings are common, and helping your child deal with them involves discussion, teaching, and reassurance. Again, if you are concerned about any of your children's feelings, speak with a social worker or psychiatrist.

How Can I Help My Children Cope?

There are many things you and your family can do to help all your children cope with JM. Here are some ideas to consider:

- Explain JM to your children in fairly simple words (see *Chapter 2, Explaining Juvenile Myositis: A Kid's Guide*). Answer their questions, and ask medical staff to help at any time. You know your children better than any healthcare professional ever will, and you probably know how to help your children learn about the changes they are experiencing in a supportive way. It may be difficult for children to express their feelings about how the illness has affected them, and this applies to brothers and sisters as well as to children who have JM. Remember to let your children know that you love them and that you understand what they are going through. This can be done with words as well as actions. Also, remember that your child's healthcare team and the hospital staff have a lot of experience with children and illness, so ask for their help if you have questions or concerns about talking to your children about JM.

- Reassure your children that JM is no one's fault and could not be prevented, that it is very rare for more than one child in a family to get it, and that it is not something that people catch, like a cold. Instead, describe it to them using an example they can relate to, such as allergies, asthma, diabetes, or arthritis.

- Allow your other children or your child's friends to come to medical appointments with you and the child with JM. This helps get rid of any sense of mystery and to dispel frightening thoughts children might have from seeing hospitals on television shows.

- Let your children's teachers know what is happening so they can provide extra support and attention to your children. Keeping the situation secret can be harmful and can give your children the idea that JM is something to be ashamed of.

- Try to continue family traditions as much as possible. These traditions might include where meals are eaten and with whom, having other children sleep over on weekends, or renting movies and watching them as a family, etc. Children are reassured by routines. This can be difficult, especially if the child with JM is hospitalized or if you are a single parent with few supports. Do the best you can, and consider adding some new routines that will be continued after your child's health improves, such as having a relative spend time with the children one night a week or having a special family outing once a month.

- Keep the child with JM involved in regular family life as much as possible. To do this, some chores or other activities might have to be modified (for example, if a child usually sets the table alone but is too weak to lift a stack of dishes, an adult can bring the dishes and silverware to the table and have the child place them from there). It is very important for your child to feel needed and useful. An illness is not an excuse or a reason to get out of chores! If you have more than one child, a family meeting might be helpful so that everyone has a chance to share ideas and contribute to a family chore plan.

• Try to set aside time with each child every week. This does not have to be what is traditionally called "quality time." Instead, it can be time that you and your child have together, alone, so that your child can discuss recent events and any concerns about his or her own life. Examples of this time can be walking the family pet together or spending time in the car during a long drive or even watching a television show together.

• Look for opportunities for your children to learn about the illness and to teach others. School projects and presentations can be an opportunity for children to learn more about a health problem, and most health professionals would be quite pleased to be interviewed by your child. Presenting the information to others also gives children an opportunity to be an expert at something that other children know nothing about. Your child may not want to do this, but it is an option that they might be interested in at some point in the future.

• Speak with other parents whose children have JM or other long-term illnesses. Perhaps they will have ideas or suggestions that you can adapt to your situation to help your whole family cope well. This can also serve as a good reminder that you are not the only parent dealing with these issues!

• If you see changes in your child's mood or behavior, let the healthcare staff know, because it might be related to the medications. For example, prednisone can cause mood swings and irritability that can be challenging for the family and the people at school. One parent had a funny and accurate name for it...she said her son had developed PMS, her nickname for prednisone mood swings. Changes that result from the disease, such as not being able to play sports, alterations in physical appearance, and time away from friends, can also cause depression in children. Discuss any concerns with your child's healthcare providers, and they will help your child and family to receive the attention needed to address your concerns. It is not unusual for children who are really sick to start to act much younger than their actual age. (Sometimes we adults act like children when we're sick too!) The sick child's brothers and sisters might also start to act younger, usually to get more attention from parents. This behavior in the face of illness is expected, and the sick child's behavior usually changes back to normal as she starts to feel well again. If your other children start acting younger, too, usually to receive more attention from you, speak with them about how they are feeling and reassure them. Some children respond well to being given a specific role or job that helps them feel like they are contributing to the family. If these things don't work, meet with a psychiatrist, psychologist, social worker, or other mental health professional to help get you or your child back on track.

How Will JM Affect Our Extended Family?

JM affects not only the child, but also the family, the extended family, and potentially anyone involved in that child's life. Grandparents face a unique set of challenges when a grandchild is diagnosed with an illness such as JM. Here are some issues and concerns raised by extended family members:

Traditional caregiving roles in the family often change when the primary caregivers (the parents) must spend most of their time and energy with one child. Other people, often relatives, are asked to take on the role of caring for the other children in the family. Differences in caregiving styles can lead to arguments. Depending on the nature of the family's relationships, it may not be easy for parents to give up their child's care to their own parent(s).

Because JM lasts from months to years, extended family members who were initially involved in the child's care may not be able to help on an ongoing basis. They might consequently feel guilty and helpless.

Concern, anxiety, and fear can make people impatient, and so they might say things they wouldn't normally say. Usually, clear communication can help reduce the difficulties between relatives. Speak with a social worker or psychiatrist if your relationship with your extended family is making it more difficult to deal with your child's health problems.

Extended family and friends might want to help but might not know what they can do. Discuss ideas that any of you might have. A few ways that extended family can help include babysitting, doing household chores, providing emotional support, providing transportation to appointments, accompanying the parent and child to medical appointments, answering telephone calls and giving updates to relatives, and providing financial support. It is important for friends and relatives to recognize that parents have the right to accept or refuse offers of help. If you have offered to help and have been turned down, try not to take it personally. Remember that the parents are under a great deal of stress, and let them know that your offer to help remains for whenever they need it.

Explain the goals of treatment to the whole family, especially the need for restricting salt and fat intake. Because most children with myositis take prednisone, which requires a low-salt and low-fat diet, grandparents who may be accustomed to providing treats to grandchildren could inadvertently contribute to unwanted weight gain or elevated blood pressure unless they understand these dietary restrictions (see *Chapter 7, Treatment Possibilities in the Beginning*).

Brace yourself against advice givers, especially among family members. It can feel like suddenly everyone is an expert. This is natural (it comes out of caring!) but can be exhausting. Bring all the "advice" in the form of questions to your medical appointment. The bottom line is this: if there were an easy cure, your doctor would have prescribed it instead of prescribing medications with potential side effects.

The same principles that apply to parents also apply to grandparents and relatives. Learn as much as you can about the illness, and most importantly, take good care of yourself so that you will be able to help the child and the family as they learn to live with an illness that will last awhile.

What Are the Special Needs of Families Facing Separation or Divorce?

Parents and children from separated or divorced families face many challenges that can become even more complicated by an illness such as JM. Here are some suggestions to consider:

Communication is vital. Both parents should be given medical information and should know about the child's treatment plan. This can be very stressful if the relationship between the parents is strained. Some parents attend their child's medical appointments together, but others find that taking turns coming to appointments works better.

Consistency is very important. If a child lives with one parent during the week and lives with the other parent on weekends, routines for getting medication and physiotherapy should be maintained. Because it can be difficult for children to keep track of which medications to take and when to take them, they depend on their parents for help with that. Written guidelines provided by the doctor or pharmacist can be a neutral reminder to both parents about when and how medication should be given.

Both parents need to learn about the exercises your child should do to maintain muscle strength (see *Chapter 13, Rehabilitation of the Child with Myositis*) and assist with them, about applying sunscreen before going outside, and about being involved with a school 504 plan (see *Chapter 36, School Issues*).

Many organizations help families deal with separation and divorce. They can provide counseling, support, mediation, and legal advice that can help ensure that issues between separated adults do not have a negative effect on your child's health and treatment. If your child's illness has made the relationships in your separated family more difficult, get in touch with an organization near you.

How Will My Child's Friends and Classmates React?

Your child's friends and classmates might not understand what is happening to your child. They probably will have some of the same feelings as your children. They might withdraw from your child because of fear or ignorance about your child's condition or the medications. Helping them understand what is happening can prevent potential problems. Children who are hospitalized might not see their friends and classmates for a long time. When younger children are absent for a long time, they might fear that their classmates and friends will forget about them and will not recognize them when they return because of differences in their appearance because of the prednisone. Sometimes high school students who are absent for several months learn that there are ugly or frightening rumors about them circulating around school. Most children who are absent from school for more than a few weeks worry that they will fail and will have to enter a new class with children they don't know. Teenagers may worry about not being able to graduate with their friends. Here are some ideas that you and your child can consider:

- Good communication may help prevent or minimize problems. Ask your child's doctor to write a letter to your child's school. This letter should describe the disease in simple language, reassure them that the condition is not contagious, describe treatment, and describe how the disease and treatment might affect the child's ability to perform regular school activities. If necessary, the letter can ask that specific accommodations be made to help your child continue to succeed. Ask the school to keep the letter in your child's student file. Keep copies of the letter, and ask your child to give a copy to her new teachers at the beginning of the school year. If you have a good information sheet on JM, include that with the doctor's letter. Try to keep this information package fairly small. Teachers are busy, but they do appreciate getting the necessary information (see also *Chapter 36, School Issues*).

- Children in elementary school might benefit from having a public health nurse give a presentation on JM or on chronic illnesses in general. You and your child might want to be a part of this presentation. If you are interested and your child agrees, speak to your child's teacher and nurse to see what can be arranged.

- Some communities have agencies that make presentations to classrooms about issues such as physical differences, teasing, or health problems. Your teacher's principal, nurse, or social worker might know whether such an organization exists near you. School staff should also help your child deal with teasing or bullying that takes place at school.

- If your child is in the hospital for more than a week, ask the hospital staff if there is a teacher in the hospital who can meet with your child regularly.

- If your child is too ill to attend school, arrange to get homework. If the doctors say your child is well enough, encourage your child to do some homework every day.

- Encourage your child's friends to visit your child at home and, if possible, at the hospital.

- If your child is too ill to attend school for an extended time, speak to your child's teacher, principal, and social worker about other options. Home instruction or homeschooling may be possible to help your child keep up with school work (see *Chapter 36, School Issues*).

- If your child has concerns about being forgotten by classmates or if there are significant changes in your child's appearance because of prednisone, consider other ways to keep your child's classmates informed and in touch. Letters and pictures to and from school can make a big difference to your child's self-esteem. Recreational therapy staff in the hospital may be able to help your child make a video to send to school. This video will help ensure that your child is remembered and that the other children can learn about what is happening, so that they are not scared. It can also help prepare peers for changes in your child's physical appearance. Some hospitals and schools have technology that allows the child in the hospital to be connected by camera with their classmates every day during regular school hours.

There are many other creative ways to minimize or even prevent problems with your child's friends or classmates. Good communication with your child, with your child's school staff, and even with the parents of your children's friends is the key.

Life Lessons from Living with JM

Living with JM can bring positive changes to your life as well. Here are some of the benefits that families and children and teenagers with this illness shared with us:

- The whole experience often brings many families closer together.

- Many young people with long-term illness say that they are nicer than they would have been if they had not gotten sick. Specifically, they say that they are more compassionate to others and do not make fun of people who are different because they understand what it's like to be different.

- Several young adults have told us that they make better, healthier choices for themselves because they have a better appreciation of health and are more careful about how they treat their bodies. For some, this means they do not drink, smoke, or use drugs. For others, it means they have healthy eating and exercise habits and have made healthy habits an important part of their lives.

- Many family members tell us that as a result of learning to live with a longstanding illness, they feel stronger and have more faith in themselves and in their ability to deal with difficulties in the future.

- Young people who are sick for awhile can be more mature in some ways than others their age as a result of their experiences. This can help them make good choices about how to live each day and what they want to do in the future.

- Many people say that their experiences with illness inspired them to pursue a career in a field they would not have otherwise considered. These people bring with them an intimate understanding of illness and a passion about their work, and this benefits the children and families they work with.

- Children of all ages say they appreciate small things more. Teenagers especially say that they take fewer things for granted after dealing with a chronic illness, and they feel that their appreciation of things and people around them makes them better people.

- One family said that the illness enabled them to understand who the real heroes are in life. Before the illness, they thought that heroes were sports personalities, but after the illness, they felt that heroes were the kids and families who endured the worst and the doctors and nurses who helped their patients. Living with a chronic illness made them see the people around them in a different way.

Does this show that there is a silver lining to each dark cloud? Maybe. More likely, it shows us that we learn from our experiences and that in the long run we can benefit from experiencing many different kinds of challenges.

Key Points

- You and your family will survive this illness, and the situation will eventually get better.

- You must take care of yourself. This will make you healthy enough to care for your children, and even more importantly, it will teach your children to take good care of themselves.

- You are not alone in this. Many have been through this before you, and until a cure is found, many will follow. Do not allow this disease to isolate you from those around you.

- If you have questions or if you are struggling, ask for help. Healthcare professionals, other families living with JM, books, and credible Internet sites are a few of the many resources that are available to you.

Acknowledgment

Heartfelt thanks to Dr. John J. Miller for sharing his important work in this area and for helpful comments on the manuscript.

To Learn More

The Myositis Association.

Living with Myositis. Available from: www.myositis.org/jmbookresources.cfm or 800-821-7356.

> Information and articles on how families have dealt with different situations arising from having a child with JM.

Coping with Myositis as a Family. JM Companion. 2004 Summer. [Order a copy at tma@myositis.org or 800-821-7356.]

Cure JM Foundation.

The Family Support Network. Available at: www.curejm.com/family_support/index.htm.
Allows families to connect and share knowledge and support with others who share their challenges.

Band-aides and Blackboards.

Joan Fleitas, EdD, RN, Associate Professor of Nursing, Lehman College, CUNY, Bronx NY 10468; Internet: www.lehman.cuny.edu/faculty/jfleitas/bandaides. Email: fleitas@optonline.net.
Information and stories about living with chronic illness, especially for children and teenagers.

For more information on these and other organizations, see Resources for Children and Family Support *and* Books and Online Diaries *in the Resource Appendix.*

Additional Information:

Brewer EJ, Angel KC. *Parenting a Child with Arthritis: A Practical, Empathetic Guide to Help You and Your Child Live With Arthritis.* CA: RGA Publishing Group, Inc.; 1992, 1995.
Common issues for parents of children with a longstanding illness.

Huegle K. *Young People and Chronic Illness: True Stories, Help, and Hope.* Minneapolis: Free Spirit Publishing; 1998.
Written by a young woman with Crohn's disease. Covers all aspects of living with a chronic illness, especially from teenager's perspective.

Meyer D, Vadasy P. *Living with a Brother or Sister with Special Needs: A Book for Sibs.* 2nd ed. Seattle: University of Washington Press; 1996.
Focus on range of emotions brothers and sisters may experience and suggestions for explaining special needs to siblings.

Tucker LB, DeNardo BA, Stebulis JA, Schaller JG. *Your Child with Arthritis: A Family Guide for Caregiving.* Baltimore: Johns Hopkins University Press; 1996.
Information on how arthritis and other similar illnesses affect all family members and how it can affect relationships within the family.

Reports in the Medical Literature

Miller, JJ 3rd. Psychosocial factors related to rheumatic diseases in childhood. *Journal of Rheumatology Supplement.* 1993 Jul;38:1–11.

Following Your Child's Progress

CHAPTER 10

Charting Your Child's Progress

Lisa G. Rider, MD; Clarissa M. Pilkington, MBBS;
Nicolino Ruperto, MD, MPH; and David A. Isenberg, MD, FRCP

In this chapter...

We summarize the approaches your child's doctor may use to tell how well your child is recovering from juvenile myositis (JM) and if myositis is causing any long-term problems for your child. We outline the new tools that researchers use to determine whether children with myositis are getting better.

From the family's point of view...

"At each appointment, the doctors went through a series of strength tests, blood tests, and more to determine whether, and by how much, our daughter's condition was improving after starting her treatment. We kept our own records at home, too, noting how she felt each day, especially after certain activities. We used a scale from 1 to 10 to rate her strength, overall tiredness, and more. This helped us remember a lot more when talking to the doctor about how her muscles may be recovering since the last appointment."

How Does a Doctor Know Whether Your Child Is Getting Better?

Your child's myositis doctor will check your child's progress to see how well the medicines are working and whether your child is recovering from juvenile myositis (JM). Trying to determine how children with myositis are responding to treatment can be much harder than it might seem. Muscle strength might improve slowly. Stress and other factors can affect how fast your child heals, and sometimes the side effects of the medicines can cause more problems than the illness itself! In addition, frequently what troubles you and your child the most is not what your child's doctor is concerned about. For example, you and your child with JM might be most concerned about the severe tiredness and inability to do everyday activities, whereas the doctor might be worried about weakening of the muscles, skin, joints, digestive system, lungs, and heart.

What Are Disease Activity and Disease Damage?

There are two major areas that your child's myositis doctor will track to see whether your child is improving. The first area, disease activity, refers to the problems in the illness that result directly from the ongoing myositis and its associated inflammation. For your child, myositis disease activity can include things like muscle weakness, elevated blood levels of muscle enzymes, skin rashes, arthritis, or other active problems from the myositis. Generally, disease activity is a problem early in the course of illness, but also during flares or later on if the illness does not respond fully to treatment. Disease activity usually requires treatment with anti-inflammatory and immunosuppressive medicines.

The second area your child's myositis doctor will track is disease damage. Over a longer period, some children continue to have problems, even though the myositis itself is no longer active. Disease damage, then, consists of the continued changes that are not due to active inflammation. These continued changes result from previous disease activity or from long-term side effects of the medicines used to treat JM. Damage can include such things as calcinosis, thinning of the muscles (muscle atrophy), growth impairment, or a delay in reaching puberty, which tends to last a long time, even after the myositis is no longer active. Damage can be thought of as a scar. It is often irreversible or permanent, but in children with JM, some scars can be repaired and eventually go away or be less noticeable. Damage usually takes time to develop (more than six months or even several years). If it does occur (not all patients develop damage), it tends to increase over a longer period of time.

It is important for your child's myositis doctor to distinguish between disease activity and damage, because the effects of disease activity will usually be helped or reversed by using medicines to control the inflammation. If the problem is from disease damage, then increasing the anti-inflammatory medicines will not help and could cause more problems because of potential side effects. Many children with JM have a combination of disease activity and disease damage. Also, damage may increase in some patients over time if the disease is still active. This can make it more difficult to detect small amounts of ongoing disease activity, which requires anti-inflammatory therapy.

How Does the Doctor Follow Your Child's Progress?

When your child returns to see the myositis doctor, the doctor might check muscle strength and physical function. Different doctors use different tests to determine whether your child is recovering from JM. Doctors will also examine your child and order blood tests and possibly other tests to tell how your child is doing, and they will use this information to adjust the medicines.

Strength and Function

Two areas of great importance in the assessment of myositis are muscle strength and physical function. Muscle strength is how much force the muscles can exert in a defined position. In patients with JM, the muscles are weakened in the beginning because of the inflammation. For example, your child might not be able to climb stairs or comb her hair if the proximal muscles are weak. Later, that kind of loss of strength may be due to the muscles becoming thin (atrophied) or scarred, rather than from inflammation.

Physical function is the ability of the muscles to do work. Function is also usually decreased in children with JM. Physical function is measured by muscle endurance (the ability to sustain activities over time) and tiredness (fatigue), as well as the ability to do everyday activities. For example, if your child has problems with muscle endurance, she might be able to hold her head off the bed for only a few seconds instead of a few minutes. She might have difficulty with everyday activities, such as dressing, riding a bicycle, or climbing onto the school bus. In *Chapter 11, Assessing Muscle Strength, Endurance, and Function*, you will learn about several different measures that your child's doctor might use to assess these important elements at the time of diagnosis or to monitor your child's progress over time.

Tests of muscle strength and physical function are very important for monitoring your child's progress. However, these tests cannot help the doctor tell whether your child has active myositis that would benefit from more medicine or whether there are residual deficits in strength and function that might benefit from physical therapy.

Blood Tests

Often your child's doctor will order blood tests to follow the progress of your child's myositis over time. Blood tests that measure muscle enzyme activity are most helpful for assessing whether the myositis is still active. These include the level of creatine kinase (CK, also known as CPK), lactate dehydrogenase (LDH or LD), aldolase, and transaminases (AST or SGOT and ALT or SGPT). You have already learned how doctors use these tests to establish a diagnosis of myositis (see *Chapter 6, Tests Your Child's Doctor Might Order*). Your child's doctor will continue to monitor several of these enzyme levels through occasional blood testing. When JM is no longer active, these enzyme levels will return to normal. However, occasionally some aspects of JM can still be active even though the enzyme levels are normal or only mildly elevated. The enzymes, then, are not 100% reliable, and other aspects of the illness and its activity must also be assessed to decide how best to treat your child.

There are other limitations in using blood levels of muscle enzymes to determine ongoing disease activity. For example, the CK level frequently returns to normal quickly, then doctors must use other enzyme levels to find out whether the myositis is still active. Furthermore, each child might have a different muscle enzyme that is elevated when all the other enzymes are within normal limits. Some doctors find that the LDH level is particularly good to follow because it can reflect activity not only in the muscles, but also in other body systems. The enzyme levels can get better before muscle strength and function improve, and they can increase several weeks before a clinical relapse, signaling a potential flare. The muscle enzyme levels can increase with vigorous exercise on the day before the blood is drawn, and certain drugs can increase CK levels. Some of these enzymes are released into the blood not only from inflamed muscle tissue, but also from liver and other body tissues. It is important to have the blood enzyme levels tested by the same lab over a period of time because different labs use different tests, which might influence the results.

Other Tests Used to Follow the Myositis

Myositis doctors also recognize that other body systems, not just the skeletal muscles, may be involved. Many of the same tests used for diagnosis also help assess changes in the inflammation during the disease course (see *Chapter 6, Tests Your Child's Doctor Might Order*). For example, your child may also have troubles with generalized tiredness, skin rashes, arthritis, swallowing difficulty, voice changes, or difficulty breathing. Your child's doctor will ask you several questions to see whether your child is having trouble in any of these areas and also do a thorough physical exam to evaluate possible involvement of some of those body systems. If other systems are involved, your child's myositis doctor might order additional tests to evaluate some of those other body systems more completely. Those tests are discussed in specific chapters in *Section 6: Important Issues on the Road to Recovery*. Sometimes, the doctor will want other health professionals with special expertise in one of the body systems to become involved in your child's care and to help evaluate or plan specific treatments for some of these problems.

Sometimes, despite a complete evaluation by your child's doctor, it remains unclear whether your child's myositis remains active. In this situation, additional testing may be available, particularly at certain specialized medical centers, which can help piece together this puzzle of disease activity. Additional tests are used at certain centers or clinics that are not discussed here. Some tests are available only if you are part of a research study, and undoubtedly new tests will be available in the future.

The most commonly used and helpful specialized test is a magnetic resonance image (MRI) of the muscles. The MRI takes pictures of your child's muscles by using a strong magnet that reveals the water content of the muscles. In *Chapter 6, Tests Your Child's Doctor Might Order*, you learned how the MRI is used to help establish a diagnosis of JM. The MRI can also be useful at critical treatment decision points because it is one of the few tests that can show the differences between active myositis and damage to the muscles that will not be helped by medicines.

Doctors can see how bright the muscles and tissues around the muscles are on the STIR (short tau inversion recovery) or fat-suppressed T2-weighted images of the MRI. This brightness usually means that there is ongoing inflammation in those tissues. The T1-weighted image shows the muscle bulk (to see whether the muscles are thinned or atrophied) and whether there is scar tissue in the muscle. (See Figures 6.1a [color plate 4 on page 227] and 6.1b in *Chapter 6, Tests Your Child's Doctor Might Order.*) Some medical centers use ultrasound (sound waves) to look at the muscles. With inflammation, there is an increase in water content of the tissues, so more sound is bounced off the tissue and makes them brighter. A myositis flare can be seen by an increase in the muscle brightness. Ultrasound is also good at showing calcinosis within the tissues. However, ultrasound is dependent on the experience of the person operating the machine, and it is not as definitive as an MRI.

Sometimes additional muscle enzyme levels measured in the blood can also be helpful to see whether there is ongoing myositis disease activity. These include CK-MB level, a portion of the total CK activity that reflects the development of new muscle fibers; creatine, which is produced and released into the bloodstream when a muscle breaks down; and isoenzymes of LDH, which measure the LDH level in specific tissues, such as liver and muscles.

Other specialized blood tests that examine activation of the immune system or blood vessels can also be helpful indicators of active juvenile dermatomyositis (JDM) (see *Chapter 6, Tests Your Child's Doctor Might Order*). Some medical centers that use these tests a lot find that they are excellent indicators of active JDM and that they take longer to return to normal than other tests, such as the muscle enzymes. These specialized blood tests might include neopterin, a product of some of the immune cells; von Willebrand factor antigen, which is released from the blood vessels when they are injured; and flow cytometry of circulating lymphocytes (also called FACS analysis). In this test the levels of B lymphocytes and activated T lymphocytes (two types of immune cells involved in muscle inflammation) are often increased in the peripheral blood when JM is active. This test can be difficult to perform because the medicines used to treat JM can interfere with the results and also because of the need to compare the levels in children with JM to those of healthy children.

In all of these tests active JDM can increase the levels of these markers, but they can be increased for other reasons, including a recent viral infection. They are difficult tests to perform and are best performed at specialized centers.

Assessing Myositis Disease Activity and Damage in Research Studies

Because it is so difficult to tell whether children with myositis have disease activity or damage and whether they are really improving with treatment, groups of doctors got together to work on these issues. These collaborating doctors, known as PRINTO and IMACS (see *To Learn More* at the end of this chapter), have developed specific ways to monitor the various parts of the body that can be affected in myositis. They have also agreed to include certain important measures in all research studies (called core set measures). Finally, they have developed rules that combine the core set measures in order to tell whether patients with myositis are really improving in a meaningful way. These rules that define improvement (called response criteria) will be useful for telling whether patients are truly better after they take part in drug studies. This will help doctors decide whether a new medicine is helpful for children with JM and will allow them to compare how well different medicines work. These advances will also help doctors take better care of children with myositis who are not in research studies.

Core Measures to Assess Disease Activity in Research Studies

IMACS and PRINTO have agreed on the general areas and specific essential measures that are needed to assess myositis disease activity in clinical and drug studies (Table 10.1). This agreement on a standardized approach enables doctors around the world to compare each other's studies to see how patients are improving with treatment. It also provides a structured approach that doctors can use when taking care of children with JM.

Table 10.1. Ways doctors determine how your child is recovering from juvenile myositis (JM) and how they will decide how much disease activity is present.*

Area of evaluation	What your child may be experiencing	How your child's doctor might assess this area of disease activity	How this will be determined in clinical research studies (Core Set Measures)
Physician Global Activity	Any of the problems listed below	Your child's doctor obtains an overall impression of how active the JM is by talking to you, examining your child, and examining the results of certain tests.	Physician global disease activity assessment
Patient/Parent Global Activity	Any of the problems listed below	You and your child have overall impressions of how active the JM is and talk to your child's doctor about this.	Patient/parent global disease activity
Muscle Strength	Weak muscles—cannot climb stairs, comb hair, lift head off bed, get out of bed easily	Your child's doctor or physical therapist sees how much resistance or force your child can apply when the muscle is held in a certain position and pushed against.	Manual Muscle Testing (MMT), to include proximal, distal, and axial muscles.+

(continued)

Table 10.1. (continued)

Area of evaluation	What your child may be experiencing	How your child's doctor might assess this area of disease activity	How this will be determined in clinical research studies (Core Set Measures)
Physical Function	Your child may not be able to dress independently, get up from bed, cut her own food, write well at school, or run and play. Your child may have difficulty keeping up with sports and everyday activities (becomes tired). She may not be able to get up off the floor without your help.	You complete a questionnaire about how well your child can dress, reach for things, perform eating activities, bathe and groom, grip objects, and be active. Your child's doctor or physical therapist watches your child perform different tasks and scores them. These include raising her head or leg off the exam table, getting onto and up off the floor, getting up from lying down, and picking up a pencil off the floor.	Validated patient/parent questionnaire of activities of daily living, Childhood Health Assessment Questionnaire (CHAQ)** Validated observational tool of function, strength, and endurance; Childhood Myositis Assessment Scale (CMAS)**
Laboratory Assessment	Not applicable	Your child will have periodic blood testing to monitor the levels of some of these muscle enzymes.	At least two serum muscle-associated enzyme activities from the following: creatine kinase (CK), aldolase, lactate dehydrogenase (LD), aspartate amino transferase (AST), or alanine aminotransferase (ALT)
Extra-skeletal Muscle Disease	Nothing or any of the following problems: Tiredness Fevers Weight loss Skin rashes Joint pain, stiffness, or swelling Difficulty swallowing Stomach pain Change in voice (hoarseness) Shortness of breath or difficulties breathing Heart beating fast or skipping beats	Your child's doctor will talk to you and your child and perform a detailed physical exam. This will include looking at your child's skin for rashes, joints for arthritis, and stomach. The doctor will ask about swallowing difficulties, hear your child speak to find out about voice impairment, find out if there is any shortness of breath, and listen to your child's lungs and heart. In some cases additional tests may be ordered to look into a specific body system in more detail.	A validated approach that is complete and assesses skin, swallowing and digestion, joints, and heart and lung activity. The Myositis Disease Activity Assessment Tool, consisting of the MITAX and MYOACT, has been developed and is being tested.
Global Disease Activity Tool	Muscle weakness Skin rashes	Your child's doctors will perform a detailed exam that sees how strong some of the muscles are and how the rashes are affecting your child's skin.	Disease Activity Score (DAS), Myositis Disease Activity Assessment Tool (MDAAT)
Health-Related Quality of Life	Having difficulty performing schoolwork due to tiredness. May be feeling sad, depressed, anxious, or worried about looks or friends.	You or your child will answer a questionnaire about your child's physical abilities, emotions, and relationships.	Child Health Questionnaire (CHQ)

*Note that there are no standard ways of assessing myositis activity for doctors taking care of juvenile myositis patients. Your child's doctor may use only some of these tests to follow your child's progress or may even use different tests. For research studies, Core Set Domains and Measures have been modified from those recommended by international collaborating groups of doctors who are studying myositis.

+ Not recommended for children less than four years of age.

**One validated tool is recommended for adults and children more than four years of age, and two tools for children less than four years of age.

Your child's myositis doctor, as well as you and your child, might want to develop an overall rating of how active the myositis is (called a global activity assessment). This score is simply an overall impression of how severe JM is at the moment or how much the JM is affecting your child. (You can make it a game with your child by asking her each day where she is on a scale of 0 to 10.) Your child's doctor makes a global activity assessment by using certain key signs of illness and lab results. Some of the types of things your child's myositis doctor looks for during an exam to assess disease activity are:

- Your child's general energy level or degree of tiredness
- Sore or tender muscles
- Muscle weakness or endurance problems caused by active myositis
- Skin rashes
- Joint pain or swelling
- Swallowing, digestive system, or breathing problems that are part of the active illness

The assessment of muscle strength and physical function are two important areas in the assessment of myositis activity (see also *Chapter 11, Assessing Muscle Strength, Endurance, and Function*). The cooperating groups of doctors, IMACS and PRINTO, have recommended including certain tools (Manual Muscle Testing, the Childhood Myositis Assessment Scale, and the Childhood Health Assessment Questionnaire) in all clinical studies (Table 10.1). This is because these specific tools have been studied most thoroughly, can be used worldwide in many settings, and can be used in both adults and children with all different forms of myositis.

Of the blood tests used to follow your child's progress, the collaborating groups of doctors have recommended that at least two tests of muscle enzyme activity be included in research studies (Table 10.1).

A new tool called the Myositis Disease Activity Assessment Tool was developed to measure disease activity in the skin, joints, swallowing and digestive system, lungs, heart, as well as general symptoms. This tool can be used to assess the disease activity other than muscle activity in all forms of juvenile and adult myositis.

Another disease activity assessment tool is known as the Disease Activity Score. This tool was developed by Dr. Lauren Pachman's group to assess JM. It scores different symptoms and signs, with an emphasis on the skin and muscle. It has been useful in helping us understand the association between some laboratory test results and the child's physical condition. It is being compared to the Myositis Activity Assessment Tool and other measures of activity.

Assessing Disease Damage in Research Studies

Unfortunately, it is not as easy to assess damage in myositis as it is to assess myositis activity (Table 10.2). Recently, a comprehensive index, called the Myositis Damage Index, was developed to capture the persistent changes or long-term

Table 10.2. Ways doctors can determine how your child has not recovered from juvenile myositis (JM) and how they decide how much disease damage is present.*

Area of damage evaluation	What your child may be experiencing	How your child's doctor assesses this area of disease damage	How this is determined in clinical research studies (Core Set Measures)
Physician Global Damage	Any of the problems listed below	Your child's doctor makes an overall assessment of how much damage has occurred over a period of time (six months or longer), due to the juvenile myositis, the medicines your child has taken, and any other illnesses.	Physician global disease damage assessment
Global Disease Damage Tool	Any of the problems listed below	Combination of everything being assessed	Myositis Damage Index
Physical Function	Persistent difficulties with dressing, getting up from bed, cutting her own meat, writing well at school, or running and playing, that are not due to active myositis.	You complete a questionnaire about how well your child can dress, reach for things, perform eating activities, bathe and groom, grip objects, and be active.	Childhood Health Assessment Questionnaire (CHAQ)
Growth and Development	Your child may not be growing well or showing signs of developing normal pubertal changes at the usual time.	Your child's doctor will monitor your child's weight gain and height over time, as well as changes in your child's body that may indicate age-appropriate development of breasts, testes, etc.	Linear growth and sexual development
Health-Related Quality of Life	Changes that are occurring over a longer period of time. Having difficulty performing schoolwork due to tiredness. May be feeling sad, depressed, anxious, worried about looks or friends.	You or your child will answer a questionnaire about your child's physical abilities, emotions, and relationships.	Child Health Questionnaire (CHQ)
Muscle Strength	Weakness that does not change with treatment	Testing how weak your child is, which has not changed over a long time	Childhood Myositis Assessment Scale (CMAS)

*Note that there are no standard ways of assessing myositis damage when doctors take care of patients. Your child's doctor may use only some of these tests to follow your child's progress or may even use different tests. Damage is assessed over long periods of time, of at least six-month intervals. For research studies, Core Set Domains and Measures have been modified from those recommended by international collaborating groups of doctors who are studying myositis.

effects of previous disease activity that have happened in adult and juvenile myositis patients since the onset of the illness. This index has been adapted from a system to assess damage in another autoimmune disease, systemic lupus erythematosus. It has been shown in patients with lupus that developing damage early is a very worrying sign in terms of the long-term outcome. We have yet to show that the same is true of myositis, although studies to explore this possibility are underway.

In patients with myositis, damage to or scarring on several different body systems is assessed by the Myositis Damage Index. With this tool your child's myositis doctor develops a judgment about how much damage or how severe the damage is in each body system. The Myositis Damage Index does not determine the exact cause of the damage. This is because it is often difficult to be sure whether the damage was the result of the JM, the side effects of the medicines used to treat JM, or from another illness that your child had at the same time.

Because it is thought that damage accumulates relatively slowly, damage is assessed not more often than once every six months. Some examples of the types of things that your child's doctor looks for include:

- Problems with ongoing muscle weakness or endurance issues that are no longer due to active myositis
- Persistent joint contractures or inability to straighten the joints osteoporosis (brittleness in the bones)
- Calcinosis

Your child's doctor might order additional tests to evaluate some of the issues related to damage, including blood tests, imaging studies, such as an MRI of the thighs to evaluate the muscle thinning, or a bone density scan, such as dual X-ray absorptiometry (DXA) (see *Chapter 22, Taking Care of the Bones*).

Assessing Quality of Life

The effects of JM on your child's quality of life are extremely important. The use of generic health-related quality-of-life tools (the Short Form-36 in adults and the Child Health Questionnaire in children) is being encouraged in clinical studies of myositis. These tools consist of a series of questions that tries to capture the effects of the myositis on your child's lifestyle. The questions cover a variety of areas, including the effects of the illness on your child's physical and emotional well-being.

Key Points

- To follow your child's progress, your child's myositis doctor assesses several different aspects of the JM, including disease activity, disease damage, and patient-reported quality of life.

- Your child's doctor might use different indicators to see how active your child's myositis is at different points in time during the illness, including muscle strength and function, myositis activity in other body systems, and looking at blood test results of muscle enzymes.

- In certain patients, there can be times when it is not clear whether the JM continues to be active. In these situations, additional testing available at specialized centers could provide a clearer picture of the extent of active myositis. These tests may include MRI of muscles and blood tests that measure how active the immune system is and whether the blood vessels are injured.

- Doctors around the world from a number of specialties are working together to standardize measurement of disease activity and damage in children and adults with myositis for research studies.

To Learn More

International Myositis Assessment and Clinical Studies Group (IMACS).

Assessment Tools. Available from: https://dir-apps.niehs.nih.gov/imacs/home.htm. International group of myositis investigators that has developed and validated standardized approaches in the assessment of myositis, which are being utilized in a number of clinical trials.

Paediatric Rheumatology International Trials Organisation (PRINTO). Phone: 0039-010-39-34-25; Internet: www.pediatric-rheumatology.printo.it (for families; in more than fifty languages) or www.printo.it; Email: printo@ospedale-gaslini.ge.it.

Facilitates the standardization, development, and reporting of controlled clinical trials and the study of new therapeutic approaches for the treatment of rheumatic diseases.

Reports in the Medical Literature

Pilkington CM. Clinical assessment in juvenile idiopathic inflammatory myopathies and the development of disease activity and damage tools. *Current Opinion in Rheumatology.* 2004 Nov; 16(6):673–7.

Rider LG. Outcome assessment in the adult and juvenile idiopathic inflammatory myopathies. *Rheumatic Diseases Clinics of North America.* 2002 Nov;28(4):935–77.

Ruperto N, Ravelli A, Murray KJ, Lovell DJ, Andersson-Gare B, Feldman BM, et al; Paediatric Rheumatology International Trials Organisation (PRINTO); Pediatric Rheumatology Collaborative Study Group (PRCSG). Preliminary core sets of measures for disease activity and damage assessment in juvenile systemic lupus erythematosus and juvenile dermatomyositis. *Rheumatology.* 2003 Dec;42(12):1452–9.

Scott DL, Kingsley GH. Use of imaging to assess patients with muscle disease. *Current Opinion in Rheumatology.* 2004 Nov;16(6):678–83.

Sultan SM. Clinical assessment in adult onset idiopathic inflammatory myopathy. *Current Opinion in Rheumatology.* 2004 Nov;16(6):668–72.

Assessing Muscle Strength, Endurance, and Function

Adam M. Huber, MSc, MD; Robert M. Rennebohm, MD;
and Susan M. Maillard, MSc, SRP, MCSP

In this chapter...

We discuss how your child's doctors and therapists can tell how strong your child is and how your child is functioning, both of which indicate how myositis is affecting your child's muscles. We will review some of the ways that doctors and therapists assess joint range of movement, muscle strength, endurance, and physical function of children with juvenile myositis.

From the family's point of view...

"The doctor gave me a series of strength tests and asked a list of questions to get a better idea of how juvenile myositis was affecting my muscles. He said using these tests would help us measure how my muscle strength improves with the medicines and exercises and tell what I need to do now to get better."

How Does Juvenile Myositis Affect Muscles?

Children with any form of juvenile myositis (JM) have an illness in which inflammation in the muscles results in weakness and a reduced ability to use the muscles repeatedly over time (endurance, stamina, fitness). Together, these two problems affect your child's ability to do things (physical function). The words "physical function" could mean something as simple as rolling over, something harder like walking up stairs, or something very complicated like playing sports.

Although the muscle inflammation itself can cause weakness, there are several other ways that JM could affect your child's muscle strength, endurance, and physical function. First, children with myositis often become out of shape (have poor physical fitness) because of their inactivity. Children with myositis can have reduced ability to exercise and capacity for their muscles to use oxygen (called reduced aerobic fitness). Children with myositis lose their physical and aerobic fitness because they cannot do many of their usual activities, often for long periods of time, due to ongoing muscle inflammation and injury to the muscle caused by the myositis. Consequently, after the myositis is treated with medicines, it is necessary to rebuild the muscle strength and endurance that have been lost.

Second, children with myositis can develop limitations in how joints move because of tightening around joints or in the nearby muscle, called joint contractures. Not being able to move a joint also makes it hard to do things (see *Chapter 21, Maintaining Flexibility: Joints and Other Considerations*).

Third, children with myositis can have arthritis (inflammation of a joint or joints). Arthritis is often painful and can make it hard to use the joint that has arthritis.

Fourth, some children with myositis develop calcium deposits in the skin and muscles, called calcinosis (see *Chapter 17, Calcinosis*). These deposits can sometimes be painful, and if they are near a joint, can also affect how that joint is able to move.

Finally, some children who have had myositis for a long time may have permanent injury or scarring to muscles. The muscles might become thin. This is called disease damage. Muscle damage may result in muscles that are unable to regain their full strength or are permanently unable to move normally.

Muscle strength, joint range of movement, muscle endurance, and physical function are therefore very important aspects of how JM affects children. Your child's doctors and therapists will be very interested in each of these factors because they help them to understand how JM affects your child's body. Usually, children who are weaker and have worse physical function require different or stronger medicines or even physical therapy as treatments for their JM. Once your child has begun medicine, following the changes in your child's muscle strength, endurance, and physical function not only helps your child's doctor but also assists physical therapists to see the progress of your child's illness over time. Sometimes, these measurements can be a warning that your child's illness is getting worse, even before you notice that there is a problem. For these reasons, children with JM will have their joint movement, muscle strength, endurance, and physical function checked at most visits to the clinic.

How Are Joints Assessed?

Joint movement is assessed by the doctor or therapist by carefully moving each joint in a specific way to see how much it can move and whether it moves normally and through a full range of motion. Most clinicians can measure the movement by observing it and by feeling the joint when it moves. They can tell when there is a loss of movement and whether this results from the muscles becoming tight or the joints themselves becoming stiff. If some joints move less than expected, your therapist may give your child certain stretching exercises to improve how they move (see *Chapter 13, Rehabilitation of the Child with Myositis*). Your child's doctors or therapists will periodically check how well your child's joints move but not necessarily at every visit. In patients with juvenile dermatomyositis (JDM), the most common joints to be affected are the ankles, hips, knees, elbows, or shoulders, but other joints can also be involved.

How Are Muscle Strength, Endurance, and Function Assessed?

Unfortunately, muscle strength, endurance, and physical function are not easy to measure in a way that allows everyone to agree on the results. Some things, like height, are very easy to measure. It is much harder to determine how weak some-

Table 11.1. Major tools for the assessment of muscle strength, endurance, and physical function in children with juvenile myositis.*

What is it called?		What does it measure?	What will your child be asked to do?	What does the score mean?
Full name	Abbreviation			
Manual Muscle Testing	MMT	Muscle strength	Your child sits or lies in a certain position, then is asked to push against the examiner's hands with the muscles being tested.	Maximum score depends on how many muscles are tested. Higher scores mean the child is stronger. Can test a number of different muscles.
Isometric Dynamometry	None	Muscle strength	Your child sits or lies in a certain position, then is asked to push against a small device (either held or attached to something).	Scores need to be interpreted by doctor or therapist. Can be more sensitive than MMT but tests a smaller number of muscles and can be harder to interpret.
Childhood Myositis Assessment Scale	CMAS	Muscle strength, endurance, and physical function	Your child is asked to perform fourteen different activities, such as raise neck off the table, raise arm or leg, and get up and down from the floor. The doctor or therapist watches your child do these and scores how they are done.	Maximum score = 52 Minimum score = 0 Higher scores mean the child is stronger and has better endurance.
Childhood Health Assessment Questionnaire	CHAQ	Physical function	You and your child are asked about the child's ability to do thirty different daily life activities in a written questionnaire.	Maximum score = 3 Minimum score = 0 Higher scores mean the child has lower physical function.
Disease Activity Score	DAS	Muscle strength, physical function	The child is graded on eight scores of physical strength; function is rated with answers to specific questions.	Maximum score = 11 Minimum score = 0 Higher scores mean more muscle involvement. A score of 0 means normal findings.
Timed functional tests		Physical function, endurance	Your child is asked to repeatedly do certain tasks, such as sit-ups, push-ups, stair climbing, squats.	Children with better endurance can do more tasks in a shorter period of time.
Six-minute walk test		Physical function, endurance	Your child is asked to walk around a space for six minutes.	Children with better physical function and endurance can walk more steps and complete the full six-minute test.
Aerobic testing		Aerobic fitness	Your child will be asked to exercise using a stationary bicycle or treadmill.	Children with better aerobic fitness can exercise harder and longer. The amount of exercise can be compared to healthy children.

* Not all tests are used by all doctors. Following one test of strength and one test of function at the beginning and during critical points of the illness can provide essential information about your child's progress.

one is or how hard it is for a child to do everyday tasks. Because of this problem, muscle strength and physical function are measured using special questionnaires and tests (Table 11.1). There are many of these tests, and different doctors or therapists may use different ones. For example, the strength of individual muscles can be determined by manual muscle testing (MMT). Muscle strength, endurance, and physical function can be tested together by observing your child doing various activities, as in the Childhood Myositis Assessment Scale (CMAS), or by asking certain questions about activities, as in the Childhood Health Assessment Questionnaire (CHAQ).

None of these tests to assess muscle strength and function is perfect. Not all tests are used by all doctors, and the specific tests your child's myositis doctor uses to follow your child will vary among doctors around the world, especially by their training or specialty. What is important is that your child's strength, endurance, and physical function are measured and followed. By following one test of strength and one test of function, especially at the beginning and during critical points of the illness, your child's myositis doctor gains essential information about your child's progress.

These tests and questionnaires are not like the tests children take in school. Nobody fails these tests, and there aren't any wrong answers. All the different tests have one thing in common: the results are affected by how hard your child tries and your child's age at the time of testing. If a child doesn't try, the results will not tell the doctor and therapist very much about how your child is doing. As many as 25% of children with myositis are too young to perform some of the tests (for example, to do a sit-up with hands behind the head). For this reason, it is very important that children try their hardest in doing these tests so that the doctors and therapists have the best information to use in making decisions about treatment.

Manual Muscle Testing

One of the main tests used to assess strength is manual muscle testing (MMT). Muscle strength means the ability of a muscle to move a part of the body, like an arm or leg, against resistance (such as moving against gravity or lifting an object). There are many different muscles in the body, and each has a different job to do. In order for your child to have normal physical function, her muscles need to be fully strong and have good endurance.

MMT is generally done by your child's doctor or therapist by hand and should not cause your child any pain or discomfort. It is extremely important that your child is positioned correctly in order to test each muscle separately. This is done by placing your child on an examination table so that only one muscle at a time is used. It may be in a sitting position or lying on her back, side, or front. Initially, testing is done against gravity. Your child will then be asked to move in a certain way. If your child can't move against gravity, she will be repositioned to remove the effect of gravity (for example, moving her arm side to side on the table instead of lifting it off the table). If she can move against gravity without any difficulty, the examiner will then push against the muscle while it is moving in this way, and her ability to resist this push will show how strong the specific muscle is (Figure 11.1). A higher score indicates better muscle strength; scores in individual muscles range from 0–5 or 0–10, depending on which scoring system is used. MMT allows your child's doctor to see which muscles are weak and the pattern of the weakness. The scores for the individual muscles are then added to give a total score, which can be followed over time, although different examiners may use a different combination of muscles.

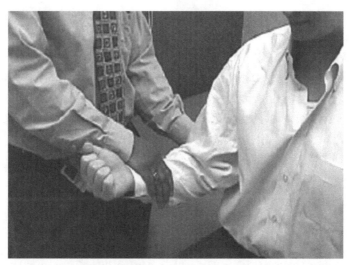

■ **Figure 11.1. Example of Manual Muscle Testing (MMT).**
This picture shows strength testing of the biceps muscle, also known as elbow flexion. The patient is positioned in a specific position, and the examiner applies resistance in a certain way. The ability of the patient to withstand the resistance determines how strong the muscle is.

Although MMT is relatively easy to do, it does have some problems. It is often difficult for young children (less than five years old) to cooperate with the testing. It is also sometimes difficult to compare results from different examiners, so it can be helpful to use the same tester each time. It can be hard to tell whether children are getting better as their strength gets closer to normal. Finally, children who appear to have normal strength on MMT might have mild weakness that persists but cannot be detected by the MMT. However, MMT remains one of the most common ways to assess strength in children with myositis and is often used by your child's doctor or therapist to follow your child's strength over time. As children get older they usually become stronger, so that must be taken into account when the test is performed.

What Other Types of Strength Testing Are Available?

Although MMT is the main test of strength, some doctors or therapists administer some of the tests described here. Occasionally, more than one test is done.

Some of these tests tend to be used more often in research studies than in clinical settings.

Sometimes muscle strength is measured by using special equipment. The most common tool is the myometer, which is a small, hand-held device that measures how hard the examiner can push against your child's movement. The advantage of this device is that it is less affected by the examiner's interpretation than the MMT. Consequently, it is easier to compare the results of different examiners. Using a myometer can also make it easier to tell whether there is any change in children whose strength is almost normal. However, the hand-held myometer is less useful when the examiner is not strong enough to overcome the child's muscle strength. This can be a problem when testing some of the large leg muscles or when testing older children who are relatively strong. Some doctors or therapists will use a rolled-up and partly inflated blood pressure cuff as a very simple way of making a myometer to assess strength in the hands.

Similar to myometry is a test called isometric dynamometry. In this test the child with myositis is asked to push against a device that cannot be moved. This device can be hand-held (like the myometer) or it can be attached to a larger structure (such as a chair or wall). This way of testing muscle strength can be more sensitive to small changes in strength, particularly in a child whose strength is almost normal, and it provides consistent results. It also has some disadvantages. Only certain muscle groups can be tested in this way, particularly when the measuring device is attached to something. Because there are many different devices that can be used, it is difficult to compare results that different examiners collect. The testing is very dependent on the position that the child is tested in—and that position may not reflect strength in other positions. Finally, if a hand-held device is used, the examiner might not be strong enough to hold the device without it moving.

Finally, some doctors or therapists will check the grip strength of children with myositis. The examiner uses either a special measuring device or a rolled-up blood pressure cuff and asks the child to squeeze it as hard as possible. This provides information about how tightly the child can hold things. Grip strength is often closely related to strength in other muscles.

Tests Used to Measure Children's Functional Abilities

Because of muscle weakness, your child might be unable to do everyday activities or be unable to use affected muscles repeatedly over time (endurance, stamina, fitness). Together, these two problems affect your child's ability to do things (physical function). The Childhood Myositis Assessment Scale (CMAS) is a test that your child's doctor may use in the clinic to observe your child's muscle strength, endurance, and muscle function. The Childhood Health Assessment Questionnaire (CHAQ) asks about your observations of your child's physical function in daily life activities. Your child's doctor may ask you to complete this while you are waiting for an appointment in the clinic or office. Some doctors do not use these two tests of function, which are commonly used in research studies, but instead use other tests described later.

CMAS Measures Muscle Strength, Endurance, and Function

Some doctors and therapists use the Childhood Myositis Assessment Scale (CMAS) to gauge your child's muscle strength, endurance, and physical function. Your child's doctor or therapist usually conducts this test during a clinic visit. The test asks your child to do fourteen different tasks that require use of different muscles. For example, while lying flat on the examination table, your child is asked to raise her head off the table and keep it in that position for as long as possible (up to two minutes). The other activities include lifting a leg off the table to touch an object, holding a leg off the table for as long as possible, rolling from back to front while lying down, doing sit-ups, sitting up from a lying position, raising the arms as high as possible, raising the arms above the head for as long as possible, sitting on the floor from a standing position, standing up from a kneeling position, standing up from sitting on a chair, stepping up on a stool, picking up a pencil off the floor, and doing a particular movement called the all-fours movement (assuming a crawling position). Your child's myositis doctor can find a copy of the CMAS on the Internet at https://dir-apps.niehs.nih.gov/imacs/docs/activity/cmas.pdf. The myositis doctor or therapist closely watches your child do each of these fourteen activities. For each activity, your child receives a score indicating how easy or difficult it was to perform. The scores for each of the fourteen activities are then added together to determine the total CMAS score.

The different activities in the CMAS were chosen for particular reasons. Some activities test the strength of individual muscles, such as lifting the arms as high as possible or touching an object with the foot. Other activities test the strength of larger groups of muscles, such as standing up from kneeling on the floor. Other activities in the CMAS, particularly the timed head, arm, and leg holds, measure endurance or the ability to use muscles and sustain a task over time. The CMAS was also designed so that it focuses on muscles near the middle of the body (like the abdominal muscle in sit-ups and the hips and shoulder muscles) because these muscles are most affected in JM. Finally, the activities in the CMAS focus more on muscles in the legs than in the arms because these muscles are so important for physical function and often regain their strength more slowly.

The highest (strongest) possible total CMAS score is 52 points, and the lowest (weakest) possible total score is 0 points. Children with moderate reductions in physical function have CMAS scores around 30, and those with mild reductions in physical function have CMAS scores around 45. An increase in as few as 3 points on the CMAS can result in recognizable improvements in physical function. There are no research data available to indicate what CMAS score children with more severe weakness have, but doctors and therapists who look after children with myositis often see children with scores less than 10.

It is important to realize that the CMAS is not a perfect test. For example, it is often difficult to get preschool children to cooperate, at least initially. (Often such children become more cooperative after the first two or three clinic visits.) The normal scores for some of the fourteen activities depend on the age of the child. For example, most four- and five-year-old healthy children are unable to maintain a head lift for two minutes and are unable to do all six sit-ups, even when they are fully cooperating with the testing. Therefore, younger children are not expected to achieve a total CMAS score of 52. On the other hand, a score of 52 does not necessarily mean that your child has normal strength, because the CMAS might not be able to detect slight weakness in some cases. Finally, some children score poorly on some parts of the CMAS because of problems other than muscle weakness, such as tightness around joints, joint pain, or tiredness.

CHAQ Measures Physical Function

The Childhood Health Assessment Questionnaire (CHAQ) tests physical function for daily life activities. You can find a copy of the CHAQ on the Internet at https://dir-apps.niehs.nih.gov/imacs/docs/activity/chaq.doc. It is different from both the MMT and the CMAS because the questions in the CHAQ ask you or your child to report what kinds of activities your child is able to do. Your child does not need to do these things in the clinic. The CHAQ was originally used for children with arthritis. However, it has been shown to work well for children with JM. In fact, the CHAQ has been used to assess physical function in children with a variety of illnesses. Because it has been used in this way, the CHAQ can be a useful way of comparing physical function in children who have different illnesses.

This questionnaire includes about thirty activities, such as removing socks, getting on and off the toilet, and writing with a pen or pencil. Some of these activities are very easy and some are harder. Only older children can do some of the activities, whereas even very young children can do others. They are arranged into eight areas: dressing and grooming, arising (getting up), eating, walking, hygiene (bathing and toileting), reaching, grip, and fun activities (like playing).

For each activity in the questionnaire, you or your child will be asked to indicate whether that activity can be done easily, with some difficulty, with much difficulty, or not at all. If your child is too young or simply has never tried the activity, then the answer is marked as "not applicable." Some questions will not be applicable to your child, because your child is not able to do them or because she has not reached a developmental milestone yet. There is also a chance to report whether your child needs assistance in order to do these things.

The questionnaire is then graded by adding up the highest scores in each of the areas and calculating an average. Children who are strong and can do things easily will have scores near 0. Children who are weak and have problems doing things will have higher scores, with the highest score being 3. This is different than MMT and the CMAS, where higher scores mean your child is doing better.

One of the biggest problems with the CHAQ is that as children get better, they will virtually all have a score of 0. Most children who still have mild reductions in their physical function will have a score of 0. This makes the CHAQ relatively less useful for tracking a child's progress when they are almost fully recovered. Currently, some researchers are trying to improve the CHAQ by adding questions that might be harder for children who have only mild problems with physical function. A modified version of the CHAQ that might be more sensitive for mild physical dysfunction has been developed and is being tested.

Other Tests Used to Assess Function

Many other questionnaires and tests could be used to help your doctors and therapists assess your child's muscle strength, endurance, and physical function. We will describe only a few of them here.

The Myositis Disease Activity Score (DAS) has a section that assesses strength and physical function. It includes questions about daily activities (such as going to school, playing with friends, walking, and climbing stairs); strength of neck, abdominal, shoulder, and hip muscles; difficulties walking; difficulties swallowing; and voice changes. This is a new questionnaire, which may become more widely used, as it has been shown to work well in children with myositis. There are many other questionnaires or muscle tests that individual doctors or therapists may use that are not mentioned here. Many of these are similar and focus on basic daily activities, such as dressing, eating, and using the bathroom.

Tests That Examine Muscle Endurance and Fitness

Children with myositis are less able to perform sustained activities; that is, they have decreased muscle endurance. They also might not be able to sustain exercise or keep up as well as friends. They might tire easily or develop muscle cramping when playing sports. If your child has these difficulties in exercise tolerance, your child's doctor or therapist might test her endurance and aerobic fitness or consider other causes of fatigue.

Assessing endurance and fitness can be done in several other ways. Some tests, like the CMAS, include questions about endurance. For example, in the CMAS your child would be asked to hold her leg off of the bed for as long as she can. However, your child's doctors and therapists might want additional information about your child's overall fitness. They might ask questions such as, "How far can your child walk before she needs a rest?" or "How many stairs can your child climb before she is out of breath?"

Your child might also be asked to do things in the clinic that assess general fitness, such as the six-minute walk test. In this test, your child is asked to walk for six minutes. Children who are more fit will be able to take more steps (i.e., go a farther distance) and walk for the full six minutes; children who are less fit may need to stop the test early or rest along the way.

Your child might also be asked to do different activities, such as repetitive squats, sit-ups, stepping up onto a stool, or stair climbing, as often and as quickly as possible. As children improve, they can do more of these activities in a limited time (often thirty seconds to two minutes).

Finally, children might be tested for their aerobic fitness, specifically their ability to exercise and the capacity for their muscles to use oxygen. In aerobic exercise, oxygen circulates briskly through the blood and supplies the muscles with an essential nutrient to create energy for the exercise. Children with myositis often have poor aerobic fitness. Aerobic fitness is tested in a variety of ways. Your child is asked to exercise, often on a stationary bicycle or treadmill. She breathes into a tube that is attached to a machine that measures how well her body uses oxygen. Depending on the kind of testing that is being done, your child will be asked to exercise until she feels tired or possibly until she doesn't think she can keep going. The person doing the test will then be able to determine the level of your child's aerobic fitness. This test takes lots of work, is not available everywhere, and cannot be done by young children—and so is not done very often.

How Are All These Tests Used?

Generally, your child's doctor or therapist will use one test of muscle strength and one test of function to follow your child over time. Occasionally, additional tests may be ordered or followed over time. Your child's doctors and therapists use these tests in several different ways. At the beginning of your child's illness, the tests are used to help understand how sick your child is and how much her muscle strength and function is affected. They are used to determine what types of things your child can do on her own; for example, is it safe for her to go up the stairs without help? Your child's doctor may use these tests to help decide whether it is safe to reduce your child's medications or whether she needs more or different medications. If your child is participating in a research study, these tests will be used to decide whether the treatment is working. All your child needs to do is to try her best.

Just as there aren't any right or wrong answers in these tests, there aren't any right or wrong tests for your child's doctors and therapists to use. They may use some of the tests discussed here. It is also possible that they will use other tests, vary the specific tests being used at different stages of your child's illness, or perhaps use even newer tests that hadn't yet been created when this book was written. What is important is that muscle strength, endurance, and physical function be assessed for your child as part of their care.

Key Points

- It is important to measure joint range of movement, muscle strength, endurance, and physical function in children with juvenile myositis at the beginning of the illness and then to monitor them repeatedly at important time points to check your child's progress.

- There are many questionnaires and tests that can be used to measure muscle strength, endurance, and physical function in children with juvenile myositis. Not all tests are used by all doctors, but using one test of strength, one test of function, and a measure of endurance provides essential information about your child's progress.

- It is important that your child try her hardest when doing these tests and questionnaires. Your doctors recognize when your child is not quite old enough or rested enough to cooperate with the testing at all the visits. There are no right or wrong answers to any of the questions.

- These tests and questionnaires will be used to make treatment decisions for your child and to determine whether she is responding to treatment.

To Learn More

American College of Rheumatology (ACR).

Practice Tools: Validated Disease Activity and Quality of Life Questionnaires. Available at: www.rheumatology.org/sections/pediatric/tools.asp?aud=mem.
Information on the various evaluation tools.

International Myositis Assessment and Clinical Studies Group (IMACS).

Assessment Tools. Available from: https://dir-apps.niehs.nih.gov/imacs/home.htm.
Information and educational materials for healthcare practitioners on the muscle strength and functional evaluation tools.

Reports in the Medical Literature

Huber AM, Feldman BM, Rennebohm RM, Hicks JE, Lindsley CB, Perez MD, et al; Juvenile Dermatomyositis Disease Activity Collaborative Study Group. Validation and clinical significance of the Childhood Myositis Assessment Scale for assessment of muscle function in the juvenile idiopathic inflammatory myopathies. *Arthritis and Rheumatism.* 2004 May;50(5):1595–603.

Huber AM, Hicks JE, Lachenbruch PA, Perez MD, Zemel LS, Rennebohm RM, et al; Juvenile Dermatomyositis Disease Activity Collaborative Study Group. Validation of the Childhood Health Assessment Questionnaire in the juvenile idiopathic inflammatory myopathies. *Journal of Rheumatology.* 2001 May;28(5):1106–11.

Jones MA, Stratton G. Muscle function assessment in children. *Acta Paediatrica.* 2000 Jul;89(7):753–61.

Rider LG. Outcome assessment in the adult and juvenile idiopathic inflammatory myopathies. *Rheumatic Diseases Clinics of North America.* 2002 Nov;28(4):935–77.

Treatment Options

CHAPTER 12

Possible Medicines During the Course

Lisa G. Rider, MD; Clarissa M. Pilkington, MBBS; Bianca A. Lang, MD, FRCPC; and Peter N. Malleson, MBBS, MRCP(UK), FRCPC

In this chapter...

We review the main medicines used to treat juvenile myositis (JM) during the course of illness, including what we know about how they work and their potential side effects. Other potential treatments for JM are discussed in *Chapter 7, Treatment Possibilities in the Beginning* and in other chapters in *Section 5, Treatment Options*.

From the family's point of view...

"She began her treatment with prednisone and continued for a period of eighteen months, but she relapsed after being off prednisone for only three weeks. The pediatric rheumatologist then offered a new course of action—we could reduce the prednisone the second time around more quickly if we added methotrexate injections. After she struggled with weight gain during her first course of prednisone, we opted for the methotrexate injections to lessen this and other side effects of the steroids. Later, we also added intravenous immune globulin (IVIG) to her regimen, and this has proven to be the best treatment for clearing up her skin symptoms and nail beds. Now, she's completely off prednisone, weaning off the methotrexate, and using IVIG only on an as-needed basis for her skin."

Many of the same medicines used to treat JM at the beginning (see *Chapter 7, Treatment Possibilities in the Beginning*) are also used throughout the course of illness. However, once the inflammation is brought under control, the treatment strategy changes, even if the actual medicines do not. It is almost like treating two different conditions. To return to the fire analogy, now it is necessary to prevent smoldering embers from flaming and to use water to put out all the embers. Some children may, in fact, experience more fire, or a relapse, when their steroid dose is reduced, particularly if steroids are reduced too rapidly, or when their illness does not appear to come under enough control with the initial treatment. These children with JM generally require longer treatment with steroids and other medicines. Each child's therapy will be tailored to her needs, so your child might not receive all of the medicines described here.

What Are the Major Medicines Used to Treat Children with Juvenile Myositis?

Several medicines are commonly used to treat children with JM during the course of illness. Of these, corticosteroids (also known as steroids) are the main treatment for JM. Other medicines, often called second-line or steroid-sparing drugs, may also be used in order to control JM while keeping the steroid doses as low as possible. Most of the current treatments for JM interfere with the function of immune cells. It is thought that immune cells are attacking the muscle, skin, and other organ tissues in JM. However, the more effectively and the earlier that the immune system is suppressed, the lower the chances that problems will occur from JM itself. Potentially less medicine will then be needed over time, thereby decreasing the risk of long-term side effects.

Today, with several choices for effective treatments, JM can often become inactive and even go into remission. *With these additional choices of medicines available for the treatment of JM, the chance of developing serious complications as a result of JM has been greatly reduced. Most children are able to function successfully with a normal childhood and life.* Exciting new treatments are also coming along that should make the treatment of JM even better.

Although almost every child with JM needs to take steroids, not every child requires second-line medicines. However, there is a recent trend for most doctors to start children with JM on these second-line medicines much earlier. Although steroids are the main medicine used to treat JM, they often have a number of side effects. Therefore, it is often helpful to add second-line (steroid-sparing) drugs to help bring the JM under control more quickly and at the same time to reduce the dose and length of treatment with steroids. For this reason, some pediatric rheumatologists now routinely start methotrexate in addition to steroids as soon as JM is diagnosed. When factors indicate the illness might be more serious or severe, these second-line medicines may be useful. They are useful later in the course of illness, if the myositis continues to be active for a long time or if a relapse occurs. These additional medicines, some of which can be used together, give the best chance for the myositis to go into remission. Finally, other medicines may work better than steroids to treat your child's particular manifestations of JM, such as certain skin rashes.

Not all of the second-line medicines are used in every patient. In fact, usually only one or two second-line drugs are used, and some patients are treated with steroids only (and associated medications, such as vitamin D, and antacids, to prevent side effects) (Table 12.1).

Table 12.1. Major medicines used to treat juvenile myositis (JM).

Drug	Special instructions	Usefulness in JM	Potential side effects
Corticosteroids* (Prednisone, Methylprednisolone) (Pill, liquid)	Take with food. Don't suddenly discontinue this medication; the dosage needs to be reduced gradually.	Always used in treating JM. Helpful for muscle, skin rashes, and all other involved body systems.	Weight gain, increased appetite, decreased growth, stretch marks, mood swings, cataracts, bone loss, diabetes, elevated blood fat levels, high blood pressure, increased susceptibility to infection.
IV pulse steroids* (Methylprednisolone) (liquid into vein, IV)		Used to treat patients with more severe illness or to gain more rapid improvement in myositis activity level. May be given once or repeatedly.	High blood sugar, altered blood pressure or heart rate, headaches, flushing of the skin, dizziness, vomiting, metallic taste with infusion, allergic reaction, mood swings. Other steroid side effects if infusions are repeated frequently.
Hydroxychloroquine* (Plaquenil) (Pill)	Take with food or a glass of milk.	Especially useful for dermatomyositis skin rashes and to reduce steroid dose requirements.	Nausea, vomiting, stomach pain, diarrhea, headache, increased sensitivity to sunlight, blurred vision. Damage to the retina in high doses (loss of color vision, depth of visual field).
Methotrexate* (Rheumatrex, Trexall) (Pill, liquid by injection under skin, by mouth, injection into muscle or into vein)	Take by mouth on empty stomach. Folic acid often helps with digestive system side effects.	Most commonly used second-line agent. May be used to reduce steroid dose or to gain better illness control. Effective in most aspects of JM, including muscle weakness, skin rashes, arthritis, lung disease, and other manifestations.	Nausea, vomiting, mouth ulcers (less with injections), hair loss, increased sun sensitivity, liver toxicity (monitor by blood tests—reversible), low blood counts, serious infection, shortness of breath.
Intravenous Immune Globulin* (IVIG) (Liquid into vein)		Second-line agent. Used to gain rapid control of most JM manifestations, including muscle weakness, skin, swallowing, and other gastrointestinal involvement. Does not suppress the immune system in fighting infections.	Infusion-related side effects: low-grade fever, chills, headache, nausea, low or high blood pressure, facial flushing, increased JDM skin rashes, fast heart rate, back pain, muscle aches, shortness of breath, and chest tightness (improved with slowing rate of infusion and with pre-administration of IV steroids, acetaminophen, diphenhydramine); severe headache, neck stiffness, fever within a few days of infusion, transmission of infectious agents (theoretical).
Cyclosporine (Neoral, Sandimmune) (Liquid, capsule by mouth, liquid into vein)	Take at same time each day, either with food or between meals.	Second-line agent. Improves muscle weakness, skin rashes, lung disease, and fevers.	High blood pressure, increased hair growth, tender or enlarged gums, mouth sores, increased liver enzymes, nausea, diarrhea, stomach pain, loss of kidney function, viral infections, tremors, numbness/tingling.

(continued)

Table 12.1. (continued)

Drug	Special instructions	Usefulness in JM	Potential side effects
Azathioprine (Imuran) (tablet)	Take with food.	Second-line agent. Effective on muscle weakness and function and perhaps in treating other JM manifestations. More experience in adult polymyositis than in JDM.	Nausea, vomiting, stomach upset, decreased blood counts, severe abdominal pain with vomiting (pancreatitis), worsening of JDM rashes, liver toxicity (usually reversible), low blood counts, tiredness, serious infections.
Cyclophosphamide (Cytoxan) (liquid into vein as monthly treatment; pill daily by mouth)	Urinate frequently. Take oral medication with food, drink. Lots of fluids throughout the day; urinate before bedtime.	Used mainly in patients with severe disease who have not responded to other medicines. Also particularly good for skin and gastrointestinal ulcerations, lung disease.	With infusion: nausea, vomiting, blood in urine (hemmorhagic cystitis), hair loss. Between infusions: low white blood cell count, severe infections. Long-term: infertility, malignancy (related to long-term dose).
Mycophenolate Mofetil (MMF or CellCept) (capsule, liquid into vein)	Take on empty stomach.	Promising for skin rashes and illness not responding to other medicines.	Nausea, vomiting, diarrhea, stomach pain, serious infections, reduced white blood cell count, elevated liver enzyme levels.
Tacrolimus (Prograf) (capsule, liquid by mouth; liquid into vein; topical cream)	Take on empty stomach.	Promising when illness is not responding to other medicines. Helps muscle weakness and lung disease.	High blood pressure, headaches, tremors, inability to sleep (insomnia), diarrhea, high blood sugar (even diabetes), and blood fat (lipid) levels, serious infections, elevated liver enzymes or low blood counts.

*These medicines are also used at the beginning of illness.

Abbreviations: JM = juvenile myositis; JDM = juvenile dermatomyositis; IV = intravenous

The medicines listed in this table may be used alone or several may be given together. All have benefits in reducing the activity of juvenile myositis and/or reducing the dose of corticosteroids to decrease steroid-related side effects.

Each child with JM will have an individualized plan of treatment. This plan depends on how the JM affects your child and how your child responds to the medicines. Side effects of treatment and any signs or symptoms suggesting that your child has severe illness requiring more intensive approaches are also taken into account. Some of the factors indicating that the illness may be difficult to control and that more intensive treatment may be needed include:

- The presence of severe symptoms at the onset
- A delay in establishing the diagnosis and in starting treatment
- A poor response to initial treatment
- Trouble swallowing
- Lung involvement
- Skin or gastrointestinal ulcerations
- The presence of some proteins in the blood called myositis-specific autoantibodies

The way different medicines are used together, when to add other medicines, and how quickly to stop medicines are decisions for which there is usually no one correct option. Doctors differ over how aggressively to treat the various signs of JM. In our experience, it is important to treat all the problems of JM, including the skin rashes of JM. If left untreated, the illness can become more severe and difficult to control over time or can lead to permanent damage (see *Chapter 10, Charting Your Child's Progress*). It is also important that the dose of medicine be adjusted as your child grows, because the dose of most medicines in children depends on your child's size.

Children with JM and their parents are often understandably concerned about the potential side effects of the medicines used to treat JM. All medications have possible side effects. In order to decide on the best treatments, your child's doctor must weigh the risk-to-benefit ratio (how bad the JM is or might become against how likely and severe the side effects from the medicines might be). Unfortunately, there are few ways to predict whether a child will respond to, or develop particular side effects, from a specific medicine, so it is important for your family to learn about the medicines your child receives. It is also important to keep in mind that most side effects are uncommon or mild, and most patients tolerate their medicines well. Your child's doctor might monitor the blood or do other tests to catch a potential side effect early.

In this chapter, we discuss medicines used during the course of illness to treat JM. Hydroxychloroquine (Plaquenil), a medicine commonly taken by JM patients, is reviewed in *Chapter 7, Treatment Possibilities in the Beginning*, and biologic therapies, which generally have very limited experience for use in patients with JM, are reviewed in *Chapter 15, New Therapies on the Horizon*.

How Long Are Corticosteroid Treatments Given to My Child?

As you learned in *Chapter 7, Treatment Possibilities in the Beginning*, most doctors will start a child who has just been diagnosed with JM on corticosteroids. Exactly how much steroid your child will need cannot be known in advance because some children have a milder illness or respond better to treatment than other children, often for reasons that we are just beginning to understand. However, within several months of starting steroid treatment many children with JM will regain muscle strength and recover the ability to do many of their normal activities. That is a sign that the amount of daily prednisone can be decreased, if the blood tests and other tests also suggest that healing has occurred.

Long-Term Treatment with Oral Steroids

Most children with JM are initially given prednisone (or prednisolone) by mouth in high doses (between 1 and 2 milligrams [mg] per kilogram [kg] of body weight per day). Some doctors divide that dose into two or three smaller doses per day.

The doses may then be consolidated, first to twice a day and then, if all is stable, to once a day. Other doctors prefer giving a single dose once a day, particularly later in the course of treatment. Although taking steroids every other day is useful in some illnesses to decrease the side effects, in our experience JM patients generally do not respond so well to doses of prednisone that are given every other day rather than on a daily basis.

As your child improves, the dose of prednisone will be decreased. Initially, large decreases, often by reducing the dose 10% at a time, may be made every few weeks, although this varies with each child's response. Once the serum level of muscle enzymes decreases to the normal range or when there is an improvement in other critical laboratory tests, as well as clinical improvement in muscle strength and other signs of illness, the dose of daily corticosteroids can be reduced slowly. Initially, small decreases in the dosage may be made monthly, although this may vary with each child's response. As the total dose of medicine is decreased, however, the amount the dose is reduced each time will be smaller, and the time between each change in dose will become longer (reductions over several months). This process of reducing the dosage is called tapering. Tapering is necessary because once your child starts taking corticosteroids, her body stops making them naturally. Tapering corticosteroids, rather than stopping them suddenly, gives the body a chance to start making them again.

Unfortunately, on this regimen of oral steroids, a significant proportion of children with JM experience a worsening of their symptoms (called a flare) after their illness initially comes under control. In this situation, the steroid dose often has to be increased again. Your child will be monitored closely for changes in muscle strength, skin rashes, and other evidence of active myositis. Worsening of symptoms is more likely to occur if the steroid dose was decreased too quickly or too soon (before your child was showing many signs of healing from the JM). In this situation, the steroid dose often has to be increased again. In other situations, if your child's JM has not responded as well as your child's doctor would like, other medicines are started along with the steroids to try to gain better control of the inflammation in the muscles, skin, or other body systems. These other medicines are discussed below.

It is very important that your child does not suddenly stop taking prednisone or fail to get the steroid into the bloodstream because of vomiting or missing doses. When a child takes steroids for more than a few days, the body stops making its own normal daily amount of steroids. The prednisone dose should always be reduced slowly to give your child's body a chance to make the natural corticosteroid hormone again. If your child has an illness that leads to vomiting, a major accident, or surgery, then she will need to receive extra corticosteroids (called stress doses), because her body cannot make the hormone on its own for as long as one year after receiving steroids. In these situations, if extra hormone is not administered right away by vein, your child's blood pressure may drop dangerously low, creating an emergency situation. You should call your child's doctor immediately if your child is not able to take steroids by mouth or is in a stressful situation requiring these additional steroid doses by vein. If your child is taking steroids each day for more than several weeks, it is a good idea to have her wear a medical alert bracelet indicating that she receives steroids. The Myositis Association has a list of sources for medical alert bracelets.

How Are Intravenous Steroids Used During the Course of JM?

Intravenous steroids called methylprednisolone (Solumedrol) are administered by letting a liquid form of steroids run into the vein over several hours to provide higher doses of steroids. The reason for using intravenous steroids is to gain more effective suppression of the myositis more quickly, while allowing lower doses of steroids to be given orally on a daily basis. This might result in fewer steroid side effects. Intravenous steroids are also given when the illness is severe or when there are complications that require immediate control, such as rapidly decreasing muscle strength, swallowing troubles, or gastrointestinal ulceration. Steroids are easily absorbed and act quickly when given by vein in high doses.

Some doctors recommend intravenous steroids with repeated and regular doses, whereas other doctors recommend intravenous steroids only when the illness relapses. The treatment schedules vary from several times a week to once weekly to once monthly or even less frequently. These treatments may be given a few times or continued for long periods, even for as long as many months. Usually, oral steroids with or without the addition of second-line drugs will be used together with intravenous steroids. In some areas, if treatments are continued for a while and your child tolerates the infusion well, a home health professional may administer the treatment at home or it can be given in a day hospital on an outpatient basis.

What Are the Possible Side Effects of Steroids and How Should My Child Be Monitored for Them?

Despite a long list of side effects, the benefits of steroids far outweigh the risks of possible side effects. Most side effects go away as the dose is reduced or the steroids are stopped. To decrease potential side effects, use a sensible approach to watching your child's diet (see *Chapter 19, Nutrition and Your Child's Weight*); try to encourage your child to be as physically active as possible; and get regular checkups with your child's doctor to follow blood pressure, blood sugar, growth, and the eyes for increased pressure and cataracts. The use of other medicines to treat JM, such as hydroxychloroquine (Plaquenil), methotrexate (Rheumatrex, or Trexall) and others discussed below, can also help reduce the side effects by enabling the dose of prednisone to be decreased sooner and more quickly than would be possible if steroids alone were used (Table 12.1).

Some side effects of steroids were discussed in *Chapter 7, Treatment Possibilities in the Beginning*, including weight gain, mood changes, infections, stomach irritation, and stretch marks. Children taking large doses of steroids also tend to stop growing while the daily dose is high. Because JM disease activity itself also causes children to stop growing, it can be difficult to know whether this problem is due to the illness itself or the steroids. If your child's JM remains controlled as the steroid doses are reduced or stopped, often the growth picks up. Her height may catch up to where it would have been if there had been no illness and no steroids (see *Chapter 20, Growth and Development*). Steroids can cause or worsen acne, which is very distressing for most adolescents, and can also cause excessive body hair growth, which disappears as the dose is reduced.

The risk of cataracts and glaucoma increases with higher dose and longer duration of steroid treatment. Cataracts are opaque deposits on the lens of the eye, but luckily it is rare for them to interfere with vision. Glaucoma is an increase in pressure inside the eye. Children receiving long-term steroids should have eye checkups twice yearly to be certain these eye problems are not developing and more frequently if they already have these eye problems (see *Chapter 27, Eye Health*).

Thinning of the bones (osteoporosis) is quite common in children with JM who receive steroids. This can sometimes result in bone fractures after only minor injury. We do not know whether the thinning of the bones gets better after the steroids are discontinued or whether it continues and results in more frequent bone fractures later in adult life. All JM patients receiving daily steroids need to receive adequate amounts of calcium and vitamin D through diet or supplements to help prevent loss of bone mass (see *Chapter 22, Taking Care of the Bones*).

Although steroids are very good at reducing the muscle inflammation and therefore help your child get stronger, occasionally the steroids can themselves cause muscle weakness (known as steroid myopathy). This occurs if your child is on high daily or divided doses of steroids for a long time. In this situation, it can be confusing as to whether the child's weakness is due to poor control of JM or to the steroid treatment.

Another very important—but fortunately rare—side effect of steroids is diabetes, which may be more frequent in children with a family history of diabetes. In this condition the child gets very high blood sugar levels. This excess of sugar in the blood can cause the child to become thirsty, urinate more than usual, and lose weight. If your child develops diabetes with use of steroids, she may need to reduce the intake of carbohydrates and sweets in the diet, temporarily use insulin injections to control the blood sugar level, or take other medicines to control the blood sugar level (see *Chapter 25, Attention to Sugar and Fat Metabolism*). Diabetes caused by steroids usually goes away once the steroid dose is lowered or stopped. High cholesterol and blood fat (lipid) levels may also result from steroid use. This can often be controlled with a low-fat diet.

High blood pressure occurs in a small proportion of children. This condition tends to be more common in patients who have a close relative with high blood pressure. A low-salt diet can help prevent this. Sometimes children have to use medicines to control the high blood pressure until it returns to normal. This side effect generally goes away once the steroids have been decreased to a low level.

How Soon Can the Steroids and Other Medicines Be Stopped?

Your child's myositis doctor will look at different aspects of the JM to see whether the disease activity is coming under control. The doctor will use findings from examining your child (such as improved muscle strength and endurance, decreased skin rashes, and other improvements) and lab test results (such as the muscle enzyme levels in the blood) to help decide whether to reduce the medications. Often, steroid doses are reduced first and then the other medicines are reduced later. It is our experience that if the doses are reduced too quickly, the illness has a greater chance of returning (relapse).

Second-Line Medicines

Doctors often have to choose between using methotrexate, hydroxychloroquine, intravenous immune globulin (IVIG), cyclosporine, and azathioprine when the JM is not responding to steroids alone or when there are signs that the illness is more severe and will require several medicines to bring it under control. As seen in Chapter 7 (*Treatment Possibilities in the Beginning*), doctors are starting to use some of these medicines more frequently as part of the initial treatment. However, they are often used in long-term treatment. Your child will not take all of these at once, but the doctor might need to try one or several of them, either one at a time or in combination to see which treatment works the best.

Who Needs to Take Second-Line Medicines in Addition to Steroids?

Many patients need to take other medicines besides steroids to treat their JM because the illness is severe at the beginning of treatment, because your child's doctor suspects that the illness course may be a difficult one, or because your child has not responded to steroids alone. These factors are all taken into account when your child's doctor decides to use more intensive treatment. Sometimes second-line medicines are used because your child develops intolerable side effects with steroids. Use of these other medicines can help bring the JM under control while allowing smaller doses of steroids to be used. Other medicines may work better than steroids to treat your child's particular manifestations of JM. Many of the second-line medicines discussed later in this chapter seem to work well in treating JDM skin rashes.

Patients receiving many of the second-line medicines, such as methotrexate, cyclosporine, azathioprine, cyclophosphamide, mycophenolate mofetil, tacrolimus, or other medicines that suppress the immune system, may be more susceptible to certain infections. This is particularly true when these medicines are taken in combination with high doses of steroids, because they too suppress or dampen the functioning of the immune system. The infections can include common and rare bacterial and viral infections, such as shingles (from herpes virus) and a pneumonia called pneumocystis (see *Chapter 29, Vaccines and Infection Protection*). Sometimes the infections may be more serious than ordinary. Perhaps surprisingly, children on these medicines usually do not seem to have more frequent common upper respiratory infections than other children. While receiving these medicines, any signs of infection require immediate attention from your child's doctors. If your child is due for an immunization, this should first be discussed with your myositis doctor. For further information on this subject, see *Chapter 29, Vaccines and Infection Protection*.

Because many of the second-line medicines suppress the immune system, there is an extremely rare chance of developing lymph node tumors (lymphoma) or other cancers. This has been seen only when several of these medicines are used together in combination along with high doses of steroids, or if they are used for a long time. With methotrexate, lymphoma occurs extremely rarely and appears to be due to reactivation of Epstein-Barr virus; it usually goes away by stopping methotrexate.

Methotrexate

Methotrexate (Rheumatrex or Trexall) appears to treat JM effectively, based on several medical reports of children having better controlled JM activity when receiving methotrexate. Methotrexate is also possibly beneficial in adult myositis patients. Patients who did not get better with prednisone treatment by itself improved significantly when the steroids were combined with methotrexate. Methotrexate can also help improve the skin rashes of dermatomyositis (DM), as well as the lung problems and arthritis associated with myositis. Methotrexate seems to work by decreasing the inflammation in the muscle, skin, and other organs, partly by changing the way your body handles a metabolite of folic acid.

Most doctors start methotrexate or other second-line medicines in patients with severe illness or those who do not respond quickly to the initial steroid treatment. Some, as you read in Chapter 7, start methotrexate from the beginning of illness. Methotrexate begins to take effect six weeks to two months after treatment is begun. Patients with JM often take six to twelve months or longer to achieve normal strength or to reduce steroid doses to very low levels while receiving methotrexate. Methotrexate is given as an injection or taken by mouth as pills or a liquid, usually in a dose given once weekly.

What are the side effects of methotrexate? Methotrexate is generally well tolerated, and serious side effects rarely occur. The most common side effects of methotrexate, including stomach upset, mouth sores, and sun sensitivity, have been discussed in Chapter 7. Your child's doctor can watch for long-term side effects of methotrexate by checking certain blood tests regularly. These tests include liver enzymes, complete blood counts, serum creatinine, and urinalysis. They might be checked more frequently when just starting methotrexate or when increasing the dose.

Liver side effects are uncommon but may be more frequent when other medicines are used that also have such side effects, including nonsteroidal anti-inflammatory drugs such as ibuprofen (Motrin), azathioprine, or cyclosporine, or, in teenagers, with regular or "binge" use of alcohol. The elevated liver enzymes could also reflect active myositis, and this can be difficult to sort out in patients with JM. Usually, liver inflammation from methotrexate is reversible, and if it develops, it goes away completely after a few doses of the medicine are withheld. Older patients should stop or limit drinking alcohol while taking methotrexate.

Methotrexate can cause a decrease in the white blood cell count and other blood cells produced by the bone marrow. This is an uncommon side effect in children and is monitored every few months with a blood test called a complete blood count. Patients with underlying kidney disease, low levels of folic acid, or who take an antibiotic called trimethoprim/ sulfamethoxazole (Bactrim, Septra) are more likely to have this problem.

Some patients develop hair loss with the use of methotrexate. Pneumonitis, inflammation in the lungs from use of methotrexate, is an *extremely uncommon* allergic type of side effect. In fact, methotrexate is usually used to treat lung problems in children with JM.

Methotrexate taken during pregnancy may result in birth defects. Teenage girls and women must not get pregnant while receiving methotrexate (see *Chapter 33, Pregnancy and Fertility*). If your child should become pregnant, then methotrexate should be discontinued and she should see her doctor. However, there is no risk of a side effect during pregnancy from the methotrexate if it has been stopped for a few weeks before pregnancy occurs. If your child received methotrexate to treat her JM during childhood or teenage years, pregnancies in adulthood do not have problems related to previous use of methotrexate.

Methotrexate can interact with other drugs that your child may also be taking, which could result in increased nausea, increased liver enzymes, or low white blood cell counts. Check with your doctor if these occur.

Intravenous Immune Globulin (IVIG)

IVIG has been a useful second-line medicine that is taken together with steroids to treat JDM long term or in certain potentially life-threatening situations, such as severe swallowing difficulties. IVIG starts working very rapidly (within hours to days). IVIG alters the functioning of the immune system without interfering with its ability to fight off infections. IVIG seems to help JM by turning down certain parts of the inflammatory or autoimmune process of JM. The exact ways in which it works in myositis, however, are not completely understood.

A number of medical reports support the use of IVIG as a treatment for JM. A controlled drug trial in adult DM found that IVIG was effective. Benefits have also been reported in a number of patients with JDM and adult polymyositis (PM).

IVIG seems to be helpful for many signs of JM. It can improve muscle strength, blood levels of muscle enzymes, skin rashes, swallowing, and other problems, and it even works well in patients who do not respond to steroids alone. In many cases, IVIG treatments can lead to decreased doses of daily oral steroids.

Usually IVIG is given by vein monthly for at least three to six months. It can be continued beyond six months if it seems to be helping, but the JM is still active. If treatments are continued over time and the child tolerates the infusion well, in some places, a home health professional can administer the treatment at home or it can be given in a day hospital on an outpatient basis. Although improvement with IVIG can sometimes be seen almost immediately, in some cases benefits may not be evident for a few months. In some patients the effectiveness of this treatment seems to decrease when it is used for more than six months. Several studies suggest that with multiple treatments the effectiveness of IVIG may last, even once it is stopped. However, some patients seem to relapse when IVIG is discontinued.

There are many different regimens for giving IVIG. One such regimen is to give 1 gram (g) per kg per day over two days (2 g/kg total) every month. Sometimes IVIG is spread out in smaller doses over five days, or it is given in two separate treatments spaced by one or two weeks. Sometimes it is given as a single infusion of 2 g/kg on one day. Some patients may require a lower dose (400 mg/kg monthly) as a replacement dose of immunoglobulin proteins in the blood to ward off infection (see *Chapter 29, Vaccines and Infection Protection*). Occasionally, patients receive the treatments less frequently (every six weeks).

What are the side effects of IVIG? IVIG is generally well tolerated. Because IVIG is made from the blood of many donors, steps have been taken to protect IVIG from carrying viruses, bacteria, and other infections. These steps include carefully screening the blood donors for infections, as well as following a manufacturing process designed to kill or get rid of infectious agents. The AIDS virus, HIV, has never been spread in IVIG, as far as we know.

IVIG has an advantage over some other second-line medicines in that it does not suppress the immune system, so it does not contribute to making your child more prone to infections or to cancers. IVIG can actually protect against certain bacterial infections by boosting the blood level of immunoglobulin G, a protein in the blood that helps fight infections. Because of antibodies in IVIG to infectious agents, live viral vaccines might not work as well if they are given shortly after IVIG treatment and therefore these vaccines may need to be delayed (see *Chapter 29, Vaccines and Infection Protection*).

The most common side effects are those associated with the infusion or treatment itself. They include low-grade fever, chills, headache, nausea, low or high blood pressure, facial flushing, an increase in JDM skin rashes, fast heart rate, back pain, muscle aches, shortness of breath, and chest tightness. These symptoms last a few minutes to a few hours to a few days. They usually improve (1) by stopping the treatment for a short time and then restarting it at a slower rate; (2) by taking certain medicines before the treatment, including intravenous steroids, acetaminophen (Tylenol or paracetomol), or diphenhydramine (Benadryl); or (3) by changing the brand or preparation of IVIG that is used, selecting one that is low in immunoglobulin A (IgA). Often, if the patient is receiving an intravenous pulse of steroids, this is given first and reduces the side effects from the IVIG infusion.

Another potential side effect is hives or a severe allergic reaction to the IVIG. This is most often seen in patients who have low levels of IgA in their blood. Using a preparation of IVIG that is low in IgA can reduce this side effect.

Some patients develop a form of meningitis (which is not due to an infection) within one to three days after the treatment. Symptoms include a very severe headache, low-grade fever, stiff neck, sensitivity to light, nausea, or vomiting. These symptoms resolve without any specific treatment, usually over the course of one to two days. Side effects may be prevented by switching brands of IVIG or by using acetaminophen or a nonsteroidal anti-inflammatory drug before the next infusion.

Cyclosporine

Cyclosporine (Neoral or Sandimmune) is a medicine that has been used to treat JM for more than a decade. It was first used to prevent rejection of transplanted organs. It also helps control illnesses caused by inflammation, such as rheumatoid arthritis and psoriasis, by stopping the activation of T and B lymphocytes (white blood cells that are involved in the inflammation in JM).

Cyclosporine helps improve muscle strength and muscle enzyme levels in patients with JM when the illness has not come under control with steroid treatment alone. Cyclosporine can also help decrease the steroid dose. It can also be especially helpful in controlling skin rashes of JDM, in treating the lung problems of JM, and for some of the general symptoms of JM, such as fevers.

Cyclosporine begins working within a few months of starting treatment, and for some symptoms (such as fever), cyclosporine can work within a few days. Cyclosporine can be used in JM in combination with steroids, as well as with methotrexate, IVIG, and cyclophosphamide.

Cyclosporine is available as a syrup or capsule, or it can be administered as an injection into the vein. It is usually given in two doses each day, and it is best to take it at the same time each day. Its absorption from the stomach and intestine varies markedly between patients, so some patients require much higher doses to achieve the proper level in the blood. Grapefruit juice and a high-fat meal increase cyclosporine absorption and so should be avoided. Its level in the bloodstream can be measured just before a dose is given. Levels are measured when there is a concern that the medicine is not working as well as possible or if there is a concern about side effects.

What are the side effects of cyclosporine? Cyclosporine has a number of potential side effects, most of which disappear once it is stopped. Side effects seem to be related to the absorption of the medicine and can be monitored by following the blood level of cyclosporine. Like steroids, it can cause fluid retention and an increase in body hair. Another common side effect is swelling of the gums, which then become tender. Mouth sores and bleeding from the gums can also be a problem. Less common side effects are tremors (mild shaking of the hands), headaches, numbness, as well as nausea, upset stomach, or diarrhea. Cyclosporine can rarely result in muscle weakness and muscle aches.

Some other side effects can be detected when your child's doctor checks your child or tests her blood. These include an increase in blood pressure, problems with kidney function, changes in body salt (electrolyte) levels, and elevated liver enzymes. These all have to be monitored on a regular basis (i.e., blood pressure measurements, blood tests, urine tests, and specific drug level) but usually return to normal when cyclosporine is discontinued. Cyclosporine also can cause high blood fat (lipid) levels (see *Chapter 25, Attention to Sugar and Fat Metabolism*).

Because the liver breaks down cyclosporine, drugs that are processed by the body using the same liver pathways can increase cyclosporine levels. These medicines can also have more side effects when used with cyclosporine. Your child's doctor will need to determine whether the benefits outweigh the risks when treatment with any of the following medicines is considered while your child is on cyclosporine: erythromycin, doxycycline, and certain other antibiotics, calcium channel blockers (such as diltiazem), nonsteroidal anti-inflammatory drugs, and statins (lipid lowering drugs), oral contraceptive pills, and methylprednisolone. A dietary supplement, St John's Wort, can markedly lower the cyclosporine level and should not be used.

Azathioprine

Azathioprine (Imuran) suppresses the immune system, possibly by preventing the T and B lymphocytes (the white blood cells in the immune system that are part of the inflammation in JM) from dividing, and it inhibits their functions. It has been used for several decades to treat organ rejection during transplantation, as well as for autoimmune diseases and cancer. Its use in JM is supported primarily by a drug study in adults with PM, in which it was shown to improve muscle strength and function and muscle enzyme levels.

There is less experience in the successful use of azathioprine for treating JM. Azathioprine can also allow your child's doctor to lower the steroid dose more rapidly. Some patients whose JM was difficult to treat have improved after receiving azathioprine.

Azathioprine is available only as a pill (not as a liquid) and should be taken once a day. It usually takes at least three months before some improvement in JM is seen, and the maximum improvements might not be seen for twelve months. Azathioprine is used less often than methotrexate, IVIG, or cyclosporine because it is less effective.

What are the side effects of azathioprine? Common side effects of azathioprine include nausea, vomiting, and stomach pain, which can be lessened by taking it after meals. Diarrhea, fevers, mouth sores, muscle aches, increased sensitivity to sunlight (with increase in JDM skin rashes), hair loss, and tiredness can also be associated with taking azathioprine. It can cause liver problems that are usually mild. Some patients lose some of their hair.

Azathioprine can reduce white blood cell, red blood cell, and platelet counts because it shuts down the bone marrow's ability to produce these cells. This usually reverses when the medicine is stopped. If your child is taking azathioprine and starts bruising easily, bleeding, or has fevers, report this immediately to your child's doctor.

Rarely, problems with severe stomach pain, vomiting, and inflammation of the pancreas (pancreatitis) can develop. An allergic type of reaction in which the JDM rashes worsen may also occur. This resolves when azathioprine is stopped. Azathioprine should not be taken if your child is pregnant because it can cause birth defects.

Cyclophosphamide

Cyclophosphamide (Cytoxan) is an effective anti-inflammatory medication that prevents all cells, particularly B and T lymphocytes (the white blood cells in the immune system that are part of the inflammation in JM) from dividing. Although it can be given daily as a pill, it is given more commonly once monthly as an infusion into the vein. The intravenous form is effective in a number of autoimmune diseases including lupus. Occasionally, the intravenous monthly dose is divided into weekly or twice monthly doses. Later on, once there is a good response to cyclophosphamide, the dosing can be spaced to once every three months.

A recent study from the United Kingdom suggests that cyclophosphamide helps improve muscle strength and function, muscle enzyme levels, and skin rashes in JDM patients. The patients in that study had severe illness that did not respond to several medicines. Because cyclophosphamide has potentially severe side effects, its use is limited to patients with severe JM or JM that has not responded to a number of medicines. It is particularly used for patients with ulcers of the skin or intestinal tract, a lung problem called interstitial lung disease, or widespread involvement of the internal organs.

What are the side effects of cyclophosphamide? The following short-term side effects are very common: lack of appetite, nausea, and vomiting. Administering an anti-nausea medicine usually eases these side effects. Cyclophosphamide causes the number of white blood cells to decrease, which occurs approximately ten days after the intravenous dose. Checking blood counts around this time allows the next dose to be reduced if the number of white blood cells has dropped to a dangerously low level. Antibody levels can also drop, and both these effects can result in the patient developing serious bacterial, viral, or other infections (see *Chapter 29, Vaccines and Infection Protection*).

Another side effect is that the bladder lining can start to bleed (hemorrhagic cystitis). This problem can be detected by testing the urine for blood. The urine needs to be monitored repeatedly for the presence of blood. If blood is present in the urine for a long time, fibrosis (scarring) of the bladder or eventually even bladder cancer can develop. To prevent this, a lot of fluid is injected into the vein with the treatment to dilute the concentration of cyclophosphamide in the bladder. A drug called mesna (Mesnex or Uromitexan) is also injected into the vein to help protect the bladder. This type of treatment is highly effective in preventing these complications. Children receiving cyclophosphamide as a pill should be reminded to drink lots of fluids regularly throughout the day and to urinate just before bed each night.

The long-term side effects of cyclophosphamide are related to its total dose over time. The pill form tends to be given for a longer time, resulting in greater side effects. With long-term use, many patients experience hair loss. The degree of hair loss varies and can occasionally be severe enough for the child to need a wig. The hair re-grows once the cyclophosphamide is stopped.

The long-term side effects of cyclophosphamide that cause the most concern are infertility and cancer. Infertility means that an individual will have difficulty or be unable to have a child. Infertility related to cyclophosphamide is mainly seen in women who are over thirty years old. It almost never is a problem in girls who are given cyclophosphamide when they are still prepubertal (have not yet menstruated), especially with the low total doses used in JM. The younger the child is when cyclophosphamide is given, the lower the chance of infertility. At higher total doses (above 25 grams), a decrease in sperm production has been seen in men, but that dose is much higher than the amount given to JM patients (see *Chapter 33, Pregnancy and Fertility*).

There are *no* reports of cancer in children receiving low total doses of intravenous cyclophosphamide, as used to treat JM. The risk of cancer appears to be greater when many doses are taken by mouth. There are some concerns about cancer developing in older patients taking much higher doses for a longer period of time. A reassuring consideration is that this treatment has been common for both adults and children with lupus for more than fifteen years, and reports of cancer in lupus patients are extremely rare.

What Newer Drugs Are Being Used to Treat JM?

Mycophenolate Mofetil

Mycophenolate mofetil (MMF or CellCept) originally was used to prevent rejection in kidney and other organ transplants. Its major effect is on T and B lymphocytes in the immune system. It has been used successfully to treat autoimmune and inflammatory illnesses, including rheumatoid arthritis, systemic lupus erythematosus, Crohn's disease, and atopic dermatitis. It has recently been reported to be useful in some cases of adult DM, including for the treatment of skin rashes that have not responded to other medicines. Mycophenolate mofetil is given as a capsule or by vein. In children the dose is divided into several per day.

What are the side effects of MMF? The side effects of MMF are nausea, vomiting, stomach pain, and diarrhea. The side effects usually improve with time. In addition, starting at small doses or dividing the total daily dose into smaller doses can lessen these side effects. Other potential side effects are decreased white blood cell and lymphocyte counts and elevated liver enzyme levels. Regular blood tests detect these changes, which usually improve within a week of stopping the drug. Rarely, problems with bleeding from the intestinal tract have been observed.

Tacrolimus

Tacrolimus or FK506 (Prograf) is a relatively new medicine, a type of antibiotic that works similarly to cyclosporine but seems to be stronger. It inhibits the functions of T lymphocytes and suppresses the immune system. It also seems to shut down other immune pathways that may be important in JM.

It has been used to prevent rejection of transplanted organs. It has also shown beneficial effects in other autoimmune diseases, including rheumatoid arthritis, systemic lupus erythematosus, and various inflammatory skin diseases. Tacrolimus has demonstrated remarkable improvement in adult PM disease activity that has been unresponsive to other medicines. In one study all patients with myositis who took tacrolimus improved. Many patients with lung disease from myositis also had improved lung function. When tacrolimus was applied to the skin as a topical treatment, the skin rashes of adult DM and JDM in some children improved (see *Chapter 16, Skin Rashes and Sun Protection*).

Tacrolimus can be taken orally as a pill or liquid or by vein. Tacrolimus should be taken on an empty stomach. A high-fat meal can interfere with its absorption and decrease the amount getting to the body tissues. Drug levels can be checked by a blood test to be certain that the dose is correct.

What are the side effects of tacrolimus when taken by mouth or vein? They include high blood pressure, headaches, tremors, inability to sleep (insomnia), diarrhea, high blood sugar levels (even diabetes), and high blood lipid (fat) levels. Nausea, constipation, stomach pain, decrease in kidney function, itchiness, increase in skin rashes, swelling, and disturbances in the balance of salts (electrolytes) in the blood have been reported. It is essential to have regular blood tests to monitor liver enzymes, electrolytes, blood counts, kidney function, and blood sugar levels, as well as to measure blood pressure.

A patient who takes tacrolimus is more vulnerable to serious infections. Tacrolimus can decrease the ability to respond to a vaccine. Women receiving tacrolimus have given birth to healthy children, and men have also fathered healthy children.

Medicines Used in Combination

Sometimes the second-line medicines used to treat JM do not work well enough by themselves and need to be used together. Sometimes several second-line medicines are used together to keep steroid doses as low as possible or to help reduce steroid doses more quickly. The second-line medicines can also be used together to minimize the risk of side effects from long-term steroid use or the total duration of treatment.

Any of the medicines discussed in this chapter can be given with daily oral steroids or intravenous steroids. Hydroxychloroquine and IVIG are also frequently used together with any of these medicines.

The aim of using a combination of second-line medicines is to get the benefit of drugs that affect the immune system in different ways so that they are not inhibiting the same pathways. For example, cyclosporine is generally not taken with tacrolimus, as they both inhibit similar pathways in T lymphocytes.

Common drug combinations include methotrexate or azathioprine with cyclosporine, or cyclosporine with cyclophosphamide. In our clinical experience, such combinations are often helpful and usually fairly safe.

The medicines discussed in this chapter are those for which there is some evidence from published medical reports in JM or adult myositis that they are effective. Mycophenolate and tacrolimus are the newest medicines and, consequently, the least amount of information is currently available about them. There are no published studies of their effectiveness in treating JM, but there is some anecdotal experience of benefit. Other drugs and biologic agents show promise and potential to treat JM, but they are still experimental agents, so you may have to be part of a research study to receive them (see *Chapter 15, New Therapies on the Horizon*). When the medicines discussed here, used alone or combined together, are still not enough, it is good to know that other options may soon be available.

Key Points

■ There is no single treatment that works for all children with JM. Different doctors treat JM in different ways, and your child's myositis doctor will help you select the best medicines for your child.

■ Treatment of JM is aimed at turning off inflammation in the muscles, skin, and other affected body systems and keeping the inflammation away until the illness goes into remission.

■ High doses of corticosteroids, administered either by mouth every day and/or by vein on varying schedules, are the main medicine used to treat JM. As the child gets better, the dose of steroid is reduced and eventually stopped. This process usually takes at least two to three years, although it can take longer.

■ If the illness is severe or does not respond adequately to steroids alone, other medicines will be required. Sometimes these drugs are also used to keep the dose of corticosteroids as low as possible or to reduce the side effects. These other medicines include:

— Commonly:
  • Methotrexate
  • Hydroxychloroquine
  • Intravenous immune globulin
  • Azathioprine
  • Cyclosporine

— Less commonly:
  • Cyclophosphamide
  • Mycophenolate mofetil
  • Tacrolimus

■ With these additional choices of medicines available for the treatment of JM, the rate of complications from JM has been greatly reduced. Many children can function successfully with a normal childhood and life.

■ All medicines have potential side effects. Most are mild and reversible, and few can be predicted. Most patients will never develop most of the side effects associated with a treatment, but it is important to learn about the side effects of medicines that your child is taking.

To Learn More

The Myositis Association (TMA).

Treatment Options for Juvenile Myositis; *Your Thoughts and Ideas on JM*; *Juvenile Myositis and Prednisone: Battling Side Effects.* Available from: www.myositis.org/jmbookresources.cfm or 800-821-7356.

Paediatric Rheumatology International Trials Organisation (PRINTO).
Drug therapy. Available from: www.printo.it/pediatric-rheumatology/information/UK/
15.htm or 0039-010-38-28-54.

General information on different medicines used to treat myositis, including possible side effects. Information is provided in different languages from the PRINTO homepage at www.printo.it/pediatric-rheumatology.

Additional Information:

Arthritis Foundation. *Medications.* In: **Raising a Child With Arthritis: A Parent's Guide.** Atlanta (GA): Arthritis Foundation; 1998. p. 29–36.

Arthritis Foundation. *2006 Drug Guide.* Arthritis Today. 2006 Jan-Feb:p. 73–90. Available from: www.arthritis.org/conditions/DrugGuide or www.arthritis.org/AFstore/CategoryHome.asp?idCat=8 [to order free brochure] or 800-568-4045.

Tucker LB, DeNardo BA, Stebulis JA, Schaller JG. *The Range of Available Medications.* In: **Your Child With Arthritis: A Family Guide for Caregiving.** Baltimore: Johns Hopkins University Press; 1996. p. 53–79.

Zukerman E, Ingelfinger J. **Coping With Prednisone and Other Cortisone-Related Medicines.** NY: St. Martin's Griffin; 1997.

Reports in the Medical Literature

Compeyrot-Lacassagne S, Feldman BM. Inflammatory myopathies in children. *Pediatric Clinics of North America.* 2005 Apr;52(2):493–520, vi-vii.

Dalakas MC. Therapeutic approaches in patients with inflammatory myopathies. *Seminars in Neurology.* 2003 Jun;23(2):199–206.

Reed AM, Lopez M. Juvenile dermatomyositis: recognition and treatment. *Paediatric Drugs.* 2002;4(5):315–21.

Rider LG, Miller FW. Classification and treatment of juvenile idiopathic inflammatory myopathies. *Rheumatic Diseases Clinics of North America.* 1997 Aug;23(3):619–55.

CHAPTER 13

Rehabilitation of the Child with Myositis

Minal S. Jain, MS, PT, PCS; Michaele R. Smith, PT, MEd; and Jeanne E. Hicks, MD

In this chapter...

Rehabilitation, including physical and occupational therapy, is a key part of the treatment that your child should receive for juvenile myositis. Rehabilitative treatments maximize your child's strength and function. Use the information in this chapter to ask your child's rehabilitation team pertinent questions about the type, frequency, and duration of rehabilitation for your child.

From the family's point of view...

"She had a lot of physical therapy appointments. The therapists tailored the exercises to her age, making them fun for a young child. She played basketball, rode a bike, and played with balls and hula hoops—all activities that encouraged her to participate without realizing she was actually exercising. We were able to take an exercise program home with us to help her regain some strength and endurance."

What Are the Physical Effects of Juvenile Myositis?

Juvenile myositis (JM), as well as the corticosteroids used to treat JM, cause physical problems that can affect daily activities. These physical problems include reduced muscle strength and endurance (ability to continue a task over a period of time), muscle thinning (atrophy), less joint motion, muscle and joint pain, overall body tiredness (fatigue), and bone loss (osteoporosis). All children with myositis do not develop all of the physical effects and problems discussed in this chapter, but most children develop some of them. With prompt and proper rehabilitation treatment, these problems can be minimized.

Your child could have problems with mobility (decreased speed and endurance in walking, running, and playing), which could hinder hobbies and sports. Other activities of daily living may be affected, including dressing, bathing, eating, speaking (see *Chapter 23, Tune to Your Voice*), and swallowing (see *Chapter 18, Swallowing and Other Digestive Problems*). Often children initially compensate for these problems by slowing down, dropping out of nonessential activities, and resting more frequently. Parents should watch for these changes in their child's routines.

Why Is Rehabilitation Treatment Important for Children with JM?

Myositis doctors have come to realize their patients can benefit from an early and expanded rehabilitation evaluation and treatment program. This approach offsets the loss of strength and endurance and prevents the development of contractures.

Studies in adults found that specific strengthening exercises in some persons with myositis are effective, without causing sustained muscle enzyme elevations or a flare in the myositis. However, therapy should begin very early rather than later. Although data from children have not yet been obtained, studies in adult myositis patients have shown improved overall endurance (conditioning) on short-term (six-week) and long-term endurance exercise programs.

Who Makes Up the Rehabilitation Team and What Are Their Roles?

Your child may be evaluated by members of the rehabilitation team, which may include a physical and occupational therapist, physiatrist (rehabilitation physician), and speech language pathologist. Physical therapists assess mobility and walking patterns, range of motion, biomechanics of joints, muscle strength, and pain. The physical therapist also recommends exercise programs, appropriate assistive devices and proper shoes for walking, heat treatments, and patient and family education. In some states physical therapists can practice independently of a physician's treatment prescription. Occupational therapists assess your child's function in areas of daily living, use of the hands and arms, and the ability to cope with functional problems. Occupational therapists offer advice on how to plan and organize activities. They make splints, recommend assistive devices, and teach your child how to conserve her energy and protect her joints. Physiatrists supervise the rehabilitation team, develop initial goals and treatment plans, and monitor the treatment program. They refer children to other team members for specialized evaluations or other types of treatment, if necessary. Some locations might not have all the members of this team available.

How Do You Find the Right Physical or Occupational Therapist and Physiatrist for Your Child?

Your child's myositis doctor will prescribe rehabilitation and refer you to the appropriate clinics or medical centers where your child can receive rehabilitation treatment. Depending on your insurance coverage, you may not be able to choose your child's therapist or physiatrist, but if you ask the right questions, you might find a qualified professional within your healthcare plan. These healthcare professionals should be either pediatric specialists and/or specialists experienced in the care of patients with JM. Individualization and communication between the rehabilitation team and your child's medical team are essential components of your child's treatment.

Make sure they have the appropriate academic credentials and are licensed in your state. Check whether they have advanced certifications. For example, pediatric clinical specialists are physical therapists who have advanced clinical knowledge, experience, and skills in the area of pediatrics. Occupational therapists also have an equivalent specialization. Some physiatrists have pediatric fellowship training. Having the specialization is not the most important criterion; it helps to assure you that the therapist has some advanced clinical skills.

As you interview prospective practitioners, there are a few specific questions you can ask to help you decide which one will be right for your child.

"What expertise do you have with myositis?" They may not have had much experience with myositis, but they should be familiar with the illness and with its clinical symptoms, physical findings, and functional impact.

"Have you worked with children with arthritis?" If they have worked with children with juvenile rheumatoid arthritis, they are at least aware of the unpredictable nature of arthritis, which is also true of myositis.

"Are you aware of the different medications related to this illness?" Knowing the medications is very important for understanding some of the side effects that can occur.

If you are satisfied with the answers to these questions, the practitioner may be a good fit for your child. In some areas of the country you will not have many choices in your selection of a physical or occupational therapist. A positive answer to some of these questions is helpful; however, if the therapists are not familiar with myositis, they may wish to consult with therapists at larger medical centers who are experts in the rehabilitation of JM. These experts can be located by contacting the associations listed at the end of this chapter or in the *Resource Appendix* at the end of the book.

What Assessments and Treatments Are Completed by the Rehabilitation Team?

Your child is evaluated for the presence and degree of physical and daily function problems and how they cope with them. Individualized treatment plans can be developed using this information, as well as information about your child's illness (the level or severity of myositis activity, damage, and medications) provided by your child's myositis doctor. A number of areas may be evaluated, which may include manual muscle strength, muscle function, and endurance (see *Chapter 11, Assessing Muscle Strength, Endurance, and Function*), and joint motion (range of motion, ROM). Sometimes a special biomechanics lab assessment of walking and how joints move may be necessary. In this chapter we have concentrated on assessments and therapies delivered by physical and occupational therapists.

For problems with muscle weakness or loss of the range of motion of joints, graded muscle strengthening, and joint stretching (range of motion) exercises may be prescribed. For each functional problem, treatments may be prescribed, which may include: training in walking and devices to assist with walking, instruction in daily life activities, and how to use assistive devices to substitute for loss of function, instruction in ways to conserve energy and protect joints from the stress and strain of activities, and education about modifying the home and school environment for safety and ease in engaging in activities, recreation, leisure, and sports.

Why Is Rehabilitation Treatment Important for Children with JM?

Doctors taking care of patients with myositis have come to realize that these patients can benefit from an early and expanded rehabilitation evaluation and treatment program. This more aggressive approach is to offset loss of strength and endurance and to prevent the development of contractures.

What Do Scientific Studies Show About Rehabilitation Evaluations and Treatments for Myositis?

Patients with JM have decreased strength and endurance, decreased ability to move the joints fully, and overall decreased body endurance (conditioning). They have slower walking speed, which may progress with increasing weakness (becomes slower as the muscles become weaker) and abnormal walking patterns, which can take more energy.

Studies in adults document that specific strengthening exercises in some persons with myositis are effective, without causing sustained muscle enzyme elevations or a flare in the myositis. However, therapy should begin very early rather than later. Studies in adult myositis patients have shown improved overall endurance (conditioning) on short-term (six-week) and long-term endurance exercise programs, but data from children have not yet been obtained.

What Are the Important Characteristics of Rehabilitation Treatments for the Child with JM?

They should ideally begin *early* in the course of the illness. Early treatment offers the best chance of preventing or minimizing loss of function.

The treatments are *individualized* for each child, based on the types and severity of the impairments, the disease activity, and damage present (see *Chapter 10, Charting Your Child's Progress*), and the level of the child's understanding and ability to follow directions.

Like medicines, the treatments are prescribed and *monitored* on a regular and ongoing basis by your child's myositis doctor and the rehabilitation team members. After reading this chapter or other materials, parents should not decide on the exercise program for their child because inappropriate exercise treatments can harm the child.

The treatments are *adjusted* from time to time depending on the degree of myositis disease activity and the response the child has had to the previous treatment schedule.

Some of the treatments need to be ongoing throughout the illness course.

The treatments need to be *practical* and *focused* on prevention of functional loss, on the particular impairments the child has, and integrated into the child's daily activities, play, and sports routines as much as possible.

Treatment should incorporate the assistance of the *parents* and *caretakers*, if possible. This helps the child know that the treatment is important and necessary.

Rehabilitation Through Exercise

The goals of exercise for patients with JM include maintaining or improving muscle strength and endurance, joint motion, and tendon flexibility; improving overall endurance (conditioning); as well as maintaining or improving the ability to function in activities. Exercise is important for muscle health, because muscles, tendons, and joints work together to help you move. They act as shock absorbers during our daily activities. Normally, they can withstand the stresses and strains of moving, walking, bending, and twisting motions. However, in JM the muscles are weak, and the joints are stiff or have limited motion, so they are less able to stand up to these stresses and strains and are injured more easily. If the joints are stiff, it takes more muscle power and energy to move them, which tires the muscles more quickly. You need both good muscles and good joints to function. For example, if a joint has normal motion but a muscle is very weak, the joint can't be moved by the muscle. If the muscle is normal but the joint is contracted, the muscle can't move the joint.

All the joints and muscles of the body work together. For example, when we walk, the muscles of the spine keep our posture straight, the muscles on the side of the pelvis keep the pelvis level so it doesn't wobble, the arms swing, and the leg muscles move to propel us forward. Muscles work together in pairs and are attached to the joints by tendons. Each muscle has a different action on the joint. For example, the knee is a hinge joint, and the muscle on the front of the thigh (the quadriceps) straightens the knee and holds it stable when we step. The muscle on the back of the leg (hamstring) bends or flexes the knee when we walk. Myositis sometimes causes muscles on one side of a joint to be stronger than those on the opposite side. The stronger muscle can exert a bigger pull on the joint and cause a contracture. That's why it is necessary to strengthen the weaker muscle and stretch the stronger one. If the hamstring muscle behind the knee is stronger than the quadriceps, it can pull too much and cause a flexion contracture at the knee. This can also happen at the ankle: if the calf muscle pulls too much and the Achilles tendon gets tight, the ankle will flex down. The therapist can design an individualized stretching and strengthening program for each child depending on which muscles and tendons are tight.

How Much Muscle Strength and Joint Motion Are Needed to Perform Activities Independently?

If your child can comb her hair but cannot resist the push of someone trying to push her arms down, this indicates that her muscle strength is at a critical level. The muscles can move against gravity, which means that she is still able to do some activities independently or with some assistive devices or adaptive strategies. If her strength drops below this level of movement against gravity, then she will need more help to do the activities involved in daily living. Therefore, it is important to try to maintain your child's strength at or above this critical level of motion against gravity.

JM can affect all the muscles of the arms and legs, neck, spine, stomach, chest, and sometimes the tongue and throat. JM most commonly affects both right and left upper arms and legs more than muscles of the lower arms and legs, including the hands and feet. The muscles in the neck, back of spine (extensors), and the stomach wall (abdominal) are commonly affected by JM. These muscles are important for keeping balance while sitting, bending over, and walking.

What Are the Types of Exercise Treatments?

There are three main types of exercise, which include range of motion, strengthening, and conditioning (aerobic or endurance exercise) (Table 13.1). Exercise can also be described as active (your child does the exercise by herself) or passive (someone helps your child do the exercise for her). Which types of exercise are used in the rehabilitation of your child with JM varies and depends on the level and severity of myositis activity. After initial diagnosis and treatment, all children can advance from passive range of motion exercises to basic active range of motion exercises to prevent motion loss. The therapist will advance your child's exercise program in collaboration with your child's myositis doctor, as your child's myositis disease activity decreases and her strength improves.

Range of Motion Exercises

The therapist, nurse, or parent helps your child perform passive range of motion exercises when her muscles are too weak to move the arms or legs or if her muscles are severely inflamed (at initial diagnosis or during a serious illness flare) and the doctor wants the muscle rested until the inflammation is controlled by

Table 13.1. Exercise and disease activity.*

Exercise Type	Active Assisted ROM, Passive ROM	Active Assisted ROM, Passive ROM	Isometric Strengthening Stretch, Active Assisted ROM, Active ROM	(Light) Recreational, Light Aerobic, Isometric Strengthening, Stretch, Active ROM	Recreational Aerobic, (Low Weight) Isotonic and Isometric Strengthening, Stretch, Active ROM	Recreational Aerobic, PRE, Isotonic and Isometric Strengthening Stretch, Active ROM
Myositis Disease Activity	Initial Diagnosis, Flare	Severe Activity	Moderate Activity	Mild to Moderate Activity	Mild Activity	Inactive
Muscle Strength Level	Below Gravity ⟶		Against Gravity ⟶			

*Specific exercises are modified based on bone density levels.
Abbreviations: ROM = range of motion; PRE = progressive resistance exercise.

medication. The purposes of this exercise are to keep the joints and tendons loose (flexible) and to prevent contractures of the tendons and joints. We recommend only passive range of motion (someone gently moving your child's joints for her) at the time of illness onset and during the introduction of medicines to treat JM, as well as during moderate and severe illness flares requiring medication adjustment.

Active assisted range of motion exercise is used when your child's muscles are too weak or painfully inflamed to complete a full range of joint motion. It can be used when your child is recovering from the initial acute inflammation or a flare. In this exercise, your child moves the joint as much as possible, and the therapist or parent completes motion. Children with this degree of weakness can do some range of motion exercise by themselves if the joint to be exercised is put in a position that minimizes the effect of gravity. This position eliminates the pull of gravity and lets even a very weak muscle complete a joint motion. Therapists can teach these positions to you and your child.

As your child gets stronger, active range of motion exercises can be performed when her muscles are strong enough to move the joint through its full or available motion against gravity. Some range of motion exercises are performed not against gravity but with the help of gravity (for example, in a sitting position, if you bend the neck down, you are going with gravity, not against it) (Figure 13.1). Active range of motion exercises can be done even during moderate muscle inflammation if the child is receiving medicines.

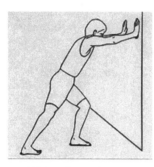 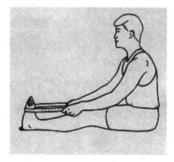 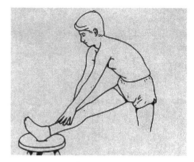

Wall heel cord stretch   **Towel heel cord stretch**   **Standing hamstring stretch**

■ **Figure 13.1. Examples of three range of motion exercises.**
These exercises might be prescribed by a physical therapist to improve the range of motion of joints. The first two are different methods for stretching the heel cord, and the third (on the right) provides an example of a stretch for hamstring tendons. These exercises should be done under the supervision of a physician or a physical therapist. Do not attempt to do these without the appropriate instructions. *Reprinted with permission from Visual Health Information, Tacoma WA. Drawings copyrighted by VHI Stretching Charts, Inc.*

Stretching Exercises to Loosen Joints or Tendons

Stretching exercises are a special type of range of motion exercise. First, the joint is moved through its range of motion. At the end of the joint range, a gradual stretch is applied for about ten seconds. This may be repeated several times. If there is reduced joint motion, a program of prolonged thirty-second stretching can be useful. Never do a quick forceful stretch, as this can harm the joint and tendon and cause pain. A parent can apply either of these stretches after instruction by a therapist. Children with myositis can do stretching exercises by themselves. The most commonly affected tendons that need to be stretched are those around the shoulder, the hamstrings, and Achilles tendon at the ankle.

If there is a marked loss of range of motion, a particular type of treatment called serial casting or splinting can be done by the therapist to try to improve the motion of a particular joint. If a joint contracture is present, it is best treated initially by the therapist in a clinic setting with hot packs and sometimes ultrasound in older children to relax tight muscles and tendons and make them easier to stretch. Visits to the clinic may be needed for several weeks during an attempt to stretch out a contracture. Home stretching programs are also provided simultaneously.

Strengthening Exercises

There are three types of strengthening exercises: isometric, isotonic, and isokinetic, which can be performed (in a clinic) under the direct supervision of a therapist. Strengthening programs may be more successful when joints are functioning as well as possible.

Isometric exercise should be the first type of strengthening exercises used in an exercise program for children with JM. Isometric exercise can be done by simply contracting the muscle. A group of contractions is done as a set. If more than one set is prescribed, then you should rest between sets. The intensity of the exercise depends on the number of contractions and sets or groups of contractions. A set of three contractions would be a mild exercise. Isometric exercise should ideally be started early in the course of illness, after the child is receiving medicines, in order to help prevent muscle thinning (atrophy) and strength loss.

Isotonic exercise can be done simply with movement against the force of gravity (the lightest form) or with movement of very light weights or Thera-bands® by The Hygenic Corporation (www.thera-band.com) held or attached to the arms or legs. A Thera-band® is a stretchy band, available in color-coded levels of resistance, that is used to strengthen the legs and arms by pulling on it. During isotonic contraction, the quadriceps muscle lengthens as the knee moves in flexion (bends) and shortens as the knee extends. Moving the limbs against gravity or with weights puts stress (force) across the joint and muscle. The heavier the weight, the greater the stress/force. If moving the weight through a full joint range of motion is uncomfortable or if reduced stress on an inflamed muscle (or joint) is needed, moving the arm or leg or a stationary object through a partial range of motion can reduce the stress/force. When the muscle is stronger, the weight can be moved through full motion.

When weights or different strength Thera-bands® are used, there are two forms of this exercise. The first is called isotonic constant low weight exercise. For this type, a light weight is chosen and lifted a certain number of times (one set of repetitions). If several sets are done, a rest is taken between each set, just like with isometric exercise. The weight remains the same, but the number of repetitions in each set and the number of sets may be increased depending on your child's progress, level of myositis activity, illness stability, and medications. This process is called adjusting the intensity of the exercise by increasing the number of repetitions. Muscle or joint pain, increased fatigue (tiredness), or increased myositis disease activity may be indications to decrease the program intensity or even stop the program for a while. This type of isotonic exercise is designed to increase muscle strength and local muscle endurance. It is not designed to build muscle bulk and may be suited for children with JM who have mild, stable, active myositis (i.e., they have had mild disease and have been on the same medications and dosage for at least several months).

Isotonic progressive resistive exercise uses a set number of repetitions, and intensity is regulated by gradually increasing the weight during the repetition sessions. It can build muscle strength and bulk but places more force on the muscle and joint. This type of exercise is recommended only when your child's myositis is stable and inactive. Even then, it should be used at low intensity and well below a body building level.

Gyms often have equipment for isotonic exercise (for example, Nautilus® machines, Nautilus, Inc., www.nautilus.com), but young children are too small to use these machines. Teenagers could have an isotonic constant low weight program or a progressive weight program (depending on disease activity and stability) designed and monitored by a therapist. It is important to limit heavy weight lifting because it can damage the muscle itself. The therapist should discuss your child's current myositis disease activity with the doctor before your child is started on an isotonic program using weights.

Conditioning Exercises

When your child's muscles have become stronger and joint motion is better, conditioning exercises can increase your child's ability to walk farther without getting as tired. The heart, lungs, and muscles all work together to produce this conditioning effect. Generally, the exercise must include a number of large muscle groups (like those in the legs). The heart rate should increase to a calculated desired level (intensity) by the exercise. This exercise can be accomplished by low-intensity walking, swimming, treadmill, and stationary bike programs individually designed by the therapist and recommended and approved by the myositis doctor. Low-intensity programs are sufficient because myositis patients most often have low levels of conditioning when they start a program. They can better prepare the child for recreational exercise programs. A child with JM should have inactive or mild, stable, active myositis to do this type of exercise, which should be approved by your child's myositis doctor before it is begun (see Table 13.1).

How Can We Fit Exercises into Our Life?

The best time to do range of motion or stretching exercises is after your child's daily bath or shower because heat relieves pain and muscle tightness. If your child's muscles are really tight, stretching exercises in the morning will make the day's activities easier. Certain play and sports routines provide excellent range of motion/stretching exercise for the joints. Children under five years old generally cannot follow directions for a formal exercise program, so their active range of motion exercises should be incorporated into play routines; for example, they may follow a parent in doing them in a "Simon says" format. If your child does not move all the joints through their range of motion daily, you can assist her to do passive range of motion and stretching when needed. These general guidelines for exercise should be followed:

- Warm up before starting any exercise.
- Stretch tight tendons to prevent injury.
- Listen to your body's signals to slow down or stop.
- Cool down after finishing exercise.
- Have a proper and safe place to do the exercises, and use a mat when appropriate.
- Do the exercise slowly and smoothly.

Research has shown that by working with another person (including family members), the frequency that the exercises are done increases, resulting in a better outcome for the patient. Your child will be more likely to work with you if there isn't too much discomfort (an hour after medications are given) and if the treatment plan is as simple as possible, such as part of a game.

The frequency of exercise treatments depends on the specific type of treatment, the level of myositis disease activity, the severity of the specific impairment, and the treatment goals. For example, a joint range of motion and stretching program to improve joint motion should be done daily to be effective. In contrast, a muscle strengthening program is effective if done three times a week. A low-intensity conditioning program can be effective if done two to three times a week. Your therapist will instruct you on how often treatments need to be done.

Can My Child Participate in Recreational Sports?

Children enjoy participating in exercise associated with recreation and sports. For the child with JM, it is best to try to get joints in good moving condition (have good range of motion), increase tendon and muscle flexibility, strengthen muscles, and improve aerobic conditioning before starting any recreational and sports activities. This plan will help prevent injuries from poor joint and muscle mechanics and lessen muscle and overall fatigue associated with these activities, thereby allowing your child to participate more fully.

Certain noncompetitive activities provide good joint motion, exercise, stretching of the joints, and some isotonic exercise. These activities include shooting basketball hoops, pitching a softball or throwing a ball or Frisbee, dancing, archery, ping-pong, and serving tennis balls. These are especially good activities for the upper body. They also provide spinal extension and abdominal exercise. Walking, swimming, stationary bicycling, bicycle riding, and Tai Chi provide good joint motion and are good for conditioning and improving balance. Duck pin bowling is also good for balance. When myositis is active and muscles are weak, the following activities should be avoided: contact sports (e.g., football), downhill skiing, jumping rope on concrete, trampoline bouncing, and riding roller coasters (and similar rides). It is especially important not to overdo sports activities while the myositis is still active. We do not recommend competitive sports during active myositis. A bone density measurement may be needed before doing any impact sports.

Children with JM often have some osteoporosis from inactivity and high-dose corticosteroids (see *Chapter 22, Taking Care of the Bones*). It is known that in adults with osteoporosis, weight-bearing exercise, such as walking, isotonic exercises of the extremities, and doing back extension exercises help increase bone mass (density) and therefore decrease bone loss. There have been no studies of this type in children with JM, but it would seem likely that these exercises could also help prevent or decrease osteoporosis in children with JM. If weight-bearing exercise is not possible, then you can use tilt tables for older children and standing frames for younger children to help promote weight bearing even if your child cannot walk. Children with moderate to severe osteoporosis are more susceptible to bone and spine fractures, which can occur with or without activity. However, activities and exercises that place more forces across their bones further increase the fracture risk. For example, bending activities (flexion) place the spine at an increased risk of fracture.

Children with mild osteoporosis can most likely perform all the exercises we described in this chapter (range of motion, stretching, isotonic low weight, isotonic progressive resistance, and aerobic). Those with moderate osteoporosis are safer using only range of motion, light stretching, isometric, and isotonic strengthening using a very low amount of weight, and aerobic walking and pool exercise. Those with severe osteoporosis are safer using only range of motion against gravity exercises (with reduced joint range and no stretching). Your child's myositis doctor should approve the level of exercise if your child has osteoporosis.

Are There Any Side Effects of Exercise?

Side effects that might occur with exercise include muscle, tendon, and joint soreness or pain and increased muscle and overall body fatigue and weakness. If these last for over an hour after exercise, the intensity and frequency of the program may need to be adjusted. Discuss with your child's myositis doctor whether the program should be reduced or even omitted for a while because inflammation increases and persists after certain exercises.

What Is the Role of the Parents in Exercise?

Parents play an important role in your child's rehabilitation: you should supervise your child's exercise programs to ensure that they are done. You can do some exercises with your child or demonstrate how they should be done. Helping small children incorporate range of motion and stretching into play routines is important. If your child is too weak for active exercise, you can do passive and assisted range of motion and stretching with your child. Monitoring your child in recreational and sports routines is necessary to prevent the side effects of too much exercise.

Where Will the Exercises Be Done?

Home: Range of motion, stretching, strengthening, and some aerobic conditioning exercise programs can be done at home after the therapist initially instructs you about use and side effects, as well as precautions. You should visit your therapist periodically to monitor the outcome of treatment, make adjustments, or advance treatment programs.

School: Federal law requires schools to provide treatment by a physical therapist if the illness interferes with a child's academic progress. The school therapist will evaluate your child and develop an Individualized Education Plan with specific goals (see *Chapter 36, School Issues*). Most children will receive private therapy as well, and so communication between the school therapist and the child's clinic therapist is necessary to ensure that the appropriate exercise routine is done in the school as well as at home. If the child is not being seen by the school physical therapist on a regular basis, the private physical therapist will develop an appropriate program to include adaptive physical education to ensure that the goals of the Individualized Education Plan are being addressed. Each state has a different set of criteria determining the level of services (consultative versus direct). In consultative services the child is evaluated on a periodic basis to determine the need for therapy; therapy is not necessarily provided by a physical therapist on a regular basis. Direct services indicate consistent hands-on services provided by the therapist for a specified period of time, i.e. four to six weeks.

It is best for the child to participate in some school recess activities and physical education programs with her classmates so she doesn't feel excluded. The regular classroom and physical education teachers should be advised in writing as to which activities and for how long the child can participate in them because often a modified physical education program is needed. In this case, your child can perform exercises prescribed by your child's physical therapist during gym class (see *Chapter 36, School Issues*).

Clinic and Rehabilitation Hospital: If strength and joint motion and function level decline or drop below a critical level, a child may need more intensive treatment in a clinic setting or occasionally in a rehabilitation hospital with the goal of restoring her previous functional level.

What Other Rehabilitation Treatments Are Effective in Children with Myositis?

Heat and Cold: Heat can reduce pain in muscles, tendons, and joints, which reduces muscle spasm and increases the stretching ability of the tendons. Hot baths and showers, spas, heated pools, and whirlpools can deliver heat. Children can do some range of motion or stretching exercises in these settings, or they can do a full range of motion or stretching program after using them. Some modern bathtubs have whirlpool features. Professional whirlpools of different sizes can be found in clinics.

Caution should be taken in using public spas and heated pools. They most often introduce chlorine into the water, which can irritate skin rashes of juvenile dermatomyositis (JDM) and areas of open calcinosis. There may also be an increased risk of skin infection from public facilities. Some spas and pools are sterilized with ultraviolet light rather than chlorine. The costs of home spas and pools may be tax deductible with a physician's justification that the child would physically benefit from exercising in them. Outdoor pools should not be used between the hours of 10 A.M. and 4 P.M. because intense sunlight at this time can aggravate the rash of JDM.

Physical therapists use therapeutic heated whirlpools and pools in the clinic setting to do range of motion and stretching of joints that have lost motion because of tight tendons and muscles. The child has the benefit of the heat treatment, and it is easier to move the arm or leg because of the buoyancy of the water and the diminished pull of gravity on the joints. Therapists also use these heated water sources to treat skin wounds that are difficult to heal or to clean infected ones. Areas of draining calcinosis sometimes respond to this type of therapy once the area is cleaned.

Occupational therapists use heat with hot packs or paraffin or heated mittens to treat hand contractures. Range of motion and stretching exercises are done after using them. Cold, via the use of cold packs (wrapped well in towels), can be used to reduce the pain and swelling of acute joint sprains.

Heat should not be used when the joints, skin, and muscle are inflamed, when sensation in the arms and legs is decreased, or when circulation is poor. When cold treatment is used in children with myositis, it should be used only over the joint and not directly over the muscle areas.

Massage Therapy: Physical and occupational therapists often use massage therapy to relieve pain from tight muscles and to reduce swelling. This may also produce overall relaxation. There are four different types of massage, and the therapist will choose the correct one according to the problem.

Assistive Devices and Mobility Aides: These assistive devices help compensate for lost function, promote independence, and reduce fatigue. They are used after an occupational therapy evaluation, on a temporary or permanent basis when muscles are too weak or joints do not have enough motion. These devices are usually needed when the shoulder, hip, or knee muscles are weak. However, children with hand weakness or arthritis that makes it hard for them to grip objects may need button and zipper hooks, scissors with wide handles, pens with wide plastic guards, large-handled utensils, and special jar and door openers. Other assistive devices can make your child's environment safer and easier to handle. These include commercially made stair blocks that can reduce stair height, stair elevators, and buses that kneel, making it easy to get on them. For more explanation of adaptive devices and strategies, see *Chapter 8, Adapting to Physical Limitations.*

When muscle strength decreases to the anti-gravity or critical level, a cane or a walker may be needed for balance or to decrease weight on one or both legs if the muscles or joints are weak and painful. The physical therapist will decide which device is necessary and when to use it. Sometimes it is hard for children to accept the need to use devices and aides.

If muscle weakness is less than anti-gravity strength, walking becomes unsafe. Walking is also unsafe if there is a severe contracture at the hip, knee, or ankle joints in one joint or several joints. A properly fitted wheelchair will be needed. Young children need custom-fitted chairs. Older children may be able to use a scooter if the back and abdominal muscles are strong enough to maintain sitting posture in the scooter seat (see *Chapter 8, Adapting to Physical Limitations*).

What Types of Orthotics Are Used for Children with JM?

Orthotics include splints and braces and may be constructed by an orthotist or pedorthotist. Orthotists are trained health professionals who create or supply supportive aids for people with disabling conditions of the limbs or spine. Orthotists create and fit patients with splints and braces to support weakened body parts and help correct physical disabilities from muscle diseases, stroke, polio, or spinal cord injury. A final check of the fit of the orthotic is made by the physician who wrote the prescription and the therapist caring for the patient. Certified pedorthotists are fully qualified to fit all types of shoe inserts and modifications. They are able to fabricate custom-made shoes for the difficult-to-fit patient in addition to providing shoe orthotics. A rehabilitation team member prescribes an orthotic device after assessing impairment and function. Some orthotics will be custom made for the child by an occupational or physical therapist, or they are ordered from commercial companies.

The purposes of orthotics include decreasing joint pain, decreasing stresses/forces across joints, decreasing motion of a joint, providing stability for an unstable joint, improving motion patterns of joints, resting joints, and improving joint function during activities. Orthotics can be functional or nonfunctional (resting). An example of a functional orthotic is a wrist splint. This can keep a painful wrist from moving while allowing the fingers to move, or it can hold a wrist in a functional position when the arm muscles are too weak to hold it up. Other functional splints can be made for the thumb and fingers. Resting splints made of orthoplast are often used at night to relieve pain in joints or to hold the joint in position so contractures do not develop. For example, a splint can be used on the wrist, knee, or elbow to prevent flexion contracture.

It is important that the orthotic device fits well. If it does not fit well, skin irritation and breakdown or nerve compression can occur. They also can be painful. The therapist or orthotist should provide your child with a "break in" wearing schedule to slowly accommodate to the orthotic. If shoe inserts are used, the feet should be inspected frequently for reddened areas that persist for more than fifteen to twenty minutes. If the redness persists, the child should stop wearing the orthotics and return for a follow-up appointment to have the orthotics adjusted.

Orthotics are made for knee, ankle, and foot problems. Braces that are used during walking are made from stronger plastic, sometimes with metal supports. For children with JM who have weakness of the ankle dorsiflexion muscles with difficulty picking up their foot while walking, a short plastic leg brace can be made. The footplate goes in the shoe, and the leg part attaches to the calf with a Velcro® strap. It holds the foot up to prevent tripping.

If the knee extensor muscle, which stabilizes the knee while walking, is below anti-gravity or critical strength, the knee will buckle, and your child could fall. A custom-made plastic brace that maintains the ankle and toes in a slightly downward direction can help stabilize the knee. It should only be worn on one leg, the weaker leg. This slightly pointed down direction is not enough to cause tripping. A physician needs to write a prescription for this type of brace.

Foot orthotics can help when the ankle muscles are weak and the ankle turns out while it is in contact with the ground while walking (pronation). This condition can cause pain. These orthotics can be made by a qualified physical therapist. For milder situations, a soft orthotic with arch support can be used inside the shoe. These can be purchased in a store. However, especially for children, custom orthotics are advised to ensure a good and comfortable fit. For moderate pronation (causing flattening of the arch when the foot strikes the ground), an orthotic made of firm plastic with padding is recommended. This fits completely in the shoe, but a half-size larger shoe may be needed. For severe pronation (in addition to the flattening of the arch, the foot may turn in toward the midline) an orthotic that comes about six inches above the shoe level and attaches to the leg with a Velcro® strap is needed.

What Educational Programs Are Taught by the Rehabilitation Team?

Occupational therapists educate children and parents about ways to conserve energy. Some suggestions include pacing your child's daily activities (don't do them too fast), planning the activities of the day ahead of time, setting priorities in the activities your child chooses, and using correct positions and postures during standing and sitting activities. There are other specific ways of conserving energy.

For muscles that are weak and joints that have decreased motion, it is good to reduce the forces on them during activities. This is called joint protection. It can help reduce joint and muscle pain, prevent injury, and conserve energy.

Joints can be protected in many ways, such as avoiding long periods in the same body position (like standing), maintaining joint range of motion and muscle strength, relieving the weight-bearing joint when it is painful (sit down or use a splint during activities), avoiding overuse of muscles and joints when inflamed or painful, modifying tasks to reduce joint and muscle stress, and using assistive devices when muscles are weak and joints lack normal motion.

Key Points

■ Rehabilitation evaluation and treatment are major components of the management of JM.

■ Rehabilitation and medications work together to achieve the goals of preserving a child's function and to help prevent impairments, handicaps, and disabilities.

■ All professionals need to communicate about the best treatments for your child, to monitor the outcome of that treatment, and to make treatment adjustments when necessary.

■ Parents play a critical role in the treatment process, to ensure monitoring and compliance with treatments. Support is also necessary to ensure good functional outcome for the child with JM.

To Learn More

To find a rehabilitation physician or therapist, see *Finding a Rehabilitation Specialist* in the *Finding a Doctor or Specialist* section of the *Resource Appendix*, specifically:

     American Physical Therapy Association (APTA)

     American Occupational Therapy Association, Inc. (AOTA)

     American Academy of Physical Medicine and Rehabilitation (AAPMR)

     Association of Academic Physiatrists

     Canadian Physiotherapy Association (CPA)

     Canadian Association of Occupational Therapists (CAOT)

     UK Chartered Society of Physiotherapy (CSP)

Additional Information:

Tucker LB, DeNardo BA, Stebulis JA, Schaller JG. *Physical and Occupational Therapy.* In: *Your Child with Arthritis: A Family Guide for Caregiving.* Baltimore: Johns Hopkins University Press; 1996. p. 80–110.

Reports in the Medical Literature

Alexandersson H, Lundberg IE. The role of exercise in the rehabilitation of idiopathic inflammatory myopathies. *Current Opinion in Rheumatology.* 2005 Mar;17(2):164–71.

Hicks JE, Drinkard B, Summers RM, Rider LG. Decreased aerobic capacity in children with juvenile dermatomyositis. *Arthritis and Rheumatism.* 2002 Apr 15;47(2):118–23.

Hicks JE. Role of rehabilitation in the management of myopathies. *Current Opinion in Rheumatology.* 1998 Nov;10(6):548–55.

CHAPTER 14

Complementary and Alternative Approaches to Juvenile Myositis

Lori A. Love, MD, PhD

The statements in this chapter are those of the author and do not necessarily reflect the official views, policies, or positions of the U.S. Food and Drug Administration or the U.S. Department of Health and Human Services.

In this chapter...

I explain what complementary and alternative medicine (CAM) is, the different health practices that are considered part of CAM, why CAM might be used in juvenile myositis (JM), and what potential problems can occur with its use.

From the family's point of view...

"Our daughter's daily regimen includes the medicines her doctor prescribes, along with a healthy, balanced diet and appropriate exercise. We emphasize fresh fruits and vegetables and give her a daily multivitamin. We also follow recommendations to supplement her calcium and vitamin D. Physical exercises and fun activities make it easier for her to deal with the downsides of JDM while helping keep or increase her strength and stamina. When she was at her worst, our pastor had the entire church pray for her. The very next day, she said she noticed that the pain throughout her body was gone! She started to cry, but not from the pain—from her faith that God was with her."

What Is Complementary and Alternative Medicine?

The National Center for Complementary and Alternative Medicine (NCCAM), which is part of the United States National Institutes of Health (NIH), defines CAM as "a group of diverse medical and healthcare systems, practices, and products not presently considered part of conventional western medicine." Much of the information about those systems, practices, and products that is presented here is taken from NCCAM's Internet site. Other terms for complementary and alternative medicine include unconventional, nonconventional, and holistic medicine, which generally means that it considers the whole person, including physical, mental, emotional, and spiritual aspects. The list of what is part of CAM changes all the time as new treatments are introduced and as other therapies, which have been shown to be safe and effective, become part of conventional medicine.

Although certain types of CAM have existed for many years (some, such as traditional Chinese medicine and ayurveda, are thousands of years old), there has been very little scientific evidence until fairly recently as to their effectiveness or safety, and there are still many questions about what works, how it works, and whether it is safe. This is especially true when these therapies are used to treat rare diseases like myositis or to treat children. It is critical that you and your child's myositis doctor jointly decide about the use of CAM therapies. Doing your homework to understand CAM, being cautious about its use, and keeping your child's doctors informed of the CAM treatments your child is using are very important parts of considering CAM.

Are Complementary, Alternative, and/or Integrative Therapies All the Same Thing?

The NCCAM defines complementary therapies as those that are combined with conventional (mainstream western) medicine. For example, ginger can be used to treat nausea caused by certain drugs, or light therapy in addition to cognitive therapy might help relieve a person's depression. Alternative medicine is used instead of conventional medicine; for example, acupuncture might be used instead of drugs to reduce back pain. Integrative medicine combines mainstream medical therapies and CAM therapies. The CAM therapies used in integrative medicine usually have been shown scientifically to be safe and effective.

What Are the Major Types of Complementary and Alternative Medicine?

CAM covers a broad range of healing philosophies, approaches, and therapies. Therefore, it is difficult to fit the major types of CAM into precise categories because there are overlaps between the types. This chapter follows the classification used by NCCAM, and the major types of CAM are listed in Table 14.1. Note that other authors and CAM practitioners might use different ways to classify and define CAM therapies. Table 14.2 defines some of the terms used for CAM therapies.

Why Is CAM Used?

In general, CAM therapies are used to try to prevent illness, reduce stress, prevent or reduce side effects of medicines and symptoms of illnesses, or to control or cure disease.

The use of CAM is very common in the United States and elsewhere, and research shows that its use is increasing. Several published surveys have addressed the use of CAM in different populations and for different reasons. Because these surveys might define CAM differently and only focus on a single type of CAM

Table 14.1. Major types of complementary and alternative medicine (CAM).

Type of CAM	Characteristics	Examples	Comments
Complete system of theory and	practice of medicine Often older than and different from "conventional" medicine	Western cultures: • homeopathy • naturopathic medicine Eastern cultures: • Traditional Chinese medicine • Ayurveda	Alternative healing systems
Mind-body interventions	Use techniques that enhance the mind's ability to affect the body's function and symptoms	Meditation Hypnosis Prayer and spirituality Mental healing Stress reduction/relaxation Visualization and guided imagery Creative outlets (art, music, dance, etc.)	Mind-body interventions now considered "mainstream" and not a part of CAM include: • Cognitive therapy • Patient support groups
Biologically based therapies	Use substances found in nature that have biological activity to affect body's function and symptoms	Botanicals (including herbs) Foods Vitamins and minerals Animal tissues or glands	Although considered "natural," many of these therapies do not yet have strong evidence to support safety or effectiveness, and for certain ones there are known safety problems. Certain conventional therapies are also referred to as being "biologically based therapies"—an example would be a human monoclonal antibody approved to treat an autoimmune disease.
Manipulation and body-based methods	Based on manipulation and/or movement of one or more parts of the body	Chiropractic Osteopathic manipulation Massage Exercise alternatives: yoga, Tai Chi Chuan, Alexander, Feldenkrais and Trager	
Energy therapies	Energy therapies affect energy fields that surround the body by applying pressure or manipulating those fields. Bioelectromagnetic-based therapies use electromagnetic fields, such as pulsed fields, magnetic fields, or alternating current or direct current fields.	Energy field manipulation: Qi gong, Reiki, and therapeutic touch Acupuncture and acupressure Magnet therapy	The existence of such fields has not yet been scientifically proven.

For more information, visit NCCAM's web site at http://nccam.nih.gov/health/whatiscam.

Table 14.2. Terms used in complementary and alternative medicine.*

Term	Meaning or information
Acupuncture, acupressure	Acupuncture involves stimulating specific anatomic points (locations) on the body for therapeutic purposes, usually by puncturing the skin with a needle. In acupressure, these points are stimulated by hand pressure.
Biological therapies	Include substances from plants and animals (cells, tissues, and glands).
Chiropractic	An alternative medical system that focuses on the relationship between bodily structure (primarily that of the spine) and function (how the body works). Chiropractors use manipulative therapy as a treatment tool to preserve and restore health.
Dietary supplements	In the United States a dietary supplement is defined by law as "a product taken by mouth that contains a 'dietary ingredient' intended to supplement the diet." Dietary ingredients include vitamins, minerals, herbs or other botanicals, amino acids, and substances such as enzymes, organ tissues, and metabolites. Dietary supplements come in many forms, including extracts, concentrates, tablets, capsules, gelcaps, liquids, and powders. They have special requirements for labeling but are considered foods, not drugs.
Conventional medicine	Medicine as practiced by holders of an MD (medical doctor) or DO (doctor of osteopathy) degree and by their allied health professionals, such as physical therapists, psychologists, and registered nurses. Other terms for conventional medicine include allopathy; Western, mainstream, orthodox, and regular medicine; and biomedicine.
Herbal therapies	Use individual plants or mixtures of plants for therapeutic value. An herb is a plant or plant part that produces and contains chemical substances that act upon the body. By strict definition, an herb is only the above-ground part of a perennial plant; therefore, some people prefer the term "botanical therapies" or "botanical medicine," which includes all plants and plant parts. Another word that is used is "phytotherapy" ("phyto" means "plant").
Homeopathic medicine	A CAM system based on the belief that "like cures like" meaning that small, highly diluted quantities of substances are given to cure symptoms, when the same substances given at higher or more concentrated doses would actually cause those symptoms. Homeopathic physicians believe that the more diluted the remedy, the greater its potency. Therefore, they use small doses of specially prepared plant extracts and minerals to stimulate the body's defense mechanisms and healing processes in order to treat illness. Generally, these products are so diluted that safety is not considered a problem.
Massage	Therapists manipulate muscle and connective tissue to enhance function of those tissues and promote relaxation and well-being.
Naturopathic medicine	Naturopathic medicine views disease as a manifestation of changes of the ways in which the body naturally heals itself and emphasizes health restoration rather than disease treatment. Naturopathic physicians use a variety of healing practices, including diet and clinical nutrition; homeopathy; acupuncture; herbal medicine; hydrotherapy (the use of water in a range of temperatures and methods of applications); spinal and soft-tissue manipulation; physical therapies involving electric currents, ultrasound, and light therapy; therapeutic counseling; and pharmacology.
Osteopathic medicine	A form of conventional medicine that emphasizes diseases arising in the musculoskeletal system. There is an underlying belief that all of the body's systems work together and that disturbances in one system can affect function elsewhere in the body. Some osteopathic physicians practice osteopathic manipulation, a full-body system of hands-on techniques to alleviate pain, restore function, and promote health and well-being.

* See the NCCAM web site for a complete list: http://nccam.nih.gov/health/whatiscam/#4.

therapy, such as the use of botanicals (herbal remedies), or only look at a defined population (pregnant women), it is difficult to summarize this information as it applies to the whole population and especially how it applies to children with myositis. There are currently no published studies on the use of CAM in myositis, and there are only a few studies of CAM used in children with other conditions. There are, however, several studies of the use of CAM in other chronic diseases, including cancer and arthritis, and some have shown benefit for some therapies.

There are a number of things that CAM can do:

- CAM can help you play an active role in your child's healthcare.
- It can ease certain symptoms (especially pain, stiffness, stress, anxiety, depressions), thus improving your child's attitude, outlook, and quality of life.
- It may enhance the effects of conventional medicine.

However, CAM does not generally:

- Treat most acute illnesses (such as infections, which require antibiotics)
- Replace proven medical remedies (chemotherapy for cancer)
- Cure longstanding illnesses (including JM)

How Do We Know That a Particular CAM Therapy Works and That It Is Safe?

There are two parts of CAM therapy—the practitioners or therapists and the products or techniques that they might use. Both of these can affect the quality, safety, and effectiveness of a CAM therapy.

In the United States, healthcare practitioners are generally regulated (controlled) by the state governments. Thus, physicians, nurses, pharmacists, and certain other healthcare practitioners must be licensed or registered by the state in which the person is working. They must show evidence that they have the required professional training and experience, and to keep their license, they must show that they stay current in their chosen field (by continuing professional education and other means).

For practitioners of CAM the situation is more complex. Some CAM therapies are regulated and some are not. A doctor of osteopathy (DO), for example, has essentially the same training as a medical doctor (MD). For other types of CAM, the requirements for practitioners may vary from state to state. Thus, certain states recognize (license or register) those who practice naturopathic medicine or acupuncture and have very specific requirements for these professions, whereas other states have no specific or minimal requirements for training and expertise and do not regulate CAM therapies.

It is important to find out about the professional training and experience of any practitioner of CAM that you are considering for treatment of your child. Specific questions you might ask include:

- What is your professional background and training in (type of CAM therapy)?

- Are you licensed or registered to practice (type of CAM therapy) in my state?
- How many years have you been practicing (type of CAM therapy)?
- What are the good points about this type of treatment? What are the problems or downsides to this treatment?
- Have you used this therapy for myositis or other autoimmune conditions before? What were your results in those illnesses?
- What is your experience in using (type of CAM therapy) in children? Are there special issues or problems when this therapy is used in children?
- How will (type of CAM therapy) affect the medicines that my child's doctor has prescribed?
- In making your treatment plan, will you work with our child's myositis doctor and us?

Safety: What's in the Bottle?

How a product is regulated in the United States is determined by the claims that the manufacturer makes about the product and not necessarily what the product is, how the doctor prescribes it, or how you use it. This regulatory classification (i.e., drug versus dietary supplement versus food product) is important because it determines what safety and effectiveness standards apply to the product, what kind of information is needed to assess safety and effectiveness, and which regulatory agency oversees that product.

Products that claim on their labels or package inserts that they can treat, cure, prevent, or lessen symptoms or be used in the diagnosis of disease are considered drugs in the United States. Drugs must be shown to be safe and effective before they can be marketed, and the Food and Drug Administration (FDA) makes that decision. There are very specific requirements for how drugs are manufactured, including standards for purity, strength, and form of the ingredients in the finished drug, and the kinds of information that can or must appear on the product label (for example, what kind of claims the product can make, safety information, or warnings).

Conventionally, foods are items ingested for flavor, taste, aroma, or nutrition. The standards for foods primarily involve the safety and suitability of the food to meet nutritional needs rather than safety and effectiveness as a form of treatment. Furthermore, the standards for manufacturing or storing foods are mainly sanitation (cleanliness) standards.

Dietary supplements are a special category of foods. Unlike prescription and over-the-counter medicines, the FDA does not review dietary supplements before they are marketed. Also, manufacturers do not need to register their products with the FDA before producing or selling them. Under the law, manufacturers of dietary supplements are responsible for making sure their products are safe before they go to market, and the FDA has the responsibility to take action against unsafe dietary supplement products after they reach the market. Except in the case of a new dietary ingredient, where premarket review for safety data and other information is required by law, a firm does not have to provide the FDA with evidence showing that its product is safe and effective. The FDA is currently writing minimum standards for manufacturing dietary supplements that will focus on practices ensuring product quality, including the identity, purity, strength, and composition of dietary supplements.

Even though many supplements are advertised as being "natural," this does not make them automatically safer or better than drugs or synthetic (man-made) ingredients. In many cases there is much less credible information about the effects of particular natural products, and there is less uniformity in the products. Natural products can contain anything found in our environment, including pesticides, bacteria, molds, heavy metals, and other poisons. There have also been numerous reported cases where a so-called natural product has been found to contain illegal drugs. If you want to know more about a particular dietary supplement, ask the manufacturer to supply information to support the claims being made for their products, information on the safety or efficacy of the ingredients in the product, and whether they have received any adverse event reports (i.e., reports of side effects or safety problems) from consumers using their products.

Which CAM Approaches Might Work in Juvenile Myositis?

There are no published studies on the use of CAM therapies for any form of myositis or any published surveys about how children with myositis might use CAM. Nevertheless, certain CAM therapies may be helpful. Two particular types of CAM, in which there is some evidence from scientific studies in other diseases to support their use in JM, are mind-body interventions and manipulation and body-based methods (see Table 14.1).

Mind-body interventions target the human mind-body-spirit and include meditation, hypnosis, prayer and spirituality, mental healing, stress reduction or relaxation, visualization and guided imagery, and creative outlets (art, music, dance, etc.). These therapies increase your mind's ability to affect your body's function and hence your symptoms. They are particularly useful for symptoms such as pain, stiffness, stress, anxiety, altered mood, and altered sleep patterns, which are common in myositis. Use of these therapies also places your child back in better control of what is happening in her life, which is very important for the quality of a child's life and that of the family. Certain types of mind-body interventions, such as patient support groups, have proven their worth and are no longer considered CAM but rather are mainstream health practices now. Exercise and physical therapy prescribed by health professionals and done under supervision are also considered mainstream or conventional health practices for children with myositis (see *Chapter 13, Rehabilitation of the Child with Myositis*).

Several small studies have used massage, relaxing baths, and related therapies to prevent muscle soreness after exercise, including one that evaluated the effects of starting physical exercise shortly after an acute flair of dermatomyositis or polymyositis. In another study healthy athletes who received a massage after exercise had less soreness and lower creatine kinase levels (which normally increase after strenuous exercise) compared with healthy people who rested after exercise but had no massage.

What Are Biologic-Based CAM Therapies?

The terms "biologic-based therapies" and "biologic therapies" are used both in conventional medicine and by CAM. In CAM they refer to substances found in nature that have biologic activity (i.e., they can affect living organisms and their vital processes). Included in this class of therapies are botanicals (herbs such as ginseng, echinacea, or chamomile), foods (such as ginger or garlic), vitamins and minerals (such as vitamin C and zinc), and animal tissues or glands (such as adrenal, pancreas, or brain preparations) (Table 14.2). Routine use of some biologic CAM treatments, such as vitamin and mineral supplements, is considered part of conventional medicine (see *Chapter 19, Nutrition and Your Child's Weight*). When doses of vitamins and minerals are used at higher levels than normally would be present in the diet or used by the body (i.e., megavitamin therapy) or when substances not traditionally considered a part of the diet (such as medicinal plants or animal extracts) are used, these are considered CAM practices.

Using products that contain large doses of vitamins and minerals (levels far above the recommended intakes) has not been shown to be helpful in JM and may be harmful. Of particular concern are products that contain high doses of the fat-soluble vitamins (A, D, E, and K), which are stored in the body and therefore can reach toxic (unsafe) levels with continued use. For example, very high levels of vitamins A and D can affect bone growth and development and cause liver problems. (For further information on appropriate vitamin D supplementation, see *Chapter 7, Treatment Possibilities in the Beginning* and *Chapter 22, Taking Care of the Bones*.) Because both the myositis itself and its treatments may have an effect on nutritional status, it is important to discuss your child's diet and nutritional needs with your child's myositis doctor and to ask for additional advice, if desired, from a registered dietician.

Table 14.3 lists some CAM therapies (and their possible side effects) that have been used in other autoimmune disorders and that might also be useful in JM. It is important to remember that these therapies have not been tested for safety and effectiveness in myositis and that often the appropriate doses for children are not known. Although there is much interest in the use of certain of these substances for myositis, the currently available information does not give us enough assurance that all of these substances can be used safely in JM. In fact, some of these can cause harm to children (see Table 14.4). Table 14.5 lists potential interactions between CAM products and the drugs used to treat children with myositis, as drug interactions are also an important consideration in the safe use of a particular product. These interactions can cause the medicines that your child is already taking for myositis to have side effects or not to work as well. Before starting any CAM, it is important to become educated about these treatments and their potential problems and to discuss this information with your child's doctor.

Table 14.3. CAM biologic-based therapies juvenile myositis patients frequently consider.

Ingredient	What is it? What does it do?	Possible problems
Coenzyme Q10 (CoQ10)	• CoQ10 is a vitamin-like substance that is important in energy metabolism and that has antioxidant properties. • Lowered CoQ10 blood levels are reported in some heart and muscle diseases (heart attacks, cardiomyopathy, and muscular dystrophies). Clinical studies in these disorders are promising but do not conclusively prove effectiveness.	• CoQ10 may decrease the effectiveness of the blood thinner warfarin. • It is generally well tolerated when taken by mouth, but high doses may cause digestive discomfort in some. • A specific CoQ10 formulation (UbiQGel) is FDA approved for the treatment of certain mitochondrial disorders, another type of muscle disease that is different from JM.
Creatine	• Used orally to improve exercise performance and to increase muscle bulk in athletes and older people.	• *Cases of muscle weakness or flares of myositis have been reported with the use of creatine.* There are reports of contamination of certain creatine products (they contained illegal hormones). • At high doses, creatine can affect the liver and kidneys. Reported side effects include stomach pain, nausea, diarrhea, fluid retention, and muscle cramping.
Fish oil (omega-3 fatty acids)	• Omega-3 fatty acids, eicosapentaenoic acid (EPA) and docosahexaenoic acid (DHA), are typically derived from oils of salmon, sardines, anchovies, or mackerel. These act to decrease inflammation and cytokine production.	• May increase the blood-thinning effects of anticoagulants and nonsteroidal anti-inflammatory drugs (NSAIDs). May be harmful in children with myositis who have clotting problems. See Table 14.4 for product interactions. • High doses can cause nausea and loose stools.
Ginger (*Zingiber officinale*)	• Can help with nausea related to the use of other drugs. • Inhibits formation of certain pro-inflammatory substances and has pain-relieving effects.	• Can increase bruising and bleeding; see Table 14.4 for product interactions.
Glucosamine	• Glucosamine is required to make proteins found in muscles, tendons, cartilage, ligaments, and blood vessels. It has been used orally for osteoarthritis, where studies have shown an improvement in symptoms.	• Glucosamine may increase blood sugar levels in diabetics. Side effects are generally mild and include stomach upset. • Use of multi-ingredient products that also contain manganese may result in ingestion of too much manganese, which can cause nervous system problems.

(continued)

Table 14.3. (continued)

Ingredient	What is it? What does it do?	Possible problems
Turmeric (*Curcuma longa*)	• Contains curcumins, which have anti-inflammatory properties. Also contains turmerin, which has antioxidant effects and can contribute to anti-inflammatory action.	• At doses higher than used in cooking may increase bruising and bleeding (see Table 14.4). • When taken by mouth, it may cause diarrhea and nausea; topically, it can cause allergic rashes.
Salicin-containing botanicals: Cramp bark Willow bark Wintergreen	• Salicins, which are similar to aspirin, have anti-inflammatory and anti-pain properties, so they can help with muscle aches and pains.	• May increase bruising and bleeding (see Table 14.4). • Do not use these botanicals if also taking methotrexate or other drugs that suppress the immune system. • We generally know much less about the effects of these botanicals in children than we do about aspirin and other NSAIDs. Do not use these if your child has a virus-like illness because of concern for Reye's syndrome.
Evening primrose oil	• Contains gamma linoleic acids (GLAs), which can decrease inflammation. • GLAs are also found in black current and borage oils.	• May increase bruising and bleeding. May be harmful in children with myositis with clotting problems (see Table 14.4). • GLA use may be associated with mild digestive side effects (nausea, vomiting, soft stools, diarrhea, gas, and belching).
Vitamin C and N-acetyl cysteine (NAC)	• NAC is an amino acid important for sulfur metabolism in the body. Both vitamin C and NAC are used for their reported antioxidant effects.	• Orally, high dose NAC can cause digestive side effects (nausea, abdominal pain, vomiting, and diarrhea). It has an unpleasant odor, which may make it difficult to take. • No studies are available on the effects of these substances for treating myositis. Their use in JM is not recommended. One study showed higher levels of muscle enzymes and markers of oxidative stress in those using NAC and vitamin C (indicating more cell damage than with no treatment at all).
Vitamin C	• A water-soluble vitamin used for its reported antioxidant effects in a variety of ailments. Although the use of vitamin C is supported by scientific studies in deficiency states like scurvy, its usefulness in other conditions has not yet been proven.	• Side effects are dose related and can include stomach upset, heartburn, tiredness, headache, and difficulty sleeping. High doses of vitamin C can result in very severe diarrhea and gastrointestinal upset in children and can cause certain types of urinary system stones. Scurvy can occur when high dose, chronic vitamin C intake is suddenly decreased.
Vitamin E	• A fat-soluble vitamin used for its antioxidant effects in a number of conditions (including those of heart, blood vessels, and muscles, and in cancer). Its usefulness for treating these conditions has not yet been proven.	• Generally well tolerated. • May increase bruising and bleeding. May be harmful in children with myositis who have clotting problems (see Table 14.4).

For more information, visit NCCAM's web site at http://nccam.nih.gov/health/whatiscam.

Table 14.4. CAM biologic-based therapies that probably *should not* be used in juvenile myositis because of safety concerns.

Ingredient	What is it? What does it do?	Possible problems
Androstenedione (andro)	• Andros are male-sex hormones that have been used to increase muscle bulk or enhance athletic performance.	• Products containing androstenedione and related hormones should not be used in children. They can cause masculinization of girls and growth failure in boys. Long-term use is associated with increase in the rates of several different cancers and can cause liver disease.
Carnitine	• An amino acid that is important for energy metabolism in muscle. Very low levels of muscle carnitine are associated with muscles that do not function well. However, supplementation with carnitine has not been shown to correct or improve muscle function or enhance athletic performance. Pharmacologically, doses of carnitine can have immunomodulatory effects similar to glucocorticoids (prednisone).	• DL-carnitine should not be used in children with myositis. Side effects include nausea, vomiting, stomach cramps, gastritis (inflammation of the stomach lining), body odor, and seizures. DL-carnitine, but not L-carnitine, has been associated with severe muscle weakness, muscle wasting, and discolored urine (myoglobin in the urine). • May interact with blood-thinning drugs at high doses.
DHEA (dehydroepi-androsterone)	• DHEA is a hormone that has been used as a drug in lupus as a steroid-sparing agent, so that prednisone dose can be reduced. It may improve bone mineral density in lupus patients treated with high-dose steroids. Taking DHEA by mouth doesn't appear to improve muscle bulk or muscle strength in elderly patients. • It has also been used to improve feelings of well-being.	• DHEA should not be used in children with myositis based on current information. • DHEA may cause liver damage if taking azathioprine or methotrexate. It can increase insulin resistance or sensitivity in diabetics. Other side effects include acne, hair loss or increased facial hair, changes in blood cholesterol and other blood fats, liver disease, and stomach pain. • Note: the DHEA found in dietary supplements may not be the same quality as that used in the drug trials for lupus.
Echinacea	• This is a medicinal herb, which is taken by mouth to prevent colds or shorten viral symptoms.	• Echinacea and other substances that stimulate (boost) the immune system should not be used in autoimmune disorders, including JM. There are reports of new onset disease or flares of disease with these substances.
L-tryptophan (LT), 5-hydroxy tryptophan (5-HTP)	• These are amino acids important for serotonin metabolism; they have been used to help with mood and sleep disorders.	• The issue of exactly what caused an epidemic of L-tryptophan-associated Eosinophilia Myalgia Syndrome has never been resolved. • *The FDA received case reports of Eosinophilia Myalgia Syndrome and myositis associated with both LT and 5-HTP.*

(continued)

Table 14.4. (continued)

Ingredient	What is it? What does it do?	Possible problems
Thunder god vine (*Tripterygium wilfordii*)	• Has been used by mouth for its immunosuppressive effects in several autoimmune diseases, including rheumatoid arthritis (RA) and lupus. In RA, it is also applied on the skin over swollen joints.	• Thunder god vine suppresses the immune system, so it should not be used with other drugs with this effect (see Table 14.5) because of the potential for increased side effects. • Long-term use may cause decreased bone density. Other side effects include gastrointestinal upset, hair loss, headache, infertility, and skin reactions.
Melatonin	• Melatonin is a hormone that helps regulate sleep and hormone secretion patterns.	• Melatonin should not be given to children. Melatonin appears to boost the immune system, so should be avoided by people with autoimmune diseases. May also affect normal sex development in children. • Other side effects may include headache, fleeting depression, daytime tiredness, mild tremor (shaking), anxiety, confusion, nausea, vomiting, and lowered blood pressure.
Frankincense (*Boswellia* species) or Myrrh (*Commiphora* species)	• Gugguls from the gum resin have anti-inflammatory properties and have been used to treat osteoarthritis. They are also used for their cholesterol-lowering effects.	• May increase the blood-thinning effects of anticoagulants and NSAIDs. May be harmful in children with myositis who have clotting problems (see Table 14.5 for product interactions). • Gugguls may also cause headaches, stomach upset, and rashes.

For more information, visit NCCAM's web site at http://nccam.nih.gov/health/whatiscam.

Table 14.5. Potential interactions between drugs used to treat juvenile myositis and CAM.

Class of drug	Names of drugs	Possible botanical / supplement interaction	Possible problem	What to watch for and what to do
Anti-inflammatory/ pain	NSAIDs (aspirinibuprofen, naprosyn,COX-2 inhibitors)	Ginkgo, Bilberry Black cohosh Boswellia, serrata Bromelain (Pineapple enzyme) Cat's Claw Chamomile, Danshen Dong quai Feverfew, Fish oil (omega-3 fatty acids) Garlic, Ginger Ginseng, Melatonin Rue Stinging nettle Tumeric, Uva ursi Vitamin E, Willow	Increased bleeding	Look for increased bruising and bleeding. If any increased bruising or bleeding occurs stop use and call your doctor. Note: Use of multiple botanicals *or* supplements in this list by themselves can also result in increased bruising and bleeding.
Blood thinners	Dipyridamole Clopidogrel eptifibatide Ticlopidine Tirofiban Heparin Warfarin			

(continued)

Table 14.5. (continued)

Class of drug	Names of drugs	Possible botanical / supplement interaction	Possible problem	What to watch for and what to do
Cholesterol-lowering drugs	Of particular concern are statin-type drugs (i.e. ritonavir, saquinavir, pravastatin, etc.)	Red yeast (Cholestin)	May cause myopathies	Watch for muscle tenderness, pain, cramps. Do not use these products together.
Corticosteroids	Prednisone prednisolone	Aloe Cascara Celery seed Horsetail Juniper Licorice Senna Yellow dock	Increased potassium loss	Watch for signs and symptoms of low potassium levels (muscle weakness, myalgia, cramps, and heart palpitations).
Corticosteroids	Prednisone Prednisolone	Panax ginseng	Increased side effects	Increased stimulation and insomnia may occur.
Immunosuppressive agents	Azathioprine Cyclosporine Methotrexate	Astralagus Echinacea Melatonin	Can potentially counteract effect of drug	Possible disease flares or increased symptoms. Do not use these botanicals if on methotrexate or another immunosuppressive agent.
	Methotrexate	Cramp bark Thunder god vine Willow Wintergreen	Increase blood levels of methotrexate, increased toxicity.	Do not use these botanicals if on methotrexate or another immunosuppressive agent.
	Methotrexate	Folic acid	Can decrease methotrexate effect	Ask your doctor how to take folic acid.
Photosensitizers (increase sensitivity to sun)	Antimalarials: hydroxychloroquine Certain antibiotics tetracycline, ciprofloxacin, sulfa drugs Diogoxin (heart meds) Certain blood pressure meds	Angelica fennel Rue St. John's Wort	Increase likelihood and severity of photosensitive rashes	Ask your doctor before using these products together. Remember the need to practice "sun precautions."

For more information, visit NCCAM's web site at http://nccam.nih.gov/health/whatiscam.

Key Points

■ Complementary and alternative medicines (CAM) consist of a variety of approaches not presently part of conventional western medicine.

■ Few studies of CAM therapies have been performed, and none is now scientifically proven to be safe and effective in treating children with myositis.

■ Do your homework to know as much as you can about a therapy that you might choose for your child. You need information on what the therapy is, what it can do or might be able to do for your child, and what possible problems could occur.

■ For CAM therapies where a therapist or practitioner is involved, find out about the training, experience, and licensure of this person.

■ For therapies where products are taken (by mouth or other means), learn about the product's ingredients and how the product is regulated, as this can affect its safety and quality.

■ Tell your doctor about everything that your child is using. The choice to use CAM in your child's therapy should be made jointly with your child's doctor.

■ If your child has any adverse (bad) experience with a product, stop the product and tell your doctor about the problem; also report serious problems to the FDA (see *To Learn More*).

To Learn More

U.S. Food and Drug Administration (FDA).

Dietary Supplements. Available at: www.cfsan.fda.gov/~dms/supplmnt.html or 888-463-6332.

Links to many topics related to supplements, from details on specific supplements to recent FDA announcements and warnings.

Reporting problems with CAM products or medicines. Available at: www.fda.gov/medwatch/index.html or 800-FDA-1088.

Tips for the Savvy Supplement User. Available from: www.cfsan.fda.gov/~dms/ds-savvy.html.

National Institutes of Health, National Center for Complementary and Alternative Medicine (NCCAM).

Health Information. Available at: http://nccam.nih.gov/health/ or 888-NIH-6226.
Definition of CAM, finding alternative treatments and supplements.

Links to Other Organizations. Available at: http://nccam.nih.gov/health/links/.

CAM on PubMed. Available at: www.nlm.nih.gov/nccam/camonpubmed.html or 888-346-3656.

A special search engine for CAM at the National Library of Medicine (NLM), which gives access to research articles and other information.

In addition to the government sources of information listed above, there are numerous other sources of information on CAM. Generally, information provided by recognized public health and consumer groups or by academic medical centers is considered more reliable, but you need to determine whether the information is current and how these organizations obtain and evaluate any information they might provide.

Arthritis Foundation (AF).

Arthritis Today's Supplement Guide. Available from: www.arthritis.org/conditions/supplementguide or 800-568-4045.

Alternative Therapies, Supplement Guide. Available from: www.arthritis.org/conditions/alttherapies/default.asp.

2006 Drug Guide. Arthritis Today. Available from: www.arthritis.org/conditions/DrugGuide or 800-568-4045.

Natural Medicines Comprehensive Database. Available from: www.naturaldatabase.com.

Paid subscription for information [ask your doctor or local library about access]. Comprehensive evaluation of potential benefits and side effects of CAM therapies, interactions with drug medications, and description of commercial products.

Longwood Herbal Task Force (LHTF). Internet: www.longwoodherbal.org; Email: PaulaGardiner2000@yahoo.com.

Organized in the fall of 1998 by faculty, staff, and students from Children's Hospital, the Massachusetts College of Pharmacy and Health Sciences, and the Dana Farber Cancer Institute to learn more and teach other clinicians about herbs and dietary supplements. Provides extensive information on their web site. Published a number of scientific articles in the area of CAM.

Reports in the Medical Literature

Lee AN, Werth VP. Activation of autoimmunity following use of immunostimulatory herbal supplements. *Archives of Dermatology.* 2004 Jun;140(6):723–7.

Treating children with alternative medicine. *Pediatric Annals.* 2004 April;33(4). [This issue is dedicated to CAM and children.]

CHAPTER 15

New Therapies on the Horizon

Frederick W. Miller, MD, PhD, and Daniel J. Lovell, MD, MPH

In this chapter...

We discuss some potentially promising new treatments for myositis called biologic therapies. They include proteins called monoclonal antibodies and the use of stem cells from the bone marrow to replace the immune system. These treatments are still being tested in myositis patients, and we have limited information to know if they work in juvenile myositis. Until more information has been obtained, they should generally be used only after the standard treatments have failed and by doctors who have experience with them.

From the family's point of view...

"'Ow!' I said. I couldn't sit on the floor. I was four years old, and I felt frustrated because I had a disease called JDM. No matter how hard I tried to move certain ways, it always hurt. One day my mom came home with a bunch of syringes and a small bottle (Enbrel). She said I needed a shot twice a week. I wasn't so sure about this, but I did it. The shot hurt, but as soon as it was over, I was okay...the medicine worked! Two weeks later, I could run faster and sit on the floor, and I felt better overall."

What Are the Possible New Treatments for Myositis?

Although the pace of discovery of new treatments for myositis has been slow in the past, exciting new therapies have recently resulted from the types of clinical research described in *Chapter 39, How We Learn About Juvenile Myositis*. Hope for more rapid progress to develop new medicines also comes from new designs for drug studies that will require fewer patients to determine if a new drug is safe and effective. Hope for progress also comes from cooperation from doctors around the world to develop a single standard to evaluate people with myositis in clinical trials so that doctors can all agree when a participant in a study has or has not improved (see *Chapter 10, Charting Your Child's Progress*).

The United States Food and Drug Administration (FDA) recently approved many new medicines for other autoimmune diseases, especially for adult and juvenile rheumatoid arthritis (RA and JRA). These medicines are called biologic agents because they are made by biologic processes using living cells. They block the immune system in specific ways by binding to a specific target or by blocking the cell's metabolism (see Figure 15.1). Most of these biologic agents are proteins called monoclonal antibodies, which recognize only one specific structure and are made by cells in large numbers in special laboratories. Monoclonal antibody treatments are becoming more popular because they can be custom made to block specific parts of the disease process that might be causing inflammation and have less effect on other parts of the body.

■ **Figure 15.1. (See color plate 8 on page 229.) Monoclonal antibody.** Example of how a monoclonal antibody can bind to a specific target and block its function to decrease inflammation and thereby result in less myositis.

These new treatments also have side effects. Some patients are allergic to these biologic treatments. Furthermore, because most of these new treatments block important parts of the immune system, they increase the risk for certain infections. Doctors have used these monoclonal antibodies to treat only a few children with JM in the whole world, so these treatments are not yet ready for routine use in the treatment of JM. Several studies are planned or ongoing to begin to test their safety and effectiveness in adult and juvenile myositis (Table 15.1).

These new biologic therapies can be divided into groups based on the part of the immune system they affect. These groups, which are described in more detail below, are called anti-tumor necrosis factor alpha (TNF-α) agents, anti-B-lymphocyte agents, anti-T-lymphocyte agents, anti-complement agents, and autologous stem cell therapies.

It is wonderful to have so many potentially helpful new therapies, particularly for patients who continue to have difficulties with myositis after trying the standard drugs. It is important to keep in mind, however, that some new therapies could eventually prove to be safe and effective for use in myositis patients, and some might even be a big breakthrough in treatment, but others might not be. By the time you read this chapter, some of the medicines discussed here might have failed these tests in myositis and other patients, but others that are not yet available at this time might soon be tested. *It is important that you talk with your child's doctor about the possible risks and benefits of all treatments before considering these agents.*

Since we will only know if these and other new therapies are safe and effective in treating myositis by doing clinical research on children with myositis, it is important to consider enrolling your child in research studies (see *Chapter 39, How We Learn About Juvenile Myositis*). Treatment studies can allow your child to have access to newer treatments that might not otherwise be available and are the only way that we will learn more about the effectiveness of these new treatments. These

Table 15.1. New therapies being studied for juvenile myositis.*

Treatment name	Treatment type	How it works	Potential side effects	Experience in juvenile and adult myositis
Etanercept (Enbrel)	Combines part of a monoclonal antibody with part of a TNF-α receptor	Blocks TNF-α, a promoter of inflammation	Injection site reactions (pain, swelling, and redness at site of injection), tuberculosis and other infections that can be very serious or, rarely, fatal. Other autoimmune diseases, such as lupus or multiple sclerosis. Seizures.	Case reports of improvement and Phase 1–2 studies are ongoing in adults with dermatomyositis; one study of 10 JDM patients showed mild improvement. Approved for the treatment of adult and juvenile rheumatoid arthritis.
Infliximab (Remicade)	Monoclonal antibody	Blocks TNF-α, a promoter of inflammation	Infusion reactions (headache, dizziness, muscle aches, low blood pressure, fever, itching, flushing, rash during intravenous treatment), tuberculosis, fungal and other very serious infections, or rarely fatal. Other autoimmune diseases, such as lupus or multiple sclerosis.	Case reports of improvement in adults and children with dermatomyositis and polymyositis, including possibly improvement in calcinosis; Phase 1–2 studies ongoing in adult myositis. Approved for the treatment of rheumatoid arthritis and Crohn's disease.
Adalimumab (Humira)	Monoclonal antibody	Blocks TNF-α, a promoter of inflammation	Injection site reactions (pain, swelling, and redness at site of injection), tuberculosis and other very serious infections or rarely fatal.	None reported. Approved for the treatment of rheumatoid arthritis.
Rituximab (Rituxan)	Monoclonal antibody	Kills and blocks functions of B cells, which are a form of lymphocyte important in the inflammation in myositis	Fevers, rashes, and other reactions to the injections, low white blood cell counts and infections that can be very serious or fatal.	Case reports of improvement in small numbers of children and adults with myositis; a larger Phase 1–2 study is ongoing. Approved for the treatment of non-Hodgkin's lymphoma and rheumatoid arthritis.
Campath 1H	Monoclonal antibody	Blocks T cell functions and may kill T cells	Infections	A single patient with juvenile polymyositis was treated and showed some improvement. A trial in inclusion body myositis is ongoing. Not approved by the FDA for any disease.
Eculizumab (anti-C5)	Monoclonal antibody	Blocks activity of complement protein C5, a possible promoter of muscle damage in dermatomyositis and JDM	Muscle/joint aches and pain, upper respiratory infection (colds), and headache.	A small number of dermatomyositis patients showed improvement of rash, but not in strength. Not approved by the FDA for any disease.
Immune stem cell therapy	Cell therapy	Resets the immune system with new stem cells from the bone marrow	Severe infections possibly resulting in death.	Case reports and Phase 1–2 studies ongoing in children and adults with myositis and other autoimmune diseases.

* All these treatments involve injections of medications into the skin or infusions by vein; none are now proven to be helpful in juvenile myositis, and all are likely to increase the risk for infections and have other serious side effects. Phase 1–2 studies are clinical trials that are designed to begin to understand the safety and effectiveness of new medicines before the Food and Drug Administration (FDA) licenses them as treatment for a particular disease.

Abbreviations: TNF-α = tumor necrosis factor alpha; JDM = juvenile dermatomyositis treatments are carefully reviewed by many experts to ensure that the studies are done in the safest and most careful ways. If your child is not doing well using standard treatments, you should discuss with your child's doctor the possibility of being involved in research studies.

Anti-TNF-α Agents

Inflammation is caused by the direct actions of cells of the immune system called lymphocytes or by the actions of proteins called cytokines, which are made by one type of cell and affect other cells. Cytokines are sometimes called the hormones of the immune system.

The most studied biologic agents are those that block the action of an important protein called tumor necrosis factor alpha (TNF-α). TNF-α is a cytokine that is produced by immune cells and generates inflammation. TNF-α is increased in the muscles of children with myositis and might indirectly cause the inflammation in muscles or directly kill the muscle cells themselves, as described in *Chapter 3, The Pathways to Juvenile Myositis.*

Several monoclonal antibodies (called infliximab [Remicade] and adalimumab [Humira]) block the bad effects of TNF-α by binding to it directly so it cannot harm the tissues. These drugs have been shown to be effective for treating rheumatoid arthritis (RA) and other autoimmune conditions. Another anti-TNF-α agent (called etanercept [Enbrel]) is made by combining parts of an antibody molecule with the TNF-α receptor. Etanercept also binds TNF-α so that it cannot do bad things inside cells and tissues. Each of these treatments is given differently. Etanercept and adalimumab are given as a shot under the skin (called a subcutaneous injection), varying from twice a week to twice a month. Infliximab is given as an infusion by vein every two to eight weeks. Only a few children with myositis have been treated with these therapies.

Some adults with myositis and children with juvenile dermatomyositis (JDM) have received infliximab. Their muscle strength and possibly the calcinosis improved. These patients tried this treatment because they had not responded to many of the other medicines.

One carefully performed study of etanercept treatment was done using ten children with JDM who had active myositis for more than thirty-six months. One child's symptoms (arthritis, rash, and weakness) got worse, and she stopped taking the medication. The other nine children had a significant but minimal (only about 10%) improvement in total Disease Activity Score (see *Chapter 10, Charting Your Child's Progress* for details about the Disease Activity Score). Muscle enzymes did not change significantly during the study. The researchers concluded that etanercept was tolerated well by most children with chronic JDM, but it did not benefit this group of children much. Studies are now in progress to see if these anti-TNF-α treatments are helpful in a larger number of patients with adult and juvenile myositis (see Table 15.1).

Anti-TNF-α agents are powerful suppressors of the immune system, and they can potentially cause many unintended problems. The most common side effects of anti-TNF-α agents include reactions at the injection site (including redness, itchiness, and pain at the injection site that lasts several days). For the intravenous form, infliximab, reactions during the infusion are common and include headache, dizziness, muscle aches, low blood pressure, fever, itching, flushing, sweating, rash, wheezing, shortness of breath, and nausea or vomiting.

A major side effect of concern is that your child could develop serious infections (including bacterial, fungal, and tuberculosis infections that can require intensive antibiotic treatment and rarely cause death) after using anti-TNF-α agents. This side effect is important to children with myositis for at least two reasons. The first reason is more theoretical. If juvenile myositis is triggered by an infection, then the myositis could be intensified by an increase in the infection after anti-TNF-α treatment. The second reason is that the calcifications in some children with JDM are associated with infection that is sometimes hard to bring under control. These biologic agents that dampen your child's defense system might be associated with further infection. If your child is taking one of these anti-TNF-α treatments and develops fever, cough, sore throat, ear pain, redness and warmth in the skin, or other symptoms of infection, it is important that you contact your child's doctor immediately and that your child is seen and evaluated for an infection. Doctors should be sure that children with myositis do not have infections, and they should do a skin test called a PPD for tuberculosis before giving your child anti-TNF-α agents. Other rare side effects of anti-TNF-α drugs include seizures and the development of new autoantibodies or new autoimmune diseases such as multiple sclerosis and lupus.

Anti-B Lymphocyte Agents

Another monoclonal antibody called rituximab (Rituxan) binds to and inactivates cells of the immune system called B lymphocytes. B lymphocytes play an important role in producing antibodies and may help the function of other immune cells called T lymphocytes that may be harmful in myositis. B lymphocytes may play a particularly important role in the development of adult dermatomyositis (DM) and JDM (see *Chapter 3, The Pathways to Juvenile Myositis*).

Rituximab has been approved to treat a form of cancer of the B lymphocytes called non-Hodgkin's lymphoma. Early studies in adults with rheumatoid arthritis and DM suggest that rituximab might be useful for treating those conditions, but rituximab is still an experimental treatment. A few people with DM and JDM have received rituximab and have had positive responses, mainly improvement in strength, rashes, and serum levels of muscle enzymes. For rituximab, as well as all of these new therapies discussed in this chapter, the follow-up period has been relatively short, and we do not know the long-term effects of the treatment.

Rituximab is infused into a vein and usually has a long period of effectiveness. The effect of a single infusion can last up to a year. The advantage is that it requires infrequent treatment, but the disadvantage is that any side effects could also last for a long time. The main problems associated with rituximab are fevers, rashes, and other reactions when the medicine is going into the bloodstream. Some of these reactions, called infusion reactions, have been severe. In addition, white blood cell counts can drop very low for a long time (months), and sometimes this can cause patients to develop serious infections. A large study is in progress in myositis patients that will include both adult DM and polymyositis, as well as JDM patients. This treatment appears promising, and this large study should help in sorting out how well it works in myositis patients and what side effects it causes.

Anti-T Lymphocyte Agents

A form of lymphocyte called the T cell or T lymphocyte is important for controlling the immune system's response to infections, but it also attacks muscle cells in myositis. Many of our current medicines for myositis stop or slow down T cell functions. Several new biologic therapies have been developed specifically to block only the T cells rather than the other types of lymphocytes.

One of these new therapies is a monoclonal antibody called Campath 1H, which binds to T cells. This antibody is now being tested in patients who have inclusion body myositis. A single child with severe juvenile polymyositis has been treated with Campath 1H and demonstrated improved strength and quality of life measures after receiving this treatment. Because so few persons have been treated with Campath 1H, we do not know much about the side effects of this new monoclonal antibody, but it is likely that the side effects of this agent will include increased infections. This treatment is experimental and is not available for use by patients who are not part of a drug trial.

Anti-Complement Agents

Complement refers to a series of blood proteins that are important in protecting you from a wide variety of infections. But in some conditions, such as lupus, the activation of complement causes inflammation and tissue damage. In some persons with myositis, particularly adults and children with DM, complement seems to be overly active and could be causing some of the problems in their skin and muscles.

A new monoclonal autoantibody called eculizumab has been developed to bind to and inactivate a single complement protein called C5. Eculizumab might benefit some people with myositis because it helps shut off the complement pathway. Eculizumab has been studied in a small number of DM patients, and it improved the skin rash but not the muscle weakness. The main problems with using eculizumab are muscle or joint aches and pain, colds, and headache. This treatment is experimental and is not available for use by patients who are not part of a drug trial.

Stem Cell Therapy

Stem cell therapy became more common after it was used to treat certain blood cancers that developed in people with rheumatoid arthritis. Some of those individuals were cured of both cancer and their arthritis. They were treated with radiation therapy and high doses of chemotherapy, which destroyed their immune system. This was followed by restoring the immune system with the patient's own bone marrow cells, which had been collected before the chemotherapy.

That experiment opened up an entirely new type of treatment, called stem cell transplantation, for patients with a variety of autoimmune diseases. Stem cells are special cells in the blood or bone marrow that can become any type of cell in the body because they don't have a specific purpose or function. Transplantation means that the body's original cells have been destroyed and are being replaced by the new cells. In stem cell transplantation the stem cells that are used in the treatment come directly from the patient's own body (this is called autologous cells). This type of immune stem cell treatment is different from using other stem cells that can form into muscles, which has been tried in other types of muscle disease but without success so far.

Preliminary studies using high doses of chemotherapy followed by infusion of the patient's own immune stem cells (obtained from prior blood or bone marrow samples) have found that in some cases this treatment improves autoimmune disease. The hope in these cases is that by eliminating the patient's entire immune system and rebuilding it with new stem cells, the new cells will not attack the body as the old cells did. Several adults and children with myositis have been treated in clinical trials using this approach. Although some have improved, several have died from the severe infections that can occur when the immune system is weakened by the chemotherapy. Further studies are needed to determine the overall risks and benefits of this promising but potentially dangerous therapy.

Summary

Many parts of the immune system are probably involved in causing problems in JM (see *Chapter 3, The Pathways to Juvenile Myositis*). Monoclonal antibodies and other biologic agents have been developed to block these different parts. Many of these agents are being studied in other diseases now, and it is likely that some of them could be helpful when used to treat JM. These new treatments, coupled with international collaborations to standardize clinical studies in myositis, should encourage all patients with JM that more effective and safer therapies are being developed and could be available in the near future. To keep updated regarding this rapidly advancing field or to find out how to join a research study, please talk to your doctor or see the web sites and other references listed at the end of this chapter and *Chapter 39, How We Learn About Juvenile Myositis.*

Key Points

■ Many new treatments, called biologic therapies, are being developed to target specific disease processes, in order to develop more effective treatments for autoimmune diseases and to offer promise in the treatment of JM.

■ These new therapies include monoclonal antibodies and treatments with stem cells from the bone marrow that can change the immune system.

■ These powerful treatments can have many side effects, including allergic reactions, infusion or injection site reactions, and rarely severe infections that can be fatal in some cases.

■ Although studies are being done now in juvenile and adult myositis to see if these new agents can be useful, we do not know whether, in the final analysis, they help or cause harm. It is best for your child to use these treatments only if he or she is participating in a research drug study, where your child can be closely monitored, or under the care of a physician who has experience with their use.

To Learn More

The Myositis Association (TMA).

Clinical Trials and *Published Research*. Available from: www.myositis.org/jmbookresources.cfm.

ClinicalTrials.gov, a service of the U.S. National Institutes of Health (NIH).

Clinical Trials. Available at: www.clinicaltrials.gov.
> Regularly updated information about federally and privately supported clinical research in human volunteers, including a trial's purpose, who may participate, locations, and phone numbers for more details.

For more information, see the Resource Appendix.

Reports in the Medical Literature

Levine TD. Rituximab in the treatment of dermatomyositis: an open-label pilot study. *Arthritis and Rheumatism.* 2005 Feb;52(2):601–7.

Miller FW. *Myositis.* In: Smolen JS, Lipsky PE, editors. *Targeted Therapies in Rheumatology.* London: Martin Dunitz; 2003. p. 603–20.

Shanahan JC, Moreland LW, Carter RH. Upcoming biologic agents for the treatment of rheumatic diseases. *Current Opinion in Rheumatology.* 2003 May;15(3):226–36.

Important Issues on the Road to Recovery

CHAPTER 16

Skin Rashes and Sun Protection

Victoria R. Barrio, MD; Jeffrey P. Callen, MD; and Amy S. Paller, MD

In this chapter...

We describe the skin problems that children with myositis have and how to treat them.

> ### From the family's point of view...
>
> *"The first rash that appeared was on the inside of her eyelids, next to her nose. It spread down under her eyes and across her cheeks in a sort of butterfly effect. Her fingers were also red and sore around her nails. With medicines, these have cleared up over time, but we continue to avoid the sun. Her skin has always been very fair, and the JDM makes her all the more photosensitive. Sun protection has become a major part of her treatment regimen—sunscreen applied multiple times each day, sun protective film on our home's windows, a sun protective parasol and clothes, and checking the UV index daily."*

Skin rashes can be a feature of juvenile myositis (JM), particularly juvenile dermatomyositis (JDM). In some patients the rash can be more bothersome than the muscle disease. Exposure to the sun can cause the skin rashes to get much worse, so proper protection from the sun is one of the most important aspects of skin care in children with JDM.

How Is the Skin Involved in Juvenile Myositis?

There are several different forms of skin involvement in JDM. One of the early symptoms is often swelling of the eyelids, which has a red to violet hue and is called a heliotrope rash (see Figure 1.1 [color plate 1 on page 227]). Red bumps called Gottron's papules can develop on the back of the hands over the knuckles, as well as over the knees and elbows (see Figure 1.2 [color plate 2 on page 227] and Figure 16.1 [color plate 9 on page 229]). These two types of rashes are characteristic skin rashes, and their presence helps to confirm the diagnosis of dermatomyositis (DM).

Other rashes are commonly seen on the face and the tops of the ears. When the cheeks become red and the rash crosses the bridge of the nose, it is called a malar rash or butterfly rash (Figure 16.2). This rash can be mistaken for the facial rash characteristic of another skin disease called lupus, but it is present in many children with pure DM. The rash can also occur on the surface of the arms or legs or between the fingers (linear extensor erythema), in the V-shaped area of the neck ("V-sign"), or on the upper back ("shawl sign"). Small, dilated blood vessels can be seen on the upper eyelids and the sun-exposed areas of the ears, face, neck, and just behind the fingernails (called periungual telangiectasia) (Figure 16.3). The nail cuticles can become overgrown and jagged. Gums around the teeth can also show capillary dilation, breakage, and swelling, like the nailfold capillaries.

With time, any affected area tends to become more discolored with either loss or increase in skin pigment. It is important to see a doctor at the earliest appearance of a rash, so that the cause of the rash can be determined.

■ **Figure 16.1. (See color plate 9 on page 229.) Gottron's papules.**
Gottron's papules are red and raised or rough scaly patches present over the extensor surfaces of the joints. Here they are present over the knees, but they may also be seen over the finger joints, elbows, insides of the ankles, or even over the toe joints.

■ **Figure 16.2. (See color plate 10 on page 229.) Malar rash.**
Erythema over the cheeks and nasal bridge.

■ **Figure 16.3. (See color plate 11 on page 229.) Periungual telangiectasia.**
Periungual telangiectasia with dilated, tortuous capillaries along the fingernail fold, an area of bushy capillary loop formation and areas of capillary loss.

Even areas that aren't exposed to the sun can have a rash. When the scalp is affected, there can be loss of hair, redness, or scale in the scalp, as well as swelling. In severe cases, the skin develops deep breaks, called ulcers. The ulcers can be present between the eyes and on the bridge of the nose and can leave pitted scars. Ulcers in the mouth can cause discomfort during eating, particularly of spicy foods.

In children, calcium deposits can form in the skin (calcinosis) if the child has inflammation for a long time. Early and aggressive treatment can decrease the probability of calcinosis happening (see *Chapter 17, Calcinosis*).

Does Everyone Get These Rashes?

Every person is different, and so not everyone will have the same rashes. Some people will get more rashes than others. The severity of the rash can also differ.

Some people find the skin rashes more bothersome than the muscle weakness and might have a harder time treating it. Sometimes the skin rashes can be more of a problem after the muscle weakness comes under control. The important thing is to treat and prevent the skin rashes as much as possible.

What If My Child Has a Rash That Differs from the Ones Described?

There are many other rashes associated with JDM that we have not described here. We have mentioned only the most common ones. Children with polymyositis generally have no rashes or only rashes that do not result from sun exposure (as far as we know), and those rashes tend to be different from the ones described above.

Sometimes a child can have JDM and then develop symptoms of other autoimmune illnesses as well. This can occasionally happen with lupus, psoriasis, or scleroderma. As mentioned previously, lupus may result in a red rash on the cheeks, called a malar or butterfly rash. Psoriasis is a red rash that develops a thick shell-like covering. Scleroderma is an illness where the skin becomes hardened and has a waxy appearance. All of these conditions require different treatments. Anytime your child develops a new rash, she should see a rheumatologist, a doctor who specializes in connective tissue diseases. A dermatologist, who specializes in the care of the skin, can be particularly helpful if rashes are very troubling for your child.

What Causes the Skin Rashes in Dermatomyositis?

At this time we are not sure. It appears that some people inherit a predisposition, but there might also be other factors, such as a virus, a chemical, stressful situations, or simply sunlight.

Sunlight or light from artificial sources (such as tanning beds) seems to aggravate the rash that is associated with JDM. In some cases the rash develops after prolonged or intense exposure to the sun, such as after returning from a family vacation to the beach or spending time at the pool. Studies have shown that more people develop DM if they live in an area that gets more sunlight. There are also cases of people who seem to be in remission and will have a recurrence of the rash after re-exposure to the sun.

What Should I Do About My Child's Sun Exposure?

Avoiding sun exposure can help decrease the intensity or extent of JDM skin rashes. There are many ways to avoid sun exposure. These include:
- Avoid areas where your child will be exposed to the sun.
- Use sun block or sunscreen everyday.
- Use clothes and hats to cover your child's skin from exposure.

Dermatologists recommend that your child try to avoid sun exposure during the peak hours of 10 A.M. to 4 P.M., when the sun is hottest and brightest. As a minimum and to be practical, it is certainly most important to stay out of the sun from 11 A.M. to 1 P.M. This can be hard to do for children in school. Speak with your child's teacher or principal about avoiding outdoor physical education activities and staying inside for recess. Consider speaking to parent-teacher organizations or school administration about having covered areas for recess. Get a note from your child's doctor to remind teachers about protecting students from sun exposure (see *Chapter 36, School Issues*).

What About Sun Block or Sunscreen?

All sunscreens are not created equal. It is important to get a sunscreen with a high sun protection factor (SPF). The SPF is a measure of how much protection the sun block provides. The higher the number, the more protection it provides. We recommend using something with an SPF of at least 30.

It is also important to protect your child from a broad spectrum of the sun's rays. The ultraviolet (UV) light in sunlight is most harmful to children with JDM. Ultraviolet light at the earth's surface is composed of two types of rays, UVA and UVB. Not all sunscreens cover both types of UV rays. UVB rays are the ones that cause sunburn and are thought to be the most dangerous for children with DM. However, UVA rays can also aggravate skin rashes.

Sunscreens and sun blocks differ in the way that they provide protection. Sun blocks (such as those containing titanium dioxide and zinc oxide) physically block the sun's rays from reaching the skin. They reflect and scatter both types of UV light, UVA and UVB. Sunscreens are chemical agents that absorb the sun's rays and change them to a less dangerous wavelength. Most sunscreens cover the UVB spectrum, but only some cover UVA as well. As a general rule, sun blocks consistently provide the best coverage, but some people do not like to wear them because they may make the skin look pale or chalky. There are newer formulations that are not as dense, are not greasy, and are fragrance free. In addition, sun blocks are less likely to cause allergic reactions. Refer to The Myositis Association or The Skin Cancer Foundation for specific product recommendations, although any product that offers an SPF of 30 or greater and covers both UVA and UVB rays is good. You can always check with your child's myositis doctor or dermatologist to see if the one that you have selected is adequate. Another factor you may want to consider is a water-resistant variety or sports stick type for the active child. There are also spray-on sunscreens that make application easier.

Regardless of which brand you choose, it is important to apply it thickly and get good coverage of the skin exposed to the sun. Most people do not apply enough sun block to reach the intended protection factor. Apply it fifteen to thirty minutes before going outside, on a cloudy or sunny day, and then reapply it after every one to two hours of sun exposure. This frequent application is necessary because the sun can degrade sunscreen and sun block. It is also important to realize that wearing sun block does not provide sufficient protection for your child to spend a lot of time in the sun. It is only a shield for when she must be exposed to the sun.

Lastly, be sure your child always wears her sun block or sunscreen. Even on a cloudy day, the sun's rays can still filter through the clouds. If your child has naturally dark skin and never burned before having JDM, your child's skin is now more sensitive and still needs to be protected. Even in cases in which skin rashes have cleared and the myositis has gone into remission, some people have had recurrences of JDM after sun exposure. It never hurts to protect your child's skin. You should probably make everyone in your family use it as well!

What Else Can I Do to Protect My Child from the Sun?

Did you ever notice how the skin under your bathing suit doesn't tan? Clothing can be a good source of sun protection. Have your child wear a hat with a wide brim to protect her face. A baseball cap doesn't offer as much protection because your child's ears and the back of the neck can still burn. There are several manufacturers that make hats specifically for sun protection, which also have vents in the crowns to allow sweat to evaporate.

Just as sunscreens vary, so does the protection factor of clothing. A wet white cotton T-shirt, for example, offers very little protection. The tighter the weave and the darker the clothing, the more protection is offered. Clothing made to protect from the sun is rated with an ultraviolet protection factor (UPF). Here again, the higher the number, the better. A value of 25–39 is very good, and a value of 40–50 is excellent. Companies are increasingly marketing stylish clothing to provide protection from the sun, and many companies can be found on the Internet. (The Myositis Association maintains a list of some of these products.) Another option is a wash-in laundry additive called Rit SunGuard™. If you add this product to the wash for several washings, it can increase the UPF of clothing.

To block sun through your car windows, you can buy UV-protective automobile film. These products can also be found on the Internet.

What About Itchy Skin?

The rash associated with JDM can be aggravating, especially at night. Don't hesitate to ask your child's doctor for medicine to ease the itching. Topical treatments and moisturizing lotions can provide relief. Dryness that occurs with the rashes contributes to the itch. Moisturizers vary, and some are greasier than others. Emollients, oils, and creams are more effective than lotions. Oatmeal baths (e.g., Aveeno™) and calamine lotion can be soothing. There are medications, including antihistamines such as hydroxyzine, that help with the itch and are best taken at night as they can cause drowsiness; but if this isn't enough, doxepin is another medication that may be helpful. The best treatment is to control the underlying JDM, although skin rashes can be bad when the muscle inflammation is under control and vice versa.

Does the Rash Go Away?

Medicines used to treat the myositis can also be used to control the rash. The skin rash usually returns if treatment is stopped, but often the skin rash will disappear with adequate treatment of the JM. Children's rashes resolve completely more frequently than adults' rashes do. If the rash has been present for a long time, some skin changes may become permanent. In these cases, your child may get thinning of the skin, called atrophy, changes in skin pigmentation, and eventually poikiloderma, which means skin that is thinned with telangiectasias and dark and light spots, which are common in people with chronic DM. Poikiloderma can be difficult to treat.

How Can My Child Cope with the Skin Rashes?

The skin rashes of JM can be debilitating. It is common for the rash associated with DM to be very itchy. Itchy skin is not only aggravating, it can also interfere with your child's sleep and affect her mood. In addition, the rash can change your child's appearance and affect her self-esteem. It is important to follow treatment directed by your child's doctor to control the rashes. If your child is self-conscious about the rash, she can consider wearing camouflage make-up with sunscreen to conceal the rash and block the sun's harmful rays.

What Can I Expect from the Dermatologist?

JDM can have many different skin manifestations. Dermatologists specialize in the recognition and treatment of rashes and are highly qualified to treat your child's skin rashes. Try to find a dermatologist with a special interest in DM or connective tissue diseases.

The dermatologist might take a skin biopsy to aid in the diagnosis of JDM or even for certain specific rashes that your child has. A skin biopsy involves removing a small piece of skin and looking at it under the microscope. It is a quick and well-tolerated procedure. The dermatologist may mark the area of the biopsy with a pen, then numb the area with a small injection of numbing medicine. This should be the only part of the procedure that is uncomfortable. A small piece of skin will then be removed using a device that looks like a very small cookie cutter. Often a stitch or two is placed to close the site. The area should heal well within about a week or two. By looking at the skin under the microscope a pathologist can determine the diagnosis.

Treatment and Medication for Skin Rashes

Dermatologists can also help in the treatment of your child's skin rashes, by suggesting either topical medicines or medicines taken by mouth or by injection. The importance of sun protection and avoidance cannot be overemphasized. Be aware of medications that can increase your child's sensitivity to the sun, such as methotrexate, piroxicam (a nonsteroidal anti-inflammatory drug), sulfonamides, and tetracyclines. Whenever a new medication is prescribed, let the doctors know that your child is sensitive to the sun, and be sure that your child keeps up with sun protective measures.

Skin can become extremely dry. Sometimes that is a sign that your whole body is dehydrated, so it is important for your child to drink lots of water. Proper skin care includes using a mild soap only when and where needed. Soaps used should be those for sensitive skin and should be fragrance and dye free. Always apply a moisturizer after bathing. Emollients are very beneficial for the rash of DM. Reapply them frequently.

Consider using a humidifier in your home if your child has severely dry skin. Some people find that fabric softeners aggravate their skin. Softer bed sheets may be helpful. Other topical treatment of the rash can include corticosteroid creams and new nonsteroidal creams called tacrolimus (Protopic) or pimecrolimus (Elidel). Medicines by mouth or vein may also be administered, including prednisone, methylprednisolone, hydroxychloroquine, methotrexate, intravenous immune globulin (IVIG), cyclosporine, azathioprine, mycophenolate, and cyclophosphamide. Use of these systemic medicines for the treatment of myositis can also help the skin rashes. These systemic medicines have been discussed in previous chapters (see *Chapter 7, Treatment Possibilities in the Beginning* and *Chapter 12, Possible Medicines During the Course*). Here we will concentrate on topical treatments.

Topical medications can be very beneficial alone or with medicines taken by mouth or injected into the vein. Topical corticosteroids come in many different strengths and formulations. They can be used to treat the rashes on any part of your child's body. For example, oil-based preparations, such as fluocinolone acetonide, are convenient for treating the scalp. The mildest forms of topical steroids are available over the counter, but the skin rashes of JDM often require a higher concentration that requires a doctor's prescription. Stronger corticosteroids might control skin rashes, but they can also have side effects, such as thinning of the skin, stretch marks, and the formation of telangiectasias (prominent, dilated blood vessels). Their use should be monitored closely to prevent side effects. Make sure to follow your child's doctor's directions closely, and only use the medication as long as directed. Some very strong preparations are applied to areas of redness or active rash for only a few days to weeks, but milder preparations can be used for longer periods of time (weeks to several months).

Tacrolimus (Protopic) and pimecrolimus (Elidel) belong to a new class of topical therapies that don't have the same side effects as corticosteroids. These agents are currently being examined as another treatment possibility for DM. There are reports of both improvement and lack of effect of these agents. Tacrolimus can sting a little when first applied to the skin, but this discomfort usually lasts only a few days. These topical medications should not be applied to weeping or open areas. They are generally applied to areas of redness and used for several weeks to several months.

Sometimes the medicines taken by mouth or injection to treat JDM can lead to other skin problems. Oral corticosteroids can lead to stretch marks and an increased risk of bacterial and fungal infections. Anytime you see a change in your skin, point it out to your child's doctor or dermatologist. Skin infections can usually be treated with creams or ointments that combat infection.

Key Points

- JDM is a form of myositis that involves the skin. Other types of myositis, including polymyositis and overlap myositis, might also cause skin rashes. There are many different possible skin manifestations, and it is important to point out any new rashes to your child's doctor.

- The sun can aggravate your child's skin rashes, so remember to use sun protection and sun avoidance measures at all times. The importance of sun block and sun avoidance cannot be overemphasized.

- Medicines taken by mouth or injection to treat the JM might also treat the skin rashes. Sometimes, topical treatments, including corticosteroid cream and tacrolimus, are helpful for the rashes if they are more involved or are not getting entirely better with the other medicines.

- For patients with difficult-to-treat skin rashes, seeing a dermatologist experienced in myositis or in connective tissue diseases can be helpful in guiding the proper diagnosis and treatment of the skin rashes.

To Learn More

To find a physician, see *Finding a Juvenile Myositis Doctor* in the *Finding a Doctor or Specialist* section of the *Resource Appendix*, specifically:

American Academy of Dermatology (AAD)

Public Resource Center. Available from www.aad.org

Additional Information:

The Myositis Association.

Sun protective products. Available from: www.myositis.org/jmbookresources.cfm or 800-821-7356.

Department of Dermatology, University of Iowa College of Medicine.

SafeSunSavvy Tips for Adults & Kids. Available at: http://tray.dermatology.uiowa.edu/SafeSun/SafeSun-Index.html.

The Skin Cancer Foundation. 245 Fifth Avenue, Suite 1403, New York NY 10016; Phone: 800-SKIN-490; Internet: www.skincancer.org; Email: info@skincancer.org.

Sun Safety Tips: Protect Yourself and Your Family All Year Round. Available at: www.skincancer.org/prevention/index.php or 800-SKIN-490.

Sun Safety for Kids, a program of The Los Angeles Metropolitan Dermatological Society, Inc. 2625 W. Alameda Avenue, Suite 517, Burbank CA 91505; Phone: 818-845-8538; Internet: www.sunsafetyforkids.org; Email: info@sunsafetyforkids.org.

Sun Protective Clothing and Sunglasses. Available at: www.sunsafetyforkids.org/clothes+glass.htm.

Sunscreen. Available at: www.sunsafetyforkids.org/sunscreen.htm.

Internet:

Sontheimer RD. Skin Disease in Dermatomyositis: What Patients and Their Families Often Want to Know. *Dermatology Online Journal.* 2001;8(1):6. Available at: http://dermatology.cdlib.org/DOJvol8num1/information/dermatomyositis/sontheimer.html.

Reports in the Medical Literature

Callen JP. Dermatomyositis. *Lancet.* 2000 Jan 1;355(9197):53–7.

Jorizzo JL. Dermatomyositis: practical aspects. *Archives of Dermatology.* 2002 Jan;138(1):114–6.

Sontheimer RD. The management of dermatomyositis: current treatment options. *Expert Opinion on Pharmacotherapy.* 2004 May;5(5):1083–99.

Vitale A, Trail L, Felici E, Traverso F, Martini A, Ravelli A. Review for the generalist: cutaneous manifestations of juvenile systemic lupus erythematosus and juvenile dermatomyositis. *Pediatric Rheumatology Online Journal.* 2004;2(6):514-23. [Available online at http://www.pedrheumonlinejournal.org/nov-dec/review_generalist.htm.]

Werth VP, Bashir M, Zhang W. Photosensitivity in rheumatic diseases. *The Journal of Investigative Dermatology. Symposium Proceedings.* 2004 Jan;9(1):57–63.

Yoshimasu T, Ohtani T, Sakamoto T, Oshima A, Furukawa F. Topical FK506 (tacrolimus) therapy for facial erythematous lesions of cutaneous lupus erythematosus and dermatomyositis. *European Journal of Dermatology.* 2002 Jan-Feb;12(1):50–2.

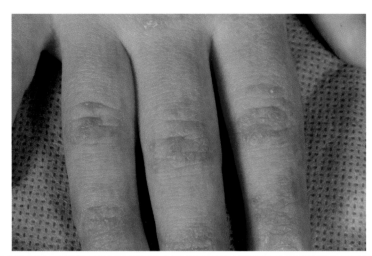

Color plate 1
■ Figure 1.1.
Gottron's papules.

Gottron's papules are red and raised or rough scaly patches present over the knuckles. They may also be seen over the elbows, knees, insides of the ankles, or even over the toe joints.

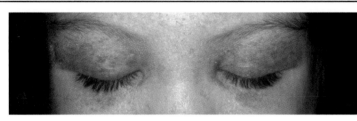

Color plate 2
■ Figure 1.2.
Heliotrope rash.

The heliotrope rash is a purple or red coloring over the eyelids that can also cause eyelid swelling. It is named after a lilac-colored flower.

Color plate 3
■ Figure 3.1. A possible sequence of events in the immune system of children with juvenile dermatomyositis.

A substance that is foreign to the body's "antigen" is processed into small pieces by one of the antigen presenting cells (i.e., dendritic cells, macrophages) so that the antigen reactive cells (T cells, NK cells) are "turned on." Sometimes B cells are turned on as well to make antibody. Many of our current medications block the activated immune cells so that target tissue damage is reduced.

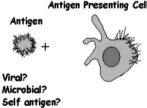

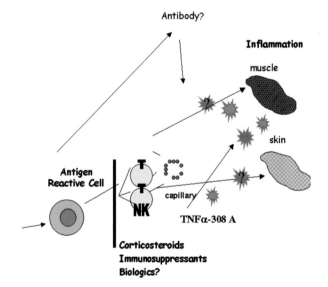

Color plate 4
■ Figure 6.1a.
T-2 weighted MRI scan of the thighs.

This is a T-2 weighted scan with fat suppression. Note that the black arrows indicate symmetrical white areas of affected muscle; the dark muscles are less affected. There is increased fascia (membrane) surrounding the muscle (white arrow).

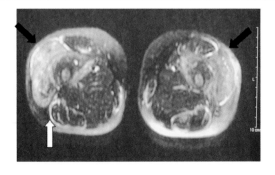

Color plate 5
■ **Figure 6.2. Normal muscle biopsy features (panels A, C, E) compared to common abnormalities seen in JDM (panels B, D, F).**

In all panels, muscle fibers (m) are displayed in cross section; a, small arteries; v, small veins. Muscle fiber diameter is normally uniform (panel A) but is very nonuniform in JDM (panel B) because of shrinkage of injured muscle fibers (arrowheads). Collections of small, round, dark inflammatory cells (arrow, panel B) are abnormal lymphocytes, which cause muscle damage in JDM. The tiny, dark-staining dots between muscle fibers (panels C and D, arrows) are capillaries, the smallest blood vessels. Capillaries are reduced in number (panel D, arrowheads) in the zone of muscle fiber shrinkage as a result of the vascular injury that commonly accompanies muscle fiber injury in JDM. Arteries also may be injured and obstructed in JDM (panel F) causing more serious reduction in blood flow.

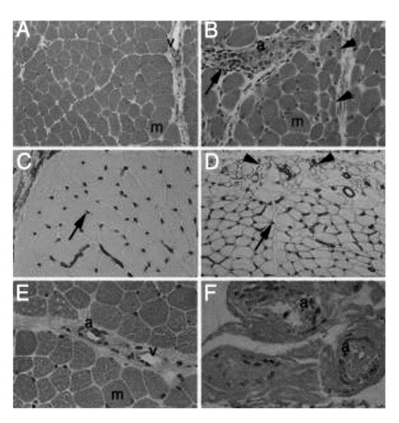

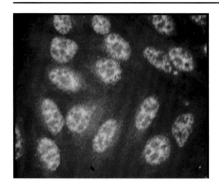

Color plate 6
■ **Figure 6.3.**
Typical ANA in children with JDM.
Typical antinuclear antibody (ANA) pattern in an untreated child with JDM, showing coarse speckled pattern of staining in the nucleus of the indicator cells.

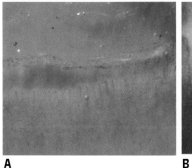
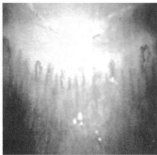

A   B

Color plate 7
■ **Figure 6.4.**
Nailfold capillary studies.
Studies of the nailfold capillaries from a normal child show an even spacing of hairpin turn capillaries that go down to the edge of the nail (A). In contrast, a child with active juvenile dermatomyositis not only has a smaller number of nailfold capillaries (dropout), but those that are there are abnormal in shape—dilated and bushy in formation (B).

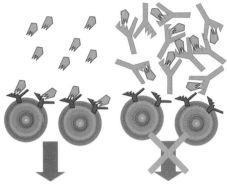

Inflammation   Inflammation

Inflammatory Protein
Antibody that Binds the Inflammatory Protein
Inflammatory Cell

Color plate 8
■ Figure 15.1. Monoclonal antibody.
Example of how a monoclonal antibody can bind to a specific target and block its function to decrease inflammation and thereby result in less myositis.

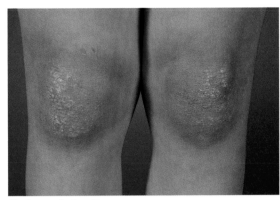

Color plate 9
■ Figure 16.1.
Gottron's papules.
Gottron's papules are red and raised or rough scaly patches present over the extensor surfaces of the joints. Here they are present over the knees, but they may also be seen over the finger joints, elbows, insides of the ankles, or even over the toe joints.

Color plate 10
■ Figure 16.2.
Malar rash.
Erythema over the cheeks and nasal bridge.

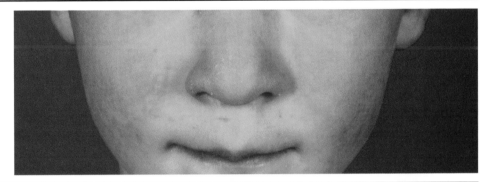

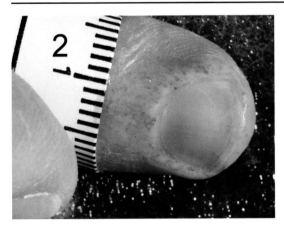

Color plate 11
■ Figure 16.3.
Periungual telangiectasia.
Periungual telangiectasia with dilated, tortuous capillaries along the fingernail fold, an area of bushy capillary loop formation and areas of capillary loss.

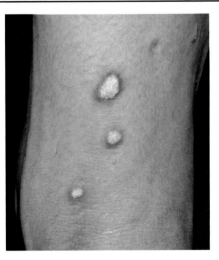

Color plate 12
■ Figure 17.1. Subcutaneous calcifications on the back of the leg.
These calcifications appear as small nodules with a white surface. Above these is a scar from a previous lesion that has extruded through the skin and resolved.

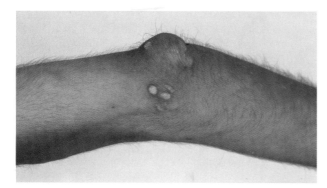

Color plate 13
■ **Figure 17.2.**
Nodular or tumoral deposit of calcinosis.
The calcinosis is over the elbow in a child with JDM, resulting in an elbow flexion contracture.

Color plate 14
■ **Figure 21.1.**
A child with juvenile dermatomyositis who has arthritis in the finger joints of the hands.
Notice the swelling of the finger joints.

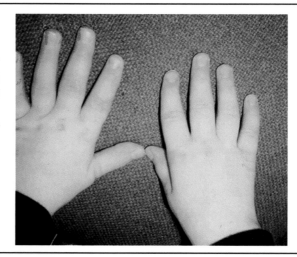

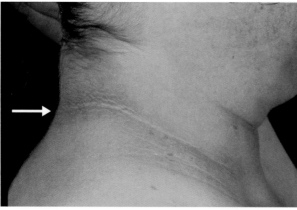

Color plate 15
■ **Figure 25.2.**
Acanthosis nigricans.
Note the pigmentation and the thickening of the skin at the back of the neck. In young individuals, acanthosis nigricans mostly reflects the existence of elevated blood levels of insulin and of insulin resistance. *Photo courtesy of Dr. H. Tildesley, Vancouver Canada.*

Color plate 16
■ **Figure 27.1.**
Posterior subcapsular cataract in a twelve-year-old girl with JM treated with prednisone, as seen through a dilated pupil with a slit lamp biomicroscope.
Note the central location of the cataract (cloudy spot in the center of the lens) with characteristic "bubbles." The background is reddish because of the reflection of light from the retina behind.

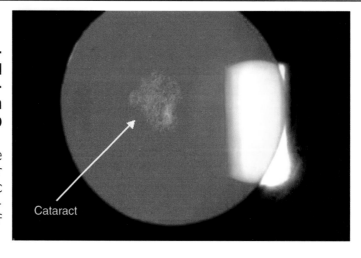

Cataract

CHAPTER 17

Calcinosis

Lauren M. Pachman, MD, and Lisa G. Rider, MD

In this chapter...

In this chapter we describe our current knowledge about one of the most trouble-some consequences of juvenile dermatomyositis (JDM)—calcifications.

From the family's point of view...

"The doctors noted mild calcinosis on her knuckles and elbow when she was first diagnosed. It had appeared early, as hard bumps, before her diagnosis. Sometimes the bumps would break open, releasing a white liquid. They caused discomfort and would often become red and inflamed. After two years of treatment with prednisone and methotrexate, they have not spread."

What Are Calcifications?

Calcifications in places that do not usually calcify are known as pathological calcifications and also as calcinosis. They are calcium-containing deposits associated with inflamed or damaged tissues. They are located under the skin in the fatty tissue or in the muscle. The calcium deposits can range greatly in size and frequency. They can be as small as the diameter of the eraser on a pencil or as large as a grapefruit. They can also be flat like coins, plates, or sheets. Unfortunately, we do not know what causes these calcium deposits or how best to treat them.

Who Gets Them?

Calcifications occur most frequently in patients with juvenile dermatomyositis (JDM) and overlap myositis, but they rarely occur in patients with juvenile poly-myositis. They can also occur in other systemic rheumatic diseases, such as systemic sclerosis.

Some children develop many deposits, some only a few, and some none at all. The number of children with JDM who have calcinosis is not exactly known. It is estimated that perhaps 30% of patients with JDM develop calcium deposits over the course of their illness, although this varies from 10% to 50%. In one study, approximately 25% of children had calcifications at diagnosis, although calcifications can develop as many as twenty years after diagnosis. We think if the inflammation that goes with the myositis is not treated adequately, these areas of calcinosis are likely to get bigger over time and even to occur in other areas.

What Do They Look Like?

Calcifications are often described as hard, sometimes mobile lumps under the skin or deeper in the muscle, or they may appear sheet-like and run along the muscles or planes of connective tissue outside of the muscle. Calcium deposits are usually painless, but sometimes they can be painful if inflamed, infected, or when they trap or pinch a nerve.

There are several subtypes of calcinosis, and they can occur alone or in combination.

- Approximately one-third of JDM patients with calcinosis have superficial plaques or nodules (calcinosis circumscripta). These are small nodules or bumps located in the skin or in the fatty tissue under the skin (subcutaneous tissues). (See Figure 17.1.)

  ■ **Figure 17.1. (See color plate 12 on page 229.) Subcutaneous calcifications on the back of the leg.**
  These calcifications appear as small nodules with a white surface. Above these is a scar from a previous lesion that has extruded through the skin and resolved.

- Larger nodular deposits that extend to deeper tissue layers, including muscle, occur in about 20% of patients (sometimes called tumoral calcinosis). (See Figure 17.2.)

  ■ **Figure 17.2. (See color plate 13 on page 230.) Nodular or tumoral deposit of calcinosis.**
  The calcinosis is over the elbow in a child with JDM, resulting in an elbow flexion contracture.

- Collections of calcium along the surfaces of muscles and tendons in a sheet-like pattern can be seen in about 15% of JDM patients who have calcinosis. These are called planar or fascial deposits.

- Widespread or generalized calcification, also known as exoskeleton, is fortunately an uncommon type, seen in no more than 10% of JDM patients with calcinosis.

A combination of these four subtypes occurs in up to one-fourth of JDM patients with calcinosis. It is not uncommon for the calcifications to change in shape, especially as they respond to therapy. For example, larger nodular deposits that are in deeper tissue layers can become plate-like and move to the areas closer to the surface, where they sometimes drain or become less detectable.

Where Should I Look for These Lumps?

Calcifications often develop at pressure points, such as an elbow, knee, edge of the foot, or even in the buttocks. However, these calcifications can also be located in protected soft tissues such as the stomach wall or the chest. They can occur virtually anywhere on the body. For some children, when the lumps first develop, the area is painful or tender to touch.

How Do I Know If My Child Has Calcinosis?
How Do Doctors Detect These Calcifications?

You might feel the hard calcium nodules like a pebble under your child's skin or in the deeper tissue layers. Larger calcifications can be seen in routine X-rays, but if they are small, they are sometimes hard to spot. We still do not have a good way to measure the change in area of calcifications over time. A procedure called computed tomography (CT) (sometimes called a CAT scan) is a very sensitive test to detect calcinosis, but it can also miss the smaller calcium nodules. Magnetic resonance imaging (MRI) is not a very good or sensitive test to detect calcinosis. When evident, calcinosis lesions show up as black spots on the MRI scan. The MRI is better at showing bright areas of inflammation, especially under the skin in the fatty tissue, before the calcium gets deposited. MRI or ultrasound can sometimes show the fluid that is trapped in the calcifications or bound by a membrane. This fluid can become infected. Drainage alone does not help because the fluid often re-accumulates. The pools of liquid often diminish slowly with adequate immuno-suppressive therapy.

Why Does My Child Have Calcinosis?

We do not understand why certain children with juvenile myositis develop calcinosis whereas others do not. We have found, however, that children whose treatment is delayed or whose inflammation is inadequately controlled are more likely to develop calcinosis. When the myositis disease process is inadequately controlled, there is continued inflammation and perhaps also one of the following circumstances:

- Inadequate treatment at the time of diagnosis
- Laboratory evidence of myositis disease activity despite improvement in clinical signs
- Clinical signs of myositis disease activity (e.g., active rash, ongoing muscle weakness) despite normal blood tests of the muscle enzymes
- Disease flare or recurrence of the inflammation

Many doctors have different opinions about what constitutes adequate treatment. Recent studies are beginning to give some important clues. Calcifications are more likely to develop in children who are given a lower dose of prednisone by mouth (< 2 mg/kg/day) that is delayed more than four months after the first symptom of JDM compared with children who receive a higher dose earlier in the disease course. Patients with long-term illness or illness that flares and then goes into remission over and over (see *Chapter 30, The Clinical Course and Outcome of Juvenile Myositis*), as well as those whose disease has been active for a long time, are more likely to develop calcinosis. Children seem to have fewer calcifications when they receive repetitive pulses of intravenous high-dose intermittent methylprednisolone at 30 mg/kg (one gram maximum) to normalize both clinical and laboratory disease activity. Early treatment with methotrexate (i.e., within six weeks of diagnosis) also may result in a low frequency of calcinosis.

The genetic makeup of the child also affects chronic inflammation, which could result in calcinosis. One factor that has been associated with calcinosis is a variation (called a polymorphism) in one of the genes for tumor necrosis factor alpha (TNF-α), a cytokine (hormone) of the immune system that promotes inflammation. Under normal circumstances, inflammation is promoted when you have a wound and the body wants to heal it. Extra white blood cells are sent to the wounded area to help clean it up. In myositis the muscle is wounded, and the body activates the pro-inflammatory cytokines. Some patients with calcinosis are more likely to have a form of this TNF-α gene, which is more likely to produce excess TNF-α. Children with JDM who develop lipodystrophy, or loss of body fat (see *Chapter 26, Too Much Body Fat Loss*), are also prone to develop calcifications.

Factors that do not seem to affect the development of calcinosis are age at diagnosis, race, gender, disease severity at onset, presence of ulcerations, or the medical center at which the patient was treated (Table 17.1). Calcium and vitamin D that are given as supplements do not seem to have an effect on calcinosis. They are taken up by the bones, helping to strengthen them, and do not deposit at the site of calcinosis. However, specific blood tests to check the levels of calcium and vitamin D should be made first, before these supplements are given (see *Chapter 22, Taking Care of the Bones*).

In summary, longstanding active illness in which appropriate initial therapy is delayed or the course of treatment is inadequate appears to be the factor that is most frequently associated with the development of calcinosis.

Table 17.1. Factors in the development of calcinosis in children with myositis.

Factor	Contributes to development of calcinosis	Does not appear to contribute to development of calcinosis
Length of untreated illness	X	
Continued disease activity	X	
Genetic factors related to inflammation	X	
Race	X	
Gender		X
Disease severity at diagnosis		X
State of residence		X
Presence of ulcerations		X
Medical center where child was treated		X
Calcium and vitamin D supplements		X

What Are the Calcifications Made Of?

Although these lumps contain calcium similar to that found in bone, they do not appear to have the same ordered structure as bone. They contain the mineral that is found in bone, called calcium hydroxyapatite, as well as several other components similar to bone and some that are different. Some of the connective tissue proteins that are found inside of bone tissue also seem to be present in the calcinosis lesions. The liquid that sometimes drains from the calcifications contains TNF-α and other pro-inflammatory cytokines or hormones of the immune system. We still need to do more research to understand exactly what is in the areas that calcify and to learn whether they change their composition over time. For example, the structure and content can vary depending on the site of the lesions, the form they take (whether they're nodules or sheets), and whether they are pushed out of the body (draining areas).

What Happens to the Calcinosis Over Time?

We have not been able to answer this question, partly because we do not have a reproducible, safe method to measure the shape of the calcium deposits over time. We do know that calcium deposits can change shape and form over time, and the changes will be different in different people. Calcium deposits may decrease or even go away, stay the same, or increase in number and enlarge over time. In many cases we cannot predict which of these conditions will occur. We cannot predict whether or when the lesions will go away, although we think this is more likely to happen in patients whose illness is under full control with adequate treatment. The lesions go away when the collections of calcium and other proteins are absorbed back into the body (called resorption) or when they work their way through the skin and drain out.

White sticky fluid sometimes drains from an area of calcification, which is called "milk of calcium." Areas that are draining can become infected, requiring antibiotic therapy. It is easy to confuse this infection of the calcification with an inflammatory reaction that frequently occurs during active deposition of the lesion, which can result in redness, warmth, tenderness, and drainage over the site and even be associated with fever. This inflammation, which is not related to infection, might require treatment with anti-inflammatory medications, such as colchicine.

Calcinosis is more likely to improve in patients with inactive myositis, those who engage in a lot of physical activity, those with superficial plaques rather than deeper or more extensive deposits, and those given aggressive treatments for JDM. In our experience, worsening of calcinosis is more likely when there is ongoing, inadequately treated muscle or skin disease activity.

Because the lesions often cross joints, some patients have difficulty fully extending or straightening joints (called joint contractures). Tumoral calcinosis lesions can also develop ulcerations or breaks in the overlying skin. When there is nerve entrapment or when a pressure point is involved, pain may be a major problem, and surgery might be required to relieve the pain. Physical discomfort of the calcifications at pressure points—where they are more likely to be hit—can also result in local pain.

How Is Calcinosis Treated?

Once calcifications have formed, their treatment is quite controversial, although most doctors agree that good initial control of the active inflammatory process is very important. Most of the treatment data are based on anecdotal reports rather than controlled clinical trials. None of the treatments is proven to work. In other words, they have not been shown to decrease the stage of the inflammatory illness nor have they been shown to decrease the size of the lesions before and after therapy.

When the calcium deposits first occur or when they increase in size, it is our experience that the myositis process is usually active and that additional anti-inflammatory approaches might be necessary. We monitor the extent of the child's immune activation and myositis activity by using tests of the immune system, such as flow cytometry of circulating lymphocyte subsets, Factor VIII-related antigen (or von Willebrand factor VIII-related antigen), and neopterin. It is often necessary to monitor these things because the routine laboratory data, including blood levels of muscle enzymes, often normalize rapidly once therapy is initiated, and routine laboratory data don't always give us an adequate picture of what is going on in the body (see *Chapter 10, Charting Your Child's Progress*). Thus, anti-inflammatory approaches can help prevent further deposits from forming, but they cannot necessarily resolve existing lesions.

Medicines for Myositis Potentially Help Calcinosis

A decrease in the size and extent of calcifications, as well as slowing in the deposition of new lesions has been reported in a few cases after treatment with certain medicines. Overall, the effectiveness of a particular drug appears to depend on its success in controlling the underlying myositis process, and many agents are potentially partially beneficial. Some of the medicines used to treat myositis that have been reported to be helpful for stabilizing or reducing the size of calcinosis lesions include hydroxychloroquine, intravenous immune globulin, cyclosporine, and most recently infliximab. Treatment is often prolonged, and can be as long as one year. Triamcinolone acetate, a steroid that is injected into the lesions, when administered monthly for up to one year, has resulted in decreased size of calcifications in several patients. Colchicine has been effective for both localized redness and warmth and for associated fevers, but it has no reported effect on the size of the lesions. There are no published data on the effectiveness of other agents. It is important to keep in mind this information on the possible benefits of such medicines is very limited, anecdotal, and not adequately scientifically tested.

Approaches to Try to Keep Calcium from Depositing in Tissues

Other therapeutic approaches for calcinosis are aimed at disrupting the mineral balance of calcium with other body salts to try to keep the calcium from depositing into the tissues. Reports using these approaches are anecdotal, and it is not clear whether any of them effectively reduce the size or extent of calcinosis lesions or prevent new calcifications from developing. The most studied of these drugs is diltiazem, which blocks calcium from entering cells. A handful of patients with JDM treated with diltiazem experienced a reduction in the size of the calcinosis lesions after receiving a high dose over a relatively long period of time of one to twelve years. Some patients have also experienced total resolution of their calcinosis without the formation of new calcifications. Potential side effects of diltiazem therapy include anecdotal reports of worsening of the myositis, low blood pressure, dizziness, headache, and nausea/vomiting.

Another approach, which is usually not successful, is to try to decrease the phosphorous level; phosphorous is the mineral that binds to calcium and helps it deposit in tissues. Drugs that decrease the level of phosphorous include aluminum hydroxide, an antacid therapy, and probenecid, which affects how the kidney excretes many substances.

Bisphosphonates (alendronate, pamidronate), which are medicines also used to treat osteoporosis (see *Chapter 22, Taking Care of the Bones*), offer another potentially promising approach. However, it is too early to know whether these drugs actually improve or prevent calcinosis. These drugs are being used as therapy for disorders associated with high blood levels of calcium, low bone density, and some other types of calcification processes. Several additional agents, including warfarin and magnesium sulfate, have been tried as treatments for calcinosis, but they have not been effective.

Physical Therapy

For some children with JDM, physical therapy approaches are helpful, including cushioning and extending the range of motion with the use of heat and gentle repeated casting to stretch out the joint that is contracted. Children are advised to avoid traumas and minor tissue injuries when the calcifications are actively depositing, because tissue injury can increase the size of existing calcinosis lesions or cause new ones to form.

Surgery

For some children with tumorous deposits, surgical removal is recommended, especially for those who have any of the following:

- Chronic or severe pain
- Loss of function
- Recurrent infections or drainage
- Ulcers that don't heal

Potential complications of surgery include problems with wound healing and recurrence of the calcinosis. Prevention of recurrence of the calcinosis after surgery requires good control of inflammation and all of the aspects of myositis disease activity before undertaking the surgery. Some physicians have found that when the child is on methotrexate during the surgery, the calcifications are less likely to recur in the operative site. Try to find an experienced surgeon who minimizes the surgical irritation and trauma. Good wound healing is helped by the use of low doses of corticosteroids, but the myositis must be well controlled. Seeking the guidance of your child's doctor in selecting an experienced surgeon and the right timing for surgery are critical for keeping the calcinosis from returning to the same site.

In summary, dystrophic calcification is a complication of JDM associated with prolonged or inadequately treated disease activity. We suspect that calcinosis can be prevented through rapid diagnosis and rapid initiation of aggressive immunosuppressive therapy for the myositis. Depositing calcinosis is also frequently associated not only with active JDM, but also with inflammation around the calcifications, too. Early intervention with immunosuppressive agents may be helpful in preventing additional calcinosis from depositing in tissues. More research in this area is needed, because a better understanding of the calcinosis process will likely help to improve its treatment and prevent it.

Key Points

■ Calcifications are deposits of calcium in or under the skin or in muscles. Most often they develop in children with JDM who started treatment of myositis late or in whom myositis has remained active despite early treatment.

■ Calcinosis or calcifications occur in up to one-third of children with JDM. They are also found in patients who have myositis associated with overlap syndromes, in which children have features of other connective tissue diseases, such as scleroderma. They are almost never seen in children with polymyositis alone.

■ Calcifications can vary from small, round, superficial lesions under the skin to deeper, larger deposits to sheet-like deposits and occur particularly over pressure points, but they can also occur in other places. The number of lesions and their size varies with each patient.

■ Calcifications can increase in size and number over time if the illness is not treated adequately.

■ Once myositis becomes inactive, calcinosis lesions may go away or shrink in size over an unpredictable period of time.

■ There are no proven treatments for calcinosis. Treating the underlying myositis to prevent new calcifications from forming is the best available treatment today for calcinosis.

Reports in the Medical Literature

Blane CE, White SJ, Braunstein EM, Bowyer SL, Sullivan DB. Patterns of calcification in childhood dermatomyositis. *AJR American Journal of Roentgenology*. 1984 Feb;142(2):397–400.

Bowyer SL, Blane CE, Sullivan DB, Cassidy JT. Childhood dermatomyositis: factors predicting functional outcome and development of dystrophic calcification. *Journal of Pediatrics*. 1983 Dec;103(6):882–8.

Fisler RE, Liang MG, Fuhlbrigge RC, Yalcindag A, Sundel RP. Aggressive management of juvenile dermatomyositis results in improved outcome and decreased incidence of calcinosis. *Journal of the American Academy of Dermatology*. 2002 Oct;47(4):505–11.

Mendelson BC, Linscheid RL, Dobyns JH, Muller SA. Surgical treatment of calcinosis cutis in the upper extremity. *Journal of Hand Surgery* [Am]. 1977 Jul;2(4):318–24.

Pachman LM, Liotta-Davis MR, Hong DK, Kinsella TR, Mendez EP, Kinder JM, Chen EH. TNFalpha-308A allele in juvenile dermatomyositis: association with increased production of tumor necrosis factor alpha, disease duration, and pathologic calcifications. *Arthritis and Rheumatism*. 2000 Oct;43(10):2368–77.

Rider, LG. Calcinosis in juvenile dermatomyositis: pathogenesis and current therapies. *Pediatric Rheumatology Online Journal.* 2003 Mar-Apr;1(2):119–33. Available at: www.pedrheumonlinejournal.org/April/calinosis.html.

Stock SR, Ignatiev K, Lee PL, Abbott K, Pachman LM. Pathological calcification in juvenile dermatomyositis (JDM): microCT and synchrotron X-ray diffraction reveal hydroxyapatite with varied microstructures. *Connective Tissue Research.* 2004;45(4–5):248–56.

CHAPTER 18

Swallowing and Other Digestive Problems

Barbara C. Sonies, PhD, CCC-SLP;
Margaret A. Marcon, MD, FRCPC; and Lisa F. Imundo, MD

In this chapter...

We describe how normal swallowing and digestion works, what can go wrong in children with myositis, and how these problems can be treated.

From the family's point of view...

"We were told that children with juvenile myositis could have swallowing problems, and our daughter did have problems at night. Luckily for us, making some simple adjustments helped—not letting her eat or drink for two hours before going to bed and having her maintain a more upright position when eating. At one time she also complained of chest pains, which frightened all of us, but we soon learned these pains were caused by reflux. Zantac helped with the discomfort, and although the reflux worsened during one flare, thankfully no other digestive problems recurred."

It is important for all children with myositis to receive good nutrition for proper growth and development and to help their bodies fight their illness (see *Chapter 19, Nutrition and Your Child's Weight*). However, many children and young adults with juvenile myositis (JM) have trouble eating and swallowing or trouble with stomach discomfort or pain. It is important for those with JM to be aware of the symptoms and causes of swallowing problems and other digestive symptoms.

What Are the Parts of the Digestive Tract, and How Do They Work?

The digestive (gastrointestinal or GI) tract is a long hollow tube that begins at your mouth and ends at your anus (the exit). Food enters at the top (mouth) and is passed from one section to another. After food is placed in the mouth and swallowed, it enters the esophagus, the tube that moves the food from the throat to the stomach. The stomach helps digestion of the food by churning it and producing chemicals that begin to break it down. The food is then pushed into the small intestine. The small intestine is where the nutrients, including sugar, protein, and fats, as well as minerals and vitamins, and many medicines, including corticosteroids, are absorbed. Lastly, the leftover material is passed to the large intestine or colon and then passed out of the body. You might think that gravity has a lot to do with the food going through the GI tract, but the GI tract actually needs to work to push the food through. This requires the nerves and muscles to work well together.

What Problems Can Develop in the Digestive Tract in JM?

The muscles in the digestive or GI tract can be affected by myositis. When the muscles become inflamed, they are not strong enough to move food through the digestive tract. If this happens, the problems that develop will depend on the specific areas involved. The two most common complaints involving the digestive tract are difficulty swallowing (dysphagia) and stomach (abdominal) pain. A large proportion of children with JM have digestive complaints during the course of the illness. Most of the difficulty with swallowing results from involvement of the muscles in the mouth and throat (oropharynx).

What Swallowing Problems Do Children with Myositis Have?

Swallowing includes several different phases involving the mouth and tongue as well as different sections of the esophagus; it is actually a complex task. When we swallow food, it is important that the food does not enter the airway. To protect the airway (trachea and lungs) from the entry of food, the epiglottis, a flap-like bit of cartilage that sits above the vocal cords, is lowered automatically. So when we swallow, the epiglottis covers this opening and creates a channel for food and liquid to pass into the esophagus, without getting into the trachea. If food "goes down the wrong way," we react by coughing to expel it from the entry into the lungs. *Aspiration* occurs if food does enter the airway, which makes it difficult to breathe. The particles of food can also cause irritation, infection, and pneumonia, an infection of the lungs that can be serious. Some parts of swallowing are under conscious control, so that we can spit out any food we don't like or that tastes bad. However, once food gets into the lower part of the throat and the esophagus, it is under reflex control and cannot be stopped voluntarily.

Dysphagia is the term used to describe swallowing difficulty that can occur in the early, middle, or late phases of swallowing. These swallowing problems make eating unpleasant or difficult. Many of these problems change in severity as the illness progresses or when a medication is altered. *Painful chewing*, although uncommon, can result from weak face or jaw muscles.

When the muscles of the soft palate are weak and do not elevate or retract sufficiently to close off the nasal passages, liquids can enter the nose causing *nasal reflux.* When this happens, not only is it uncomfortable, but also the food remains undigested. Nasal reflux or regurgitation affects up to 30% of children with JM. Frequent choking and coughing during swallowing are clear signs that food or liquid has entered the airway and is being expelled. A cough is a protective reflex that is caused by the sensation created when food or liquids enter the top of the airway. If your child coughs and chokes frequently, notify your healthcare team immediately to evaluate the possibility of the more serious problem of aspiration.

Some people have *silent aspiration*, which is when food or liquid enters the airway without causing a protective cough response. The frequency of aspiration pneumonia or infection is higher with silent aspiration because this usually means that there is a neurological or sensory impairment. A common sign of aspiration or silent aspiration is a *gurgly or wet sounding* voice after swallowing. The changes in voice are caused by food or liquid that remains in the airway just above the muscles that produce voice (the vocal folds).

Heartburn, indigestion, or acid reflux is another common problem that occurs when the stomach contents, which might include partially digested food and stomach acids, back up into the esophagus or into the throat and cause a burning sensation.

Because myositis causes inflammation of many different muscles, it can affect not only the muscles that move the arms and legs, but also the muscles of the tongue, face, throat, voice box (larynx), and all of the muscles that operate the esophagus. When these muscles become inflamed and swollen, they cause weakness, tenderness, and slowed movement. Dysphagia can occur early in the course of JM and may be associated with changes in the voice, such as hoarseness or pitch changes (see *Chapter 23, Tune to Your Voice*). Many of the muscles that produce the voice are the same ones that close off the airway; thus, swallowing and voice changes are often related. Moderate to severe dysphagia most often occurs in the acute phases of JM and places the child at higher risk for aspiration and irritation or inflammation in the lungs, resulting in pneumonitis or pneumonia. These problems can be serious if they are not treated and can create a medical emergency. For some children a change in voice or a more nasal stuffed up quality to the voice may be the initial symptom of weakness and may also be the initial symptom of a flare of JM.

Specific swallowing problems associated with the muscle weakness of myositis can affect all of the phases of a swallow. In the oral phase (when the food is in the mouth being chewed), the weakness of the tongue and facial muscles can cause food to spill from the lips or remain in the mouth passing slowly into the throat without swallowing. This can put the child at risk for food to enter the airway and be aspirated. When the tongue is weak and swallowing is uncoordinated, lowering of the epiglottis and opening of the esophagus are also impaired and food might remain in the throat after a swallow, causing further risk of it getting in the airway.

Children with profound weakness who cannot lift their heads from their pillows usually have swallowing problems that are moderate to very severe. Children who cannot swallow correctly or who have profound weakness may not need detailed testing immediately but will need testing as they recover. These children need to be watched very closely and are often hospitalized. In addition, children who cannot gag (lift the muscles of the palate) when their tongue is touched by a tongue depressor are not strong enough to eat because they cannot stop nasal reflux. Children who cannot cough or choke, who show evidence of food or liquid going into their lungs, or who have profound weakness in swallowing should not eat or drink by mouth and should receive nutrition in other ways described below. They may be able to take tiny sips of water or chew gum to keep the mouth lubricated. Ignoring this problem can lead to severe pneumonia.

Table 18.1. Signs and causes of dysphagia in JM.

Signs of dysphagia	Cause of the problem
Difficulty swallowing and chewing	• Weakness or thinning of the tongue and muscles of the floor of the mouth • Slow, uncoordinated swallow
Pain when swallowing	• Inflammation of the muscles of the throat, voice box, gums, and tongue
Difficulty swallowing pills	• Not enough saliva • Tongue weakness, reduced sensation in the mouth or throat, weakness of muscles of the throat
Heartburn, chest pain, and regurgitation of food and stomach acid	• Weakness of muscles of the esophagus (swallowing tube) and valve at the bottom of the esophagus causing reflux or backup into the upper esophagus or throat
Coughing or choking	• Reflux of food back into the throat • Food pooling on the vocal folds • Food entering the airway • Pooled food in the throat passing down to the airway after a swallow
Voice changes (hoarseness, pitch, gurgly voice)	• Weakness and inflammation of muscles of the voice box • Reflux of food or stomach acid back into the throat
Nasal regurgitation	• Failure of the soft palate to close off the nose from the back of the throat
Aspiration	• Weakness and inflammation of the muscles of the throat, voice box, and tongue • Slow, uncoordinated swallow • Failure to close off the airway • Reflux of food back into the airway • Dripping of food or liquid from the mouth into the throat

Some of the problems in the esophageal phase of swallowing occur because both the upper and lower valves of the esophagus (upper and lower esophageal sphincters) do not work properly. Early in the disease the upper sphincter or gate to the esophagus can be weak, but over time it can become thickened and not relax or open well enough to allow the food to pass into the esophagus. These problems can lead to difficulty swallowing both solids and liquids.

Reflux of acid can irritate the lower sphincter and cause it to work poorly. *Reflux* means that the acid produced in the stomach flows backward into the esophagus. The acid irritates the esophagus and can make it work poorly. In myositis, if the muscles in the esophagus are weak, the sphincter at the bottom of the esophagus doesn't do a good job of keeping the stomach contents in the stomach. The tube portion above this sphincter also cannot efficiently push the acid back into the stomach. This is called gastroesophageal reflux disease (GERD). Symptoms of GERD include heartburn, chest pain, and sour taste in your mouth. The emptying of the esophagus is slower for solids than for liquids in myositis and is associated with discomfort when myositis patients eat solid, crusty foods, such as meat or hard breads (see *Chapter 19, Nutrition and Your Child's Weight*). Younger children may simply complain of tummy aches and point to their chest or just below the breastbone, especially after eating. Some children simply stop eating mid-meal or are very irritable at mealtime. Vomiting can also be a problem. A summary of the common signs of dysphagia associated with myositis, the site or anatomy of the problem, and the reason for these problems can be found in Table 18.1.

How Are Swallowing Problems Evaluated?

A speech-language pathologist is a professional who is trained to diagnose and recommend treatment for the oral and pharyngeal problems of swallowing. Speech-language pathologists are trained to conduct the diagnostic tests (X-ray and ultrasound swallowing studies) and will work with the dietician to plan the most appropriate diet for your child and consult with your child's doctors and nurses for medical aspects of treatment.

The most common test of swallowing problems in children is the *modified barium swallow study*. Barium is a radioactive element that glows on an X-ray, allowing doctors to see what is happening inside the body. In this study various foods are coated with barium or barium of varying textures is swallowed. Then a videotaped moving X-ray study is done while your child swallows, which allows the examiner to see how well food travels from the mouth to the stomach. This study can reveal most of the problems described in the previous section. Another technique used to study the oral phase of the swallow is *ultrasound imaging*, which is available only in a few centers and is usually done by a speech-language pathologist.

Ultrasound studies use regular food and liquids, have no radiation exposure, and provide excellent views of the movement of the muscles of the mouth, larynx, and tongue during swallowing. Based on the results of these studies, the complete swallowing process can be evaluated, and progress can be monitored to see how the treatment is working.

How Are Swallowing Problems Treated?

Many swallowing strategies and techniques are used to treat children with swallowing disorders based on the specific kinds of problems that are revealed during the testing mentioned above. Swallowing strategies are classified as *direct* if they involve the use of food and *indirect* if they do not use food (Table 18.2). *Indirect strategies* used by speech-language pathologists often focus on muscle coordination and strengthening, sensory stimulation, and teaching specific swallowing maneuvers without food. *Direct swallowing therapy techniques* include proper or alternative *positioning* of the body, neck, and head when eating so that the food will be directed properly from the mouth through the pharynx and into the esophagus. Positioning affects swallowing because a child's overall muscle tone, gross and fine motor ability, and respiration all interact while eating. Some children with poor head control try to compensate by extending the head or have a floppy chin down posture. These children can use a chair with head support to keep the head in an upright midline posture.

Table 18.2. Strategies for treating swallowing problems.

Indirect strategies: No food given

1. Tongue exercises and use of devices to increase tongue pressure during swallowing
2. Lip exercises
3. Thermal (cold) and tactile (touch) application near the back of the mouth to stimulate a swallow
4. Special seating and head positioning
5. Exercises to elevate the palate and the voice box
6. Food given through a stomach tube or vein (no food by mouth)

Direct strategies: Used with food

1. Head positioning: midline, straight ahead, or tilted to compensate for weakness
2. Alternate placement of food in the mouth
3. Modification of dietary textures (smoothies, purees, grinding meats); blenderizing foods
4. Crushing pills into sauces or pudding
5. Use pills that dissolve
6. Use of cold or sour foods to stimulate a swallow
7. Alternate liquids with solids
8. Proper use of water with pills
9. Special cups and utensils for easy feeding
10. Food thickeners and thickened liquids
11. Swallow with airway protection strategies

Changing the consistency or texture of foods often makes it easier for children to swallow. Solid and crunchy foods, such as popcorn, raw carrots, stringy meat, doughy breads, and peanuts, can be difficult to eat for children who have weakness of the tongue or throat and should be avoided when possible. Solid foods can be cut into small pieces, ground, blenderized, or mixed with sauces to make them easier to swallow. If your child chokes on liquids, they can be thickened naturally with cornstarch or commercial thickening products and commercially thickened juices. Parents should consult with their child's medical team before changing their child's diet.

If your child has difficulty swallowing pills, have her try this technique: always take pills with liquids both before and after taking each pill. Take several swallows to moisten the mouth before taking the tablet or capsule. Place pills near the middle of the mouth, drink the fluid, lift the head, and then lower the chin at the time of the swallow. Since fluids improve how fast pills are dissolved and aid in moving the tablet through the gastrointestinal system, drink a half glass of water or clear fluids after taking pills. Take one pill at a time, and remain sitting upright after swallowing. At night use several pillows or a wedge at the head of the bed to ensure that both pills and foods are properly passed into the stomach. If needed, crush pills (be sure first to ask the pharmacist whether this is possible because some pills will not work properly if crushed) and mix with sauces or find out if a liquid form of the pill is available. A new way of making pills that allows them to dissolve rapidly in the mouth is being developed and might be available in the future. To help your child learn how to swallow pills, have her practice swallowing small candies.

If a child has aspirated or is at high risk for aspiration, this is a medically urgent situation. Children should not be allowed to eat or drink until weakness of the palate and tongue improves. In severe cases, children may be unable even to swallow saliva and may need airway protection provided by placing a tube in the breathing pipe (called a tracheostomy tube). In this case treatment to improve muscle strength may be given, including medications described in *Chapter 12, Possible Medicines During the Course*; these medicines are often given by vein when children have difficulty swallowing. A feeding tube, which is passed through the nose into the stomach, may be needed to supply nutrition until the child improves enough to be fed by mouth. As a preventative strategy, we suggest that children do not snack while lying with their heads down on the couch or bed, and we encourage them to eat meals and drink liquids sitting up while a caretaker observes them. Once your child has recovered to her full strength, these precautions are no longer needed.

> **If there is sudden worsening in swallowing characterized by excessive choking and coughing, fever after eating, unwanted weight loss, vomiting, or noticeable changes in voice, this is a possible medical emergency, and you need to tell your medical team immediately.**

What Other Digestive Tract Problems Can Occur in Children with Myositis?

Medications can also cause intestinal problems. Many of the medications used to treat the "itis" or inflammation are also hard on the lining of the digestive tract. Poor muscle function or irritation of the stomach by medication can increase the risk of acid reflux. If the stomach empties too slowly, it is more likely that acid will reflux up into the esophagus. A child might feel full much sooner, so she might eat less, leading to poor weight gain or even weight loss. Slow stomach emptying can also make the absorption of drugs more difficult. Stomachaches or abdominal pain can occur, as well as nausea and occasionally vomiting.

The intestines might also move too slowly and in an uncoordinated way. When this happens, your child might not be able to absorb nutrients normally. Inflammation caused by vasculitis and myositis can also decrease the absorption of important nutrients. This is called *malabsorption*, and it can contribute to poor nutrition as well as stomach pain. Problems such as constipation or difficulty emptying the bowels can also occur, and in this situation your child may need to increase her fluid, fiber, and fruit intake.

Small blood vessels in the digestive tract can sometimes be inflamed (called vasculitis), and this can contribute to the pain as well as to the poor intestinal movement or dysmotility. Small blood vessels in the skin can also be affected in these children and cause what are known as vasculitic skin rashes (see *Chapter 16, Skin Rashes and Sun Protection*). Children with vasculitic skin rashes may be at higher risk for vasculitis of the intestines, as are patients with more severe disease. Occasionally, the vasculitis can cause ulcers. These are not the same type of ulcers that someone without myositis might have. These ulcers are not caused by bacteria but by the vasculitis. They can occur anywhere along the digestive tract and cause pain where they occur. Sometimes these ulcers can bleed, even requiring blood transfusions or an operation to stop the bleeding. Blood in the stool can make it dark and tarry or sticky. Report any blood in your child's stool to your child's healthcare team. If your doctor is suspicious that your child has vasculitis or an ulcer, he or she may ask your child to use stool collection cards to test for trace amounts of blood. If the stomach pain persists or becomes more severe, then X-ray studies to look for intestinal tract problems are needed. Sometimes other intestinal problems can occur, causing severe stomach pain, and some may require surgery, whereas others can be treated with bowel rest and antibiotics.

> If severe abdominal pain develops or the pain becomes progressively worse, your child needs to be under close medical supervision. If stomach pain gets worse or becomes very severe, your child may need to see a doctor immediately or go to an emergency room.

Although it seems that the first part of the digestive tract (mouth and throat) is more often affected by myositis, careful questioning and testing often reveals that there are also problems lower down. If there are problems with weight gain or evidence of a shortage of some nutrients, the child with JM should be carefully questioned for symptoms relating to the lower esophagus, stomach, and intestines. It is not uncommon to have belly pain, constipation, or weight loss, suggesting that the lower esophagus and stomach are slow and uncoordinated.

What Tests Are Used to Examine the Esophagus, Stomach, and Intestines?

Another member of your child's medical team might be a gastroenterologist (a digestive tract specialist) or an otolaryngologist (an ear, nose, and throat doctor). There are several different tests that these doctors might perform to see whether the disease is in the digestive tract or how well the digestive tract is working. As mentioned before, the barium swallow (also called an upper GI series) can be used to show how food goes down the esophagus and out the stomach. The barium can be followed all the way through the small intestine; this is called a small bowel series.

Upper endoscopy allows the gastroenterologist to see the inside lining of the digestive tract. An endoscope is a long flexible tube with a camera on the end that allows your child's doctor to see inside the digestive tract and watch the pictures on a television screen. The child is either partially or fully asleep while this procedure is done. The doctor might check to see whether there are signs of an ulcer or gastroesophageal reflux.

What Medicines Can Be Used to Treat Problems in the Digestive Tract?

The same medicines given for the myositis in the rest of the body often treat the myositis and vasculitis occurring in the digestive tract (see *Chapter 7, Treatment Possibilities in the Beginning* and *Chapter 12, Possible Medicines During the Course*). In addition, drugs more specific to the digestive tract may also be used. Drugs that decrease stomach acid may be used if there are signs of gastroesophageal reflux. These drugs may also help decrease inflammation. They include medicines that block histamine to decrease stomach acid, such as ranitidine (Zantac), and ones that block the acid pump (called the proton pump), such as omeprosol (Prilosec or Losec) and lansoprazole (Prevacid). There are also medicines that help the stomach empty better; these are called motility-enhancing drugs. They include metoclopramide (Reglan, Maxeran) and domperidone (Motilium, not available in the U.S.).

Nutrition is also important for good intestinal tract function (see *Chapter 19, Nutrition and Your Child's Weight*). Because the myositis can make it difficult to swallow and because some of the drugs and the inflammation in the intestines can take away a child's appetite, poor nutrition can be a real problem. Sometimes, over time, the inflammation can lead to such poor motility in the intestinal tract that a child has difficulty absorbing enough nutrients to grow. Sometimes simple changes in the choice of foods allow for better absorption of nutrition.

Anxiety and worrying can also cause or worsen stomach pain. If a child becomes anxious while trying to swallow, food sticking in the throat may seem worse. Seeing a counselor or social worker, psychologist, or psychiatrist to help deal with the anxiety might help in these cases. Therapies may include relaxation, biofeedback, self-hypnosis, and certain medications. Feeling bad can be depressing. If you suspect that your child is depressed, it is important to discuss this with your child's healthcare team. It is also important to be open to the idea that some of the pain may be due to stress. Your child's healthcare providers need to address all of the issues that can make your child feel bad.

Key Points

- The digestive or gastrointestinal (GI) tract, from the mouth to the anus (exit), can be affected in patients with myositis by both muscle weakness and by inflammation in and around the blood vessels in the intestines (called vasculitis).

- Swallowing problems are common in children with myositis because the muscles of the tongue, throat, soft palate, and esophagus are often weak or inflamed. Trouble swallowing should be reported to your child's medical team and treated to prevent serious complications, such as aspiration and pneumonia.

- Other common problems are nasal regurgitation, heartburn, hoarse voice, and belly pain.

- Diagnosis of the specific swallowing and other digestive tract problems may require special procedures, such as barium swallow and bowel X-rays, ultrasound, or endoscopy.

- Treatment of the myositis often helps the digestive tract improve, but specific eating strategies and medicines for the digestive tract can also be helpful.

To Learn More

To find a specialist, see *Finding a specialist for Other Complications (Swallowing)* in the *Finding a Doctor or Specialist* section of the *Resource Appendix*, specifically:

> **American Gastroenterological Association**
>
> **American Speech-Language-Hearing Association (ASHA)**

Additional Information:

The Myositis Association (TMA).

> *Dysphagia: when myositis is hard to swallow.* Available from: www.myositis.org/jmbookresources.cfm or 800-821-7356.

Dysphagia: what you should know. Winter 2004 OutLook Extra Treatment Issue. Call 800-821-7356 or email tma@myositis.org to obtain a copy.

American Speech-Language-Hearing Association (ASHA).

For the public. Available at: www.asha.org/public.

> Provides services for professionals and advocates for people with swallowing disorders; list of board-recognized specialists in swallowing disorders; and information on support groups, speech, and swallowing.

American Gastroenterological Association.

Patient Center. Available at: www.gastro.org/wmspage.cfm?parm1=478.

Children's Digestive Health and Nutrition Foundation. Phone: 800-344-8888; Internet: www.cdhnf.org.

Information on pediatric gastrointestinal, liver, and nutritional issues. Dedicated to education and research related to understanding children's digestive problems.

Kids Acid Reflux, geared toward younger children, available at www.kidsacidreflux.org; for teenagers (age 12–21 years), www.teensacidreflux.org.

Book:

Achilles E. *The Dysphagia Cookbook*. Nashville TN: Cumberland House Publishing; 2004. Wide range of recipes and helpful hints for those with swallowing problems.

Reports in the Medical Literature

Pachman LM, Cooke N. Juvenile dermatomyositis: a clinical and immunologic study. *Journal of Pediatrics.* 1980 Feb;96(2):226–34.

Schullinger JN, Jacobs JC, Berdon WE. Diagnosis and management of gastrointestinal perforations in childhood dermatomyositis with particular reference to perforations of the duodenum. *Journal of Pediatric Surgery.* 1985 Oct;20(5):521–4.

Sonies BC. Evaluation and treatment of speech and swallowing disorders associated with myopathies. *Current Opinion in Rheumatology.* 1997 Nov;9(6):486–95.

CHAPTER 19

Nutrition and Your Child's Weight

Carol J. Henderson, PhD, RD, and Barbara E. Ostrov, MD

In this chapter...

We review how juvenile myositis affects your child's nutrition and how your child's weight may change as a result. We discuss some nutritional problems that your child may have because she has myositis. We also provide suggestions you might find helpful to tackle these nutritional problems. (If your child with myositis would like to read about food and cooking, there are child-friendly web sites like www.kidshealth.org.)

From the family's point of view...

"She's hungry all the time, and sometimes even begs for food. It's so hard to set limits on her eating since it's one of her few pleasures now that she's so weak."

Why Is Nutrition Important to My Child?

Your child's health and well-being are directly affected by how nutritious her food is and how the body absorbs and uses that food. The nutrients we get from the food we eat enable our bodies to live and grow. Like your car, which needs gas to run, our bodies need certain nutrients, including vitamins, minerals, protein, carbohydrates, and fats. If you put non-nutritional food in your body or the wrong balance of foods, it's like putting water or orange juice in your car instead of gasoline. Your car might not run too well. If your body doesn't get enough of the right nutrients, the damage caused by the inflammation can't be fixed. So nutrition is very important for your child with JM. Unfortunately, both the disease itself and some treatments for it can prevent your child from getting enough of some nutrients and too much of others. What we eat, including food, drinks, and supplements, is called "nutritional intake," and how those foods affect our overall health and well-being is called "nutritional status." As you probably know, although most food is essentially good for us, too much or too little of one kind of food can result in poor nutritional status. You should seek the advice of a registered dietitian if your child develops any nutritional problems, such as excessive weight gain or high blood pressure.

Myositis can change how your child feels about food and how well she can digest it. How we eat and what we eat is influenced by many things: the variety of food choices; the strength of our appetite; food appearance, taste, and smell; and our ability to chew and swallow easily. If food gets stuck when you swallow or if you get full too easily, then nutritional intake goes down. This can really impair your child's nutritional status.

Children with myositis often do not have a proper diet even though they are given healthy food. Sometimes they might eat too little because the effort of eating can make them tired, or they might feel full after only a little bit of food. Other times they might select foods that are poor in nutrient quality, such as fast foods or salty snack foods. These foods are often high in fat calories and salt; when eaten frequently, such foods (e.g., pizza, burgers, fries, and chips) may increase the side effects of medicine (especially steroids), including weight gain and elevated blood pressure. Consequently, undesirable weight gain and high blood pressure are common problems in patients with myositis. Instead of offering these low-nutrient snacks, provide healthier choices—fresh fruits and raw vegetables or rice cakes with low-fat cheese and low-salt salsa. Eating healthy doesn't have to be boring, so be creative. Choose wheat crackers over potato chips, low-sugar fruit smoothies over milkshakes or sodas, and low-fat frozen yogurt over ice cream.

How Does Myositis Cause My Child to Have Poor Nutrition?

There are several ways myositis affects nutritional intake and nutritional status. The first is muscle weakness. Weakness in the muscles needed for chewing or swallowing (esophageal dysmotility) makes eating difficult (see *Chapter 18, Swallowing and Other Digestive Problems*). Your child may no longer enjoy meals and thus eat less, thereby lowering her intake of proper nutrients. Weakness in the stomach muscles allows food to remain in the stomach for a long time, creating a feeling of fullness after only a few bites of food (gastroparesis). Inflammation in the muscles that run along the gastrointestinal tract can cause them not to work (contract) as well as normal. This can sometimes lead to weight loss and shrinkage (atrophy) of the muscles. When muscle weakness results in decreased physical activity, getting regular exercise becomes quite difficult. Inactivity combined with the craving for increased food intake due to steroid use, as well as boredom and anxiety, all can result in weight gain. Your doctor or physical therapist can recommend certain exercises for your child at different stages of the condition to help combat this.

Inflammation also affects nutrition. Inflammation in the intestines caused by the myositis can lead to belly pain, constipation, or diarrhea. Because the inflammation around the blood vessels prevents absorption of food from the gastrointestinal tract, weight loss is possible in children with active myositis. Weight loss can also follow complications of myositis, such as infections, intestinal problems, and, in some children, depression. If your child's bowels are inflamed, nutrients will not be properly absorbed, especially in juvenile dermatomyositis (JDM) or overlap myositis (see *Chapter 28, When Your Child Has More Than One Autoimmune Disease*). Myositis may be associated with other autoimmune illnesses, such as those that affect the bowels. Disorders with bowel inflammation, such as colitis and celiac disease, also cause poor absorption of nutrients and impair growth. Poor appetite can occur when your child just "doesn't feel good." Poor intake and absorption of vitamins and minerals, especially vitamin D and calcium, contribute to weakening of the bones or osteoporosis (see *Chapter 22, Taking Care of the Bones*). So nutrition and inflammation go hand in hand.

Myositis can also cause heartburn or acid reflux (gastroesophageal reflux disease, GERD) as a result of the weakness of the swallowing and stomach muscles. GERD symptoms are often more severe in patients taking medium to high doses of steroids (see *Chapter 18, Swallowing and Other Digestive Problems*) or who have severe symptoms of myositis.

Depression and boredom associated with a serious systemic illness can cause some children to overeat and gain weight. Conversely, depression can decrease the appetite and lead to reduced food intake for some children. Infrequently, older children and teens may intentionally avoid eating to prevent weight gain associated with steroid use. Rarely, a child will not take her steroid medicine to avoid the changes in her body that occur with steroids.

Other symptoms of myositis can affect nutritional intake. Thrush, or yeast in the mouth or esophagus, mouth sores, and stomach ulcers can decrease your child's appetite. Difficulty grasping smaller items, like forks and spoons, triggers frustration and may result in your child eating less to avoid this aggravation. Your child may feel embarrassed when eating with others; she may eat less in these situations because it takes a long time to chew and swallow even a small amount of food.

How Do Treatments for Myositis Cause Nutrition Problems?

As mentioned in earlier chapters about treatment (see *Chapter 7, Treatment Possibilities in the Beginning* and *Chapter 12, Possible Medicines During the Course*), steroid use can bring about nutrition problems. Common side effects of steroids, such as weight gain, water retention, and loss of calcium and potassium, often affect nutritional intake and status and are more likely to occur with higher steroid doses. Weight gain from steroid use increases body fat, not muscle; therefore, the nutritional status of a child who gains weight from steroid use may not be as good as you would think, if you are using the child's weight as a measure of adequate nutritional status. Increased appetite often results in increased food portions and frequent snacking. Steroid-induced appetite can generate increased interest in poor food choices, such as non-nutritional snacks and beverages (e.g., soda, fruit drinks, and sports drinks), which often contain large amounts of salt (or sodium) and calories. As you can see, routine intake of these foods contributes to excess weight gain and fluid retention. Steroids can also increase blood sugar levels, which can lead to the development of diabetes and thrush. Thrush can be visible as patches of white on the inside of the mouth—often on the inside of the cheeks, and if it extends down the esophagus, it can cause your child to experience pain while swallowing. Although the development of thrush, or yeast in the mouth, may not be preventable, you can minimize its severity by having your child brush her teeth frequently and rinse with mouthwash or other solutions recommended by your doctor after eating and drinking. Use a new toothbrush once the mouth thrush has cleared up to prevent it from coming back.

It is usually essential to control the inflammation of myositis with medicines that tone down or suppress the immune system. Immune suppression with medications such as methotrexate or cyclosporine also produces side effects that negatively influence nutritional status. For example, methotrexate can cause nausea, diarrhea, stomach pain, and loss of appetite; cyclosporine can affect your child's gums, making them more tender and sensitive. Hydroxychloroquine can occasionally be associated with abdominal pain. Sometime antacids or other supplemental therapies, such as iron taken by mouth, can also produce diarrhea and cramping. If your child has chronic diarrhea, nutrients such as proteins, vitamins, and minerals are not absorbed properly, resulting in weight loss and further muscle weakness.

How Can We Deal with These Nutrition Problems?

Achieving adequate nutritional intake that is neither too little nor excessive is desirable. Although many of the nutritional problems identified are caused by the myositis or the medications used to treat the inflammation, there are many things you can do to help minimize these problems. The following suggestions are useful to decrease nutritional problems related to myositis.

Ways to Improve Poor Nutritional Intake Due to...

Swallowing difficulties: Choose soft foods that require very little chewing and have a pudding-like consistency, such as cooked cereals (prepared with milk instead of water to boost the nutritional value), cold flake cereal softened with milk, scrambled eggs, yogurt, pudding, finely chopped egg salad, thick cream soups (soups can be thickened with instant mashed potatoes or finely crushed unsalted crackers or food thickeners that are available at most drug stores), applesauce, or ice cream. (Remember to choose low-salt, low-fat foods.) If your child has developed difficulty swallowing or has a problem with choking, do not leave your child alone when eating or drinking. Let your doctor know about this right away. Provide your child with additional head support as needed if she has difficulty maintaining head control, especially at meal times. Ask your physical therapist for suggestions on ways to do this for your child. If your child has extreme difficulties, such as swallowing her own saliva, then elevating her head off the bed by approximately 90 degrees is recommended, even when she is napping or sleeping (see *Chapter 18, Swallowing and Other Digestive Problems* for more specific recommendations).

Slow stomach emptying (gastroparesis): To help your child with this problem, offer small, frequent meals and snacks. Help your child drink fluids before or after meals and snacks. It's a good idea for your child to eat foods that are low in fat because they require less time to digest. Avoid non-nutritional foods, such as soda, sweets, and pastries, and salty, high-fat foods, such as potato chips, tortilla chips, etc.

Heartburn or GERD: Help your child to eat and drink in an upright position. Avoid foods your child associates with heartburn, such as peppermint, spicy foods, or greasy foods. Avoid napping or sleeping immediately after eating or drinking. It is best to wait at least one to two hours after eating before lying down to lessen the likelihood that the stomach's contents will back up into the esophagus.

Poor nutrient absorption from chronic diarrhea: Provide a serving or more of foods containing probiotic bacteria each day if your child has chronic diarrhea. Probiotic bacteria are commonly found in cultured and fermented foods, such as yogurt, buttermilk, fermented and kefir cheeses, tempeh, and miso, which contain active cultures. Yogurt that has been pasteurized does not have active cultures. Probiotics are beneficial microorganisms that help maintain the natural balance of organisms (microflora, which contain more than four hundred types of normal bacteria) normally present in the intestines. They aid the digestion and absorption of some nutrients and lessen diarrhea. Avoidance of fats can lessen both the volume and frequency of diarrhea episodes. Adequate hydration is very important and can be achieved with Pedialyte, apple juice diluted with water, and flavored water.

Steroids used to treat myositis: Increased appetite is a real occurrence in children receiving steroids. The higher the steroid dose, the more likely it is that your child will feel hungry all of the time, even right after eating. This is often frustrating for parents who want to prevent their child from gaining excess weight. To help curb your child's appetite, encourage her to drink six to eight ounces of non-calorie containing fluid, such as water or sugar-free drinks, before each meal or snack. Wait a full fifteen to twenty minutes from the time your child announces being hungry until the time you offer a snack. Allow her to chew sugarless gum between meals and snacks. Have low-calorie snack foods already prepared at home and readily available when your child becomes hungry in order to prevent her from eating fast foods or foods that are commercially prepackaged, which are likely to be higher in calories and salt. Examples of convenient and healthy snack foods are fresh fruits that are prewashed and cut vegetables, a small portion of dried fruits (2–3 tablespoons), miniature flavored rice cakes, small containers of nonfat yogurt, nonfat cottage cheese, nonfat pudding, applesauce without added sugar, fruit packed in its own juice, string cheese (low fat, low salt), miniature bagels, reduced-fat, low-sodium crackers (read the label to determine the serving size for different types of crackers), and one slice of angel food cake with non-fat whipped topping and fresh or frozen berries.

Other Ways to Improve Nutritional Intake

Ideally, the best way to improve your child's nutritional intake is to eat more vegetables and fresh foods rather than prepackaged or processed food, which will benefit the whole family, not just the child with JM. Vegetables are high in nutrients, including potassium, and most are relatively low in calories, fat, and sugar. Use fresh vegetables rather than frozen or canned ones, and experiment with different recipes to help your children enjoy eating them. You can also buy no-salt seasonings to sprinkle on them to add flavor. Steroids also deplete the body of certain vital nutrients, such as calcium and potassium, so foods high in these elements are important as are supplements that also contain magnesium.

It is important for you to learn to read the food labels on packages, which list the calories and the content of the food inside, to avoid unwanted calories from fat and sugar as well as excessive salt or sodium intake. Refer to the following web site to get more information about how to read and interpret food labels in both English and Spanish: www.cfsan.fda.gov/~dms/foodlab.html. While grocery shopping, you will need to budget extra time so that you and your child can read food labels and product ingredients, especially when you find new specialty food products. When you are shopping with your child, she can help you choose which kinds of foods to include on the menu for the week. Help your child recognize poor food choices, especially foods high in fat, sugar, and salt. Children are frequently offered foods for special occasions, such as birthday parties, both at school and outside the school setting. It is difficult to prevent a child from participating in food events; therefore, plan carefully and regularly to avoid undesired amounts and types of certain foods. Once again, the higher the dose of steroids your child is receiving, the more important it is to restrict calories (especially from fat) and salt in order to minimize fluid retention and weight gain. If your child has high blood sugar levels, it is also important to minimize sugar intake, such as sugar-coated cereals, sweets and pastries, and fruit juice, fruit punch, Kool-Aid, and soda that contains both natural and added forms of sugar.

Foods that contain more than 300 milligrams of salt per the serving size printed on the label are high in salt. Avoid offering these foods or using seasonings containing salt in food preparation. Limit foods high in salt, such as hot dogs, pizza, grilled cheese sandwiches, or school lunches, to once a week. You can decrease the salt and fat when serving pizza by avoiding salty toppings, such as pepperoni, sausage, and extra cheese. Use a napkin or paper towel to press the grease off each pizza slice, and allow your child to eat no more than two slices of pizza. Offer additional foods lower in fat and salt to fill her up, such as carrots, salad with limited salad dressing (approximately 2 tablespoons and preferably a low-fat variety), or plain bread sticks. Offer a piece of fruit if your child is still hungry. When eating in a restaurant, look for items marked "heart healthy" (often denoted with a ♥). These items are generally lower in fat and salt. Avoid foods described with terms such as "teriyaki," "marinated," and "sautéed," which will increase the sodium and/or fat.

Salt-free products can be substituted in several ways. For example, many children like tomato-based dishes, and some like to drown their foods in catsup. Most regular canned tomato products, including catsup, are high in sodium and need to be limited to one or two servings per week. Try unsalted canned tomato products and salt-free catsup. In order to increase the acceptability of salt-free catsup, fill a bottle halfway with regular catsup and the remaining half with salt-free catsup. Gradually replace the emptied container with a greater proportion of salt-free catsup.

How Can We Help Improve Our Child's Nutritional Status?

Ask to see a registered dietitian soon after your child is started on steroids in order to help you plan meals and snacks that are low in fat, salt, and sugar and to plan a diet that meets your child's nutritional needs.

A liquid or a chewable multivitamin is recommended once a day. Liquid vitamins can be absorbed better by the body than pills or tablets. If your child is currently receiving steroids to treat the myositis, she will require calcium and vitamin D supplementation beyond what she receives in the foods eaten. (Note: Most children's multivitamin preparations contain 400 IU of vitamin D, but 800 IU is needed for the larger child [see *Chapter 22, Taking Care of the Bones*].)

Weight gain is more common than weight loss in children with myositis because of the effect of steroids on appetite. However, some children who have complications from myositis may lose weight. Depending on the nature of the myositis complications, varying dietary interventions may be used to improve nutritional intake, such as giving high-calorie, high-protein nutritional supplements, and when necessary, providing liquid nutrition intravenously.

In addition, it is important to take care of your child's mouth and dental care. Because of the swollen gums and difficulty in chewing that children with JM may have, brushing teeth and flossing gums after each meal are useful habits to acquire. Cavities should be repaired immediately, for infection can start up the JM disease activity. Weight can be controlled with diet and also with exercise. Ask your child's doctor or physical therapist about an exercise program compatible with the activity of the myositis (see *Chapter 13, Rehabilitation of the Child with Myositis*).

Key Points

- Myositis can directly affect nutritional status due to problems with swallowing and chewing, slow absorption due to vasculitis or intestinal problems, or loss of appetite and/or depression.

- Medications used to treat myositis can affect nutritional status. Steroids cause weight gain and fluid retention, as well as loss of calcium and potassium. Methotrexate can cause nausea and loss of appetite; hydroxychloroquine can cause abdominal pain.

- Suggestions for managing nutritional problems include making better food choices; eating at proper times and in the correct position, especially if there are swallowing or stomach problems; choosing healthy snacks (avoid salty and fatty foods); planning meals and snacks; and reading food labels.

- Seek the advice of a registered dietitian as needed.

To Learn More

Internet:

U.S. Food and Drug Administration.

Guidance on How to Understand and Use the Nutrition Facts Panel on Food Labels. Available at: www.cfsan.fda.gov/~dms/foodlab.html.

The Myositis Association.

Choosing the right foods. Available from: www.myositis.org/jmbookresources.cfm or 800-821-7356.

American Heart Association.

Dietary Guidelines for Healthy Children. Available at: www.amhrt.org/presenter.jhtml ?identifier=4575.

  Recommendations for calorie and fat intake and links to other useful web sites.

Books:

Arthritis Foundation. *Medications.* In: **Raising a Child with Arthritis: A Parent's Guide.** Atlanta (GA): Arthritis Foundation; 1998. p. 29–36.

Zukerman E, Ingelfinger J. **Coping with Prednisone and Other Cortisone-Related Medicines.** NY: St. Martin's Griffin; 1997.

Organizations:

American Dietetic Association. 120 South Riverside Plaza, Suite 2000, Chicago IL 60606-6995; Phone: 800-877-1600; Internet: www.eatright.org.

  Information on healthy eating habits, dieting, and finding a nutrition specialist. For fact sheets on nutrition, see www.eatright.org/cps/rde/xchg/ada/hs.xsl/nutrition_350_ENU_HTML.htm.

International Food Information Council Foundation. 1100 Connecticut Avenue NW, Suite 430, Washington DC 20036; Phone: 202-296-6540; Internet: www.ific.org; Email: foodinfo@ific.org.

  Topics of nutrition and food safety, including information for children and adolescents.

CHAPTER 20

Growth and Development

Aida N. Lteif, MD; Wendy J. Brickman, MD;
and Patricia Woo, CBE, PhD, FRCP, FRCPCH, FMedSci

In this chapter...

We describe the usual patterns of growth and puberty and how they can be affected in children with juvenile myositis (JM). In addition, we discuss problems with thyroid function, which can occur in children with well-controlled myositis and alter their normal pattern of growth and development.

From the family's point of view...

"By the time we found out she had myositis, our six-year-old daughter had lost several pounds and had been the same size for a few months. Then she started steroids, and we were concerned this would lead her to be shorter all her life. The doctors reassured us that once she could be weaned from the higher doses of steroid medicines, her growth shouldn't be overly affected in the long run."

Overview and Definitions Used in This Chapter

The term "growth" describes the increase in height, which is one of the essential physical features of childhood. "Development" has many aspects, but in this chapter we will concentrate on sexual maturation that culminates in a person's ability to reproduce. Many conditions can cause poor growth and abnormal pubertal development in children. Any disease that is severe and long lasting can potentially suppress growth and puberty by affecting the endocrine system. The endocrine system is composed of glands that secrete hormones that influence almost every function in our bodies. These hormones regulate growth, metabolism, pubertal development, and other organ functions. Some children with myositis have problems with growth, puberty, or thyroid disease, which are all sicknesses involving hormones. A "pediatric endocrinologist" is a doctor who specializes in hormones and who can determine whether your child has a hormone problem and treat it.

Growth

Does Myositis Cause My Child Not to Grow as Fast as Other Children?

Children grow very fast during their first year of life. By 3 to 4 years of age, growth in height usually proceeds at a steady rate of approximately 2 to 2½ inches (5 to 6 centimeters) per year until puberty. A major growth spurt occurs at puberty, when growth can exceed 4 inches per year.

Growth delay, meaning poor growth in height, is often a concern in children and adolescents with myositis, as it is for many children who have long-term autoimmune diseases. Growth might slow down during the active phase of the illness, and doctors don't know why. Poor growth in childhood can result in short stature as an adult. Some children with chronic inflammation become resistant to the action of growth hormones, which promotes normal growth in healthy children. Growth can also be affected by poor nutrition, which may be made worse by the inflammation of blood vessels in the intestines.

What Is "Catch-Up Growth," and Will Every Child with JM Have This Option?

Corticosteroids (e.g., prednisone, methylprednisolone [Solumedrol]) can contribute to your child's reduced growth pattern. The mechanism of growth inhibition is not well understood but probably results from a direct effect of the corticosteroids on the epiphyses, which is the part of the bone that grows. The use of corticosteroids on an every-other-day basis in the hopes of allowing linear growth, not only is usually insufficient to control the myositis inflammation but may prolong the time the disease is active requiring medication. Usually once the corticosteroids are stopped and the inflammation is under control, children have what is called "catch-up" growth. They grow faster initially and then grow at a normal pace, reaching a final height that is expected, given their parental heights (Figure 20.1). If your child takes corticosteroids for a long time, however, she might not have enough time for catch-up growth and might not reach her expected final height. Therefore, more aggressive short-term treatment with steroids in combination with disease-modifying agents, such as methotrexate or other immunosuppressive medicines, can be used to control the inflammation more quickly and minimize the time your child has to take corticosteroids. This treatment strategy could allow children with growth potential to achieve their expected height.

How Will My Child with JM Be Monitored for Changes in Height?

Height should be monitored closely during any child's treatment of myositis. First, the height of both parents and their own pattern of growth in childhood will be checked, because this is the most important influence on your child's height in adulthood. If poor growth is noted, laboratory studies and a bone age test may be ordered. A bone age test is an X-ray of the hand (Figure 20.2). This picture, which looks different at different ages or stages of growth, helps the doctor figure out the

CDC Growth Charts: United States

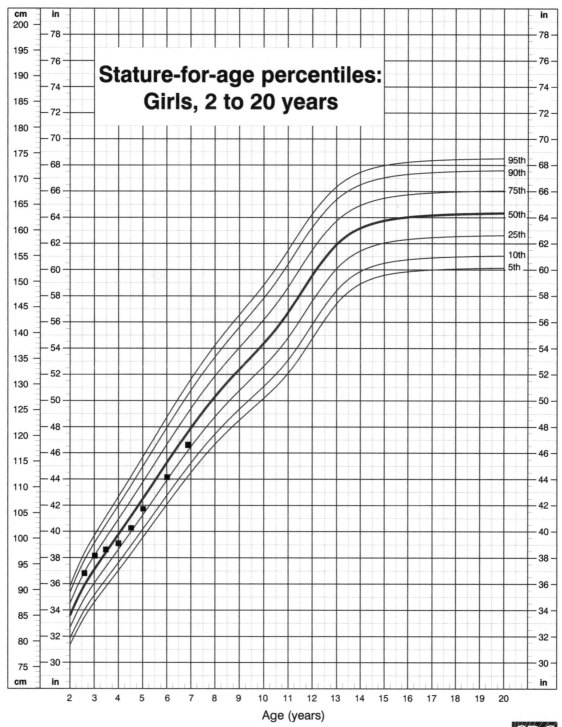

**Stature-for-age percentiles:
Girls, 2 to 20 years**

Published May 30, 2000.
SOURCE: Developed by the National Center for Health Statistics in collaboration with
the National Center for Chronic Disease Prevention and Health Promotion (2000).

CDC
SAFER · HEALTHIER · PEOPLE

■ **Figure 20.1. Growth curve of a girl with juvenile dermatomyositis, diagnosed at three years of age.**
High-dose steroid treatments were started at 3.6 years of age and gradually were decreased by six years of age. Flattening of the growth curve is noted at three years of age. With treatment of disease process and weaning of steroid therapy, growth velocity increased.

amount of each child's growth potential. During growth the bones of the hand and wrist mature until puberty is completed and the ends of the bones seal off. In the case of delayed bone age the bone maturity is less than expected for the chronologic age, suggesting that the child would likely have more potential for growth. As mentioned above, however, some children who receive higher doses of steroids for a long time or well into puberty, when the chance to catch up on growth is reduced, might not be able to experience all of the catch-up growth that the delayed bone age indicated was initially available. If the bone age test is inconclusive, laboratory studies will be done to see whether there are other reasons for the poor growth, such as an underactive thyroid. A blood test for proteins that carry out the action of growth hormone may also be obtained.

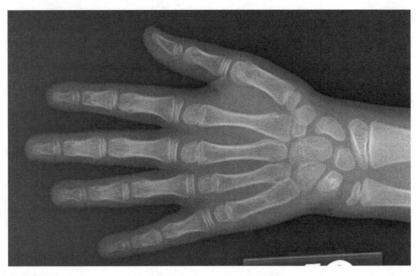

■ Figure 20.2. Left-hand X-ray of a 10-year-old girl.
Assessment of the bones in the hand and wrist suggests that this girl has a delayed bone age. Her bones are similar to those usually seen in an 8½-year-old girl. Therefore, her growth potential is more similar to that of an 8-year-old rather than a 10-year-old girl.

Why Not Give Growth Hormone to Children with JM?

Recombinant growth hormone, a synthetic hormone that resembles the growth hormone made by your pituitary gland, has been used to optimize the growth of children with a variety of illnesses. Studies performed in children with inflammatory diseases, such as juvenile arthritis, who were on steroid therapy for a long time suggested that growth hormone therapy might improve short-term growth. However, in children with juvenile arthritis, linear growth was not consistent because some of the children given growth hormone had very active inflammation, which counteracts the effect of the growth hormone treatment. In those children the long-term effect on growth and final adult height are still unknown. In children with juvenile dermatomyositis the use of growth hormone is frequently associated with a flare of the myositis (both skin and muscle), which is often difficult to bring under control. For this reason, growth hormone therapy is not suggested for children with JM. Other risks for growth hormone therapy include: 1) daily injections, 2) high cost, 3) transient high blood sugar from increased insulin resistance, especially in children with impaired glucose tolerance or insulin resistance (see *Chapter 25, Attention to Sugar and Fat Metabolism*), and 4) possible increase in the chance of getting cancer.

What Can We Do to Help My Child with Myositis Grow?

To control the myositis disease activity, your child may require high doses of steroids, which are often given by mouth on a daily basis. If so, it can be helpful for your child's myositis doctor to start additional medicines that suppress the activated immune system. Some of these medicines include intermittent pulse intravenous high-dose steroids, methotrexate, cyclosporine, or other medications (see *Chapter 12, Possible Medicines During the Course*). Adding these powerful medicines (which have much less effect on your child's growth) will help your doctor to be able to reduce the amount of daily steroid that is given, which could then help your child's growth. However, oral doses of steroids taken every other day (sometimes given to help children grow better) are *not helpful* for controlling myositis.

Puberty

What Is the Normal Pattern of Sexual Maturation?

Puberty is when your child's body changes from being a child to being an adult. Normal pubertal development begins in girls at eight to thirteen years of age and boys at nine to fourteen years of age, with mean age of menarche (onset of menstrual periods) in girls being twelve years of age. However, family patterns of maturation and growth also affect when puberty begins. Myositis doctors often ask about the growth pattern of the parents (for example, were they the shortest people in the class until eighth grade). You should also tell your child's doctor when her mother's and sisters' periods began as well. At the start of puberty in girls, follicle-stimulating hormone and leutinizing hormone trigger the production of the hormone estrogen by the ovaries. For most girls the first evidence of puberty is breast development and the growth of pubic hair. These first signs of puberty are followed one or two years later by a growth spurt. The culminating event will be the arrival of menarche. Young women might have irregular periods (less often than every five weeks) for the first two years, but then they should occur approximately once every three to five weeks. In boys, hormones give the signal to the testes to begin production of the hormone testosterone. Puberty for a boy usually starts with enlargement of the testicles and development of pubic hair, followed by a growth spurt, which occurs on average one to two years later than when girls start puberty.

How Might Myositis Affect My Child's Maturation?

Delayed puberty, where breast development, menstrual cycles, testicular growth, and/or pubic hair growth occur later than expected, has been reported in boys and girls with chronic medical conditions. Sometimes in girls with severe myositis, menstrual periods stop for a while but resume when the active inflammation resolves. The reasons for delayed puberty vary. Nutritional deficiency, chronic inflammation, and medications all could contribute to delayed puberty, irregular menses, or testicular dysfunction. Corticosteroid therapy inhibits secretion of a hormone from the brain, which can lead to delayed puberty in all children, irregular menses in females, and low testosterone production in males. The medications used to treat JM might also contribute to the delay. Cyclophosphamide, an alternative treatment for juvenile dermatomyositis, can cause transient or permanent infertility in both men and women, including irregular or absent menstrual periods. The younger the age of the child at the time cyclophosphamide is given, the lower the chance of infertility. Cyclophosphamide given to prepubertal girls is almost never a problem, especially with the low cumulative doses used in children with JM. Infertility related to cyclophosphamide is mainly seen in women who are over thirty years old. At higher cumulative doses (more than 25 grams total), a decrease in sperm production has been seen in men, but this dose is much higher than the amount given to children with JM. Another endocrine problem that can lead to irregular menses is insulin resistance, i.e., high insulin, which can be brought on by the use of steroids (discussed in *Chapter 25, Attention to Sugar and Fat Metabolism*). Irregular menses can also occur when the child with JDM has had a long period of uncontrolled inflammation

When Should I Start to Worry About Delayed Maturation?

Girls should consult their doctor if breasts and pubic hair have not developed by age thirteen years, if menstrual periods have not occurred by two years after the start of breast development, or if the frequency of the periods continues to be irregular (less than once every five weeks) 1½ to two years after the onset of menstruation. If your child is older than fourteen years, you should talk to your doctor if she is not maturing the way her peers are. You should also tell your child's doctor if your son has difficulties getting an erection or ejaculating. Your myositis doctor might then check the levels of certain hormones in the blood, hormones that could affect pubertal development, and the level of thyroid hormone. Your doctor might also order an X-ray of your child's hand to see if bone age is delayed and is contributing to the delayed puberty.

What Kind of Treatment Is Available for Delayed Development?

To obtain the best treatment for hormonal issues, your child should see an endocrinologist or gynecologist. If your adolescent daughter has breast development but no menstrual cycles, your doctor might prescribe progesterone, a hormone made in the ovaries, for five to seven days to try to stimulate a period. The doctor might also order an ultrasound of the ovaries and pelvis to document their presence and state of development. Treatment will depend on the reason for the delayed puberty or irregular periods. However, it is important for the child and the family to know that, in many instances, once the myositis is brought under control, the menses resume normally. Waiting until this occurs can eliminate worry and extra medications. Sometimes oral contraceptives are used to promote normal menstruation when they are irregular, and this should be discussed with your child's myositis doctor, too. Boys with delayed puberty might receive testosterone replacement. Depending on the reason for the delayed puberty, young men might need just a couple of doses of testosterone to jump-start puberty or might require longer-term therapy. Testosterone can be given to males as a twice-monthly or monthly injection or as a patch put on the skin, which continuously dispenses testosterone.

Both estrogen and testosterone will accelerate growth in height in the short term. Eventually, however, they will lead to closure of the growth plate and will shorten the time available for growth, so care is needed to make the best decision for your child with myositis.

What Kind of Changes in Thyroid Function Can Affect Growth and Development?

The thyroid is a butterfly-shaped gland in the neck, just below the Adam's apple. It produces thyroid hormone, which regulates your metabolism and organ function. Thyroid-stimulating hormone (TSH) is a chemical signal from the brain that controls the thyroid's production of thyroid hormone. Autoimmune thyroid disease has been reported in children with juvenile dermatomyositis.

One such disease is Hashimoto's thyroiditis, which causes your body to make antibodies in parts of your thyroid gland, leading to an inflamed thyroid and, most commonly, hypothyroidism or an underactive thyroid. Hashimoto's thyroiditis is most common in women but also occurs in men and children without myositis. Signs and symptoms of an underactive thyroid include tiredness, cold intolerance, constipation, dry skin, poor concentration, and low heart rate, as well as hoarseness and swelling of the thyroid gland (goiter). An underactive thyroid can be detected by blood tests measuring thyroid hormone and TSH and treated by giving thyroid hormone in a small, tasteless pill, which is taken once a day. Children with uncomplicated JM can have some of the same symptoms as children with hypothyroidism, so your child's myositis doctor may want to review the results of the thyroid tests.

In rare cases the thyroid may be overactive, as seen in hyperthyroidism (e.g., Graves' disease). The signs and symptoms of an overactive thyroid include weight loss, fast heart rate, tremors, anxiety, poor sleep, diarrhea, mood swings, heat intolerance, and tiredness. To make the diagnosis of hyperthyroidism, the same hormones should be measured. In the case of an overactive thyroid, thyroid hormone production can be decreased in one of the following three ways: medications, surgical removal of the thyroid, and radioactive iodine. There are benefits and risks to each method. These should be weighed carefully as you and your physicians decide on the most appropriate treatment.

Key Points

- Active JM can inhibit growth. Corticosteroids can contribute to this poor growth. However, if the corticosteroids are used with disease-modifying medications and remission is achieved, long-term growth most likely will not be affected.

- Active JM and the medications used to treat JM can both delay puberty. Hormonal supplementation is available as needed to assist with puberty. However, more research is needed to determine whether this supplementation affects disease activity.

- Autoimmune thyroid disease, leading to an underactive or overactive gland, can coexist with the symptoms of JM.

- A pediatric endocrinologist or gynecologist can assist in determining whether your child has a disorder that results in hormone imbalances and in treating these conditions.

To Learn More

To find a specialist, see *Finding an Endocrinologist* in the *Finding a Doctor or Specialist* section of the *Resource Appendix*, specifically:

American Association of Clinical Endocrinologists

The Hormone Foundation

Lawson Wilkins Pediatric Endocrine Society

National Committee for Quality Assurance

Additional Information:

The Hormone Foundation, an affiliate of The Endrocrine Society. 8401 Connecticut Avenue, Suite 900, Chevy Chase MD 20815-5817; Phone: 800-467-6663 (HORMONE); Internet: www.hormone.org.

Resource for the public; promotes the prevention, treatment and cure of hormone-related conditions through public outreach, support, education, and advocacy.

Human Growth Foundation. 997 Glen Cove Avenue, Suite 5, Glen Head NY 11545; Phone: 800-451-6434; Internet: www.hgfound.org; Email: hgf1@hgfound.org.

Helps children and adults with disorders of growth and growth hormone through research, education, support, and advocacy; helps medical science to understand the process of growth better.

CHAPTER 21

Maintaining Flexibility: Joints and Other Considerations

Brian M. Feldman, MD, MSc, FRCPC, and Angelo Ravelli, MD

In this chapter...

We describe what we know about different joint problems that can occur in children with myositis and how to potentially treat them.

From the family's point of view...

"Our son began to have difficulty getting out of bed and complained of sore wrists. He avoided pushing on the palms of his hands, instead using the backs of his hands when playing on the floor. He was diagnosed with juvenile rheumatoid arthritis and began treatment with methotrexate and indomethacin, but his arthropathy continued to worsen. His range of motion was so limited that he couldn't reach to put on his shoes or wash his hair. Soon after, he was diagnosed with juvenile dermatomyositis and given oral prednisone and etanercept. It seemed his range of motion returned almost overnight."

What Types of Joint Problems Can Occur in Children with Juvenile Myositis?

The medical word for joint problems is arthropathy, which comes from two Greek words—"arthro" meaning "joint" and "pathy" meaning "to suffer." So arthropathy means "sickness of the joints." Arthritis means "inflammation of the joints," which can result in swelling, stiffness, and limitation of motion or pain of the joints. Arthritis is one form of arthropathy.

Children with myositis often have some form of arthropathy during their illness. These joint problems are part of the myositis illness, not a separate disease. Most often, when children have trouble with their joints, the problem is arthritis. Inflammation of the joints is similar to inflammation of the muscles. The symptoms of arthritis include swelling, heat, pain, and sometimes a decrease in function of the joint (you can't bend the joint as far, and the joint is stiff to move). The pain and stiffness that go along with arthritis are usually worst in the morning; the soreness sometimes improves during the day as the joints are stretched out a bit (Figure 21.1).

■ **Figure 21.1. (See color plate 14 on page 230.) A child with juvenile dermatomyositis who has arthritis in the finger joints of the hands.** Notice the swelling of the finger joints.

Another type of joint problem is called a contracture, which means that movement is limited because of muscle weakness or inflammation in the connective tissue. Think of contracture as a shortening of muscles and tendons, causing the joint to stay bent or to stiffen, so that the joint cannot be completely stretched out. Joint contractures in children with myositis are not really a joint problem. Instead, they result in limited joint movement due to muscle weakness or due to inflammation in the connective tissue surrounding the muscles. Consequently, full use of the joint may be lost. The presence of calcinosis across joints can result in contractures (see Figure 17.2 [color plate 13 on page 230]). Joint contractures can also be caused by calcium deposits in the muscle or around the joint. The nearby joints cannot fully open or close (the range of motion is limited compared to normal joints) because the calcium deposit prevents the joint from moving fully.

Some myositis patients have tenosynovitis, an inflammation of the tendons. Tenosynovitis usually occurs at the back of the wrists and can cause wrist pain.

Although it is very rare, it is possible for children to develop problems with the blood supply to the bones as a side effect of prednisone, causing part of the bone to die. This is called avascular necrosis. This rare side effect, when it does occur, sometimes affects the bones in the hip or the knee and can lead to joint pain and swelling that is not arthritis.

How Often Does Arthropathy Happen?

Most children with myositis have arthropathy at some point in their illness. In studies of a large population of JM patients treated at The Hospital for Sick Children in Toronto Canada, most of whom had juvenile dermatomyositis (JDM), 61% of the JM patients had at least some joint problems, although they were often short-lived. The joint problems were almost all due to arthritis (inflammation).

Significant joint contractures (as a separate problem from arthritis) occurred in 27% of children with JM. In almost 10% of these children, it was already present at the time of diagnosis. Experience with other children with JM suggests that joint contractures may be more frequent than in the patients from Toronto. Ankles, hips, elbows, shoulders, and wrists are most often involved with joint contractures. Joint contractures that are caused by muscle inflammation usually improve when the myositis is treated. Joint contractures resulting from muscle scarring or calcinosis require physical therapy exercises designed to stretch the joints and to extend their range of motion (see *Chapter 13, Rehabilitation of the Child with Myositis*).

We often see swelling of the knees in children with myositis who are taking prednisone (about 25% of the Toronto patients). This swelling is cool to the touch, and the child does not have pain and stiffness. It may be an effect of the prednisone treatment itself and not arthritis.

Which Children Develop Arthropathy?

Any child with myositis could develop arthropathy as part of the illness. In the Toronto patients, none of the five children with polymyositis developed arthropathy, although other centers have documented arthropathy in children with polymyositis. Children with amyopathic dermatomyositis or overlap myositis had the same frequency of arthropathy as those with JDM, with the majority of patients having a joint problem at some point during the illness.

It is difficult to predict who will and who will not develop arthropathy. We know that certain myositis-specific autoantibodies (MSAs) may go along with an increased chance of developing arthritis. Children who have anti-Jo1 and other anti-synthetase autoantibodies and those with anti-PM-Scl antibody frequently have arthritis as part of their illness. However, these MSAs are uncommon in children (see *Chapter 1, What Is Juvenile Myositis?* and *Chapter 6, Tests Your Child's Doctor Might Order*).

In the Toronto studies, girls were just as likely to have joint problems as boys. Children in all racial groups were equally affected. Those who had positive results of lab tests, such as the antinuclear antibody (ANA) or rheumatoid factor (RF) tests, were just as likely to get arthropathy as those with negative results. Other features of the myositis did not appear more often for a child who had arthropathy than for a child without joint problems. In summary, we have not identified any reliable clues as to who will develop arthropathy or not.

When Does Arthropathy Occur?

Arthropathy usually starts at about the same time that other problems with myositis begin. About half of the Toronto children had their joint problems identified within four months of their first myositis symptoms. It is possible, however, for the arthropathy to begin a long time (even a year or longer) before or after the other myositis symptoms. In a few children the myositis goes away completely (remission), leaving only the arthritis, which can persist for years.

Which Joints Does Arthropathy Affect?

When describing arthropathy, we often use the terms "pauciarticular," which means just a few joints, and "polyarticular," which means five or more joints. Most children with myositis (about two-thirds) have pauciarticular joint problems, usually arthritis. Most often, arthritis affects the knees, wrists, or both. Less commonly, children have polyarticular arthritis. These children frequently have swelling in the small joints (fingers and toes) as well as the larger joints (most commonly knees, wrists, elbows, and ankles). In overlap myositis the small joints of the hands are frequently involved. Children with the anti-synthetase autoantibodies usually have small joints (e.g., hands) involved. Children with PM-Scl autoantibodies can have small or large joints involved.

Does the Arthropathy Cause Joint Damage?

The most common type of arthritis in children *who do not have myositis* is called juvenile idiopathic arthritis (JIA). (Idiopathic means a disease arising from an unknown cause.) Over time this type of arthritis leads to damaged cartilage and bone near the joints that have the arthritis. This damage can be seen on X-rays and is usually permanent. In contrast, the arthritis that is part of myositis is usually not that form of arthritis. Children with myositis usually do *not* develop damage to the bones and cartilage and usually have normal X-rays. In the Toronto studies only two patients had subtle damage to the cartilage, and none had bone damage.

How Long Does the Arthropathy Last?

It is hard to know how long arthropathy lasts because it is different for each person. If the arthropathy is either arthritis or tenosynovitis, it almost always goes away when the myositis is treated. However, in some children the arthritis comes back when their myositis treatment is stopped or if the illness recurs or flares. Rarely do children develop arthritis that lasts for a long time. If the arthritis comes back after myositis treatment is stopped or tapered, then the arthritis itself will need to be treated.

How Is Arthropathy Treated?

The arthritis that comes with myositis is usually milder than idiopathic forms of arthritis and usually responds easily to treatment for the myositis. There are a few children, though, who require directed treatment for their arthritis in addition to medicines for their myositis. For children whose myositis no longer needs treatment but whose arthritis is troubling, standard arthritis treatments may be used. These treatments include:

- Medications (anti-inflammatory medications, methotrexate, prednisone, hydroxychloroquine, etanercept, and others)
- Local therapy (corticosteroid injections directly into the joint)
- Physical therapy for strengthening, pain relief, and increasing the stretch of the joint

If the arthropathy is from joint contractures, a physical therapist will often prescribe physical exercises that include stretching the joints (see *Chapter 13, Rehabilitation of the Child with Myositis*).

If the arthropathy is from avascular necrosis, it will often improve on its own. However, avascular necrosis can be painful, and children might need to be treated with nonsteroidal anti-inflammatory drugs or other pain medications. Avascular necrosis can sometimes be damaging to the bones and can require rapidly lowering the dose of prednisone and sometimes even surgery. Fortunately, this form of arthropathy is rare in children with myositis.

Key Points

- Arthropathy, particularly arthritis, is common in children with myositis. It usually is mild and does not cause joint damage.

- The treatments used for the myositis usually get rid of the arthritis, and if the arthritis comes back or requires specific treatment, it is usually easily treated with standard arthritis treatments.

- Joint contractures—limited movement of a joint—result from muscle and connective tissue inflammation or calcinosis. Contractures are treated with physiotherapy stretching exercises.

To Learn More

See the *Resource Appendix* for full contact information for the following organizations:

Arthritis Foundation (AF).

Disease center: types of juvenile arthritis. Available from: www.arthritis.org/conditions/DiseaseCenter/typesofJA.asp.

Types of juvenile rheumatic diseases, including arthritis and dermatomyositis, and related information for each one.

American Juvenile Arthritis Organization (AJAO).

About the AJAO. Available from: www.arthritis.org/communities/juvenile_arthritis/about_ajao.asp.

Activities, events, and useful information for children and families dealing with arthritis and rheumatic diseases.

Paediatric Rheumatology International Trials Organisation (PRINTO).

Juvenile idiopathic arthritis. Available from: www.printo.it/pediatric-rheumatology/information/UK/1.htm.

General information about the different types of juvenile arthritis, including symptoms, tests, and treatments.

Arthritis Society.

Childhood arthritis. Available from: www.arthritis.ca/types%20of%20arthritis/childhood.

General information about the different types of juvenile arthritis, including symptoms, tests, and treatments.

Additional Information:

Lehman TJA. *It's Not Just Growing Pains: A Guide to Childhood Muscle, Bone and Joint Pain, Rheumatic Diseases, and the Latest Treatments*. Oxford: Oxford University Press; 2004.

Reports in the Medical Literature

Ramanan AV, Feldman BM. Clinical features and outcomes of juvenile dermatomyositis and other childhood onset myositis syndromes. *Rheumatic Diseases Clinics of North America*. 2002 Nov;28(4):833–57.

Tse S, Lubelsky S, Gordon M, Al Mayouf SM, Babyn PS, Laxer RM, et al. The arthritis of inflammatory childhood myositis syndromes. *Journal of Rheumatology*. 2001 Jan;28(1):192–7.

CHAPTER 22

Taking Care of the Bones

Emily von Scheven, MD; Rolando Cimaz, MD;
and Kelly A. Rouster-Stevens, MD, PharmD

In this chapter...

We describe the way that bones become weak in children with juvenile myositis (JM), as well as some of the medications that can be used to prevent bones from breaking. One of the best ways of keeping bones healthy is to control the inflammation associated with JM with medicine and to take enough calcium and vitamin D.

From the family's point of view...

"We knew that older people need to be careful about their bones, but it wasn't until she developed back pain that we realized thin bones and fractures can be a problem for children with JM."

What Is Osteoporosis? The Importance of Bone Health During Childhood

Osteoporosis means porous bone and is characterized by low bone mass and structural deterioration of bone tissue. In other words, your bones "lose weight" and become weaker—breaking more often and becoming unable to support the muscles. Osteoporosis is often called the "silent disease" because bone loss occurs without symptoms. People might not know that they have osteoporosis until their bones become so weak that a sudden bump or fall causes one to break.

In a similar way to skin cells, which die and are replaced, bone is continuously being replenished and reformed, a process called remodeling. This occurs through a delicate balance between bone-forming cells (osteoblasts) and bone-resorbing cells (osteoclasts). Resorption is the process by which bone that is in place is broken down and absorbed back into the body. During childhood, and particularly during adolescence, in addition to getting longer, bones are becoming denser. This occurs because bone formation is greater than bone resorption. By our early twenties, in addition to reaching maximum height, we also reach maximum bone density, a state called "peak bone mass." After that, you do not gain more bone density. Thus, childhood and adolescence represent a critical window of opportunity regarding lifelong bone health. As you age, bone density is lost, so if you enter adulthood with insufficient bone mass, you are significantly more likely to develop fractures.

How Do You Get Osteoporosis?

Osteoporosis can result from either not enough bone formation or from too much bone resorption. To help bone formation, you need calcium and vitamin D. Calcium is the most abundant mineral found in bone and makes the bones strong. Vitamin D helps the calcium absorption in the stomach and intestines. The body can make some vitamin D, but sunlight is needed to make it work properly. Children with JM must be sure to get adequate amounts of calcium and vitamin D, either in their diet or as a nutritional supplement, because intestinal inflammation from JM as well as the steroid therapy can hinder the absorption of these nutrients, and the use of sunscreen might decrease natural vitamin D formation. Nevertheless, it is particularly important for individuals with juvenile dermatomyositis (JDM) to use a sunscreen greater than SPF 30 to prevent exposure to ultraviolet (UVB) light, which can make their JDM worse. Vitamin D can be measured in the blood to monitor for adequate stores in the body. However, monitoring blood levels of calcium is not reliable for evaluating total body calcium stores, for the body is driven to maintain a "good" level of calcium in the circulating blood—often at the cost of stealing it from the bones.

Another risk factor for osteoporosis is decreased physical activity. Researchers have found that calcium is removed from bones when you do not move much, and several studies have shown that exercises involving standing up can improve bone density. Weight-bearing exercises are those in which your bones have to support your body weight, so walking, jogging, and dancing are examples; it does not mean that you have to lift weights, although that can be helpful, too, later on in the recovery phase of the illness. Children with evidence of active myositis should concentrate on stretching exercises rather than exercises to "bulk up" the muscles. Consult with a doctor about how much exercise is safe for your child. Bed rest is not usually recommended for children with JM—for it is important to get them out of bed and standing up.

Specific factors increasing the chance that osteoporosis will develop in children with JM include inflammation, medications, and loss of muscle mass or bulk. Many children with inflammatory diseases have decreased bone density at the time of diagnosis, suggesting that the inflammation itself might cause osteoporosis. Inflammation in the muscle is associated with chemicals in the bloodstream that slow down new bone cell formation. Medications that we use to control the inflammation can exacerbate this problem. Corticosteroids (such as prednisone), the primary medication used to control inflammation, may be associated with decreased bone density, in part by blocking the absorption of calcium from the gastrointestinal tract—which is why vitamin D is important to act as a magnet to bring the calcium into the bloodstream from the gastrointestinal tract. However, the benefit of rapidly controlling the inflammation central to myositis far outweighs the risk of using corticosteroids. Finally, the reduced muscle mass in children with JDM may also contribute to osteoporosis because the muscle normally tugs on the bones as the child moves and increases her strength. If there is less "tug," the bone becomes weaker.

Bone fractures in children with osteoporosis are not uncommon; however, the exact risk is not yet known. Fractures can develop in the vertebral body of the backbone (spinal column) and can occur spontaneously without trauma. They can also occur in other bones, such as the arm and leg bones, usually after trauma such as falling. When fractures occur, treatment includes braces, casts, and/or surgery. Calcitonin nasal spray can decrease the bone pain associated with fracture.

How to Know If Your Child's Bones Are Healthy

Bone density can be measured through several methods. The most direct method is to biopsy the bone and examine it under a microscope; however, this is rarely necessary. Occasionally, when routine X-rays are obtained, radiologists comment that the bones appear thin in children with JM. However, routine X-rays are not a reliable method for diagnosing osteoporosis because they do not quantify the bone density. There are several methods, some of which use radiation, like X-rays, that can quantify the density of bone. All are safe and not painful. The most common methods to measure bone density include dual X-ray absorptiometry (DXA), computed tomography (CT) scan, and ultrasound. DXA is commonly used in clinical practice, and CT and ultrasound are more common in research. Because bone density is continuously changing during growth, a patient's bone density measure cannot be interpreted unless it is compared with that of a healthy person of the same age. Some doctors think that it should also be compared to somebody of similar ethnic background, gender, and height, as these factors can also influence bone density measurements. Once this comparison is made, a bone density measurement for a child is converted to a standardized score called a Z-score, in which a score of –2.5 is considered by many doctors to be an indicator of osteoporosis. Bone density measurements in adults are converted to a standardized score called a T-score.

The T-score is used to determine whether an adult has normal bone density (T-score above –1), reduced bone density (called osteopenia [T-score between –1 and –2.5]), or osteoporosis (T-score below –2.5). These categories have been determined by the World Health Organization (WHO) for adults, but similar categories have not been determined for children. Thus, the terms osteopenia and osteoporosis for children are generally used to describe bone health but do not specifically relate to the Z-score.

Until recently, measurement of bone density has not been applied much to children, although its use is rapidly growing. Not all facilities have the appropriate equipment and experience with children, but new machines and standards are being developed. Also, not all facilities have the ability to compare the result to a healthy child's measurement to calculate the Z-score for the child with JM. Another limitation of our knowledge is that physicians do not know exactly how a bone density measurement relates to an estimate of fracture risk. For example, is it a linear relationship or does the risk of fracture increase exponentially with reduced bone density? Doctors can determine that your child's bones are getting stronger or weaker by comparing her bone density measurement with the value for healthy children over time. Thus, despite several limitations, measuring bone density can be very useful. For this reason many physicians recommend a DXA for children who are receiving corticosteroid therapy. If the results are abnormal or the patient continues to be at risk for osteoporosis, the measurement should be done every six to twelve months, depending on the severity of JM inflammation and the response to therapy.

Finally, blood and urine tests are used occasionally to measure calcium and vitamin D stores and to evaluate the status of bone mineral metabolism in children with active inflammation who are taking corticosteroids. Not all centers have these tests, and the cost-effective value of the various specific tests of bone mineral metabolism remains to be established in children with JM.

How Can We Prevent Osteoporosis?

Osteoporosis can be prevented by identifying the known risk factors. The recommended dietary requirement for calcium in healthy children is 800–1200 mg/day (1200–1500 mg/day for adolescents and young adults). Calcium-rich foods, such as dairy products, calcium-fortified orange juice or apple juice, certain vegetables (e.g., cabbage and broccoli), and calcium-rich mineral water, are good sources (see Table 22.1 for a comparison of foods). To maximize calcium absorption, patients need to have sufficient vitamin D stores. Supplements of 400–800 units per day are usually recommended, depending on your child's weight. This amount (400 units) is obtained in a standard multivitamin or as a separate supplement. Even if your child with JM has calcifications, her bones may be at risk for fracture, and both vitamin D and a calcium-sufficient diet are needed. If your doctor agrees, weight-bearing exercise is encouraged. In contrast, although swimming is good for strengthening and improving joint range of motion, it does not enhance bone formation. A physical therapist can recommend exercises specifically for your child. Finally, patients with JM and their families should be aware that smoking and alcohol consumption lower peak bone mass.

Table 22.1. Comparison of sources of absorbable calcium with milk.

Food	Servings needed to equal 240 mL or 8 oz. milk
Milk	1.00
Beans	
Pinto	8.10
Red	9.70
White	3.90
Bok choy	2.30
Broccoli	4.50
Cheddar cheese	1.00
Cheese food	1.20
Chinese cabbage flower leaves	1.00
Chinese mustard greens	1.10
Chinese spinach	3.30
Fruit punch with calcium citrate malate	0.62
Kale	3.20
Spinach	16.30
Sweet potatoes	9.80
Rhubarb	9.50
Tofu with calcium	1.20
Yogurt	1.00

Modified from Weaver CM, Proulx WR, Heaney R. Choices for achieving adequate dietary calcium with a vegetarian diet. *American Journal of Clinical Nutrition.* 1999 Sep;70(3 Suppl):543S–548S. Review.

If Bone Density Is Low, How Is It Treated?

Although it is best to prevent childhood osteoporosis, if severe bone loss or fracture has occurred, drug treatment is sometimes recommended. At this time there aren't many studies of treatments for childhood osteoporosis. In general the underlying condition, degree of inflammation, child's age, level of maturation, and degree of osteoporosis must be considered before choosing a treatment (see Table 22.2).

The medicines used to treat osteoporosis can be divided into those that promote bone formation (anabolic) and those that decrease bone resorption. However, those two processes are tightly linked. Some medicines, such as growth hormone, have helped children with other diseases, but growth hormone is *not recommended* for JDM because there have been many cases in which the JDM was worsened by this therapy. Calcitonin is another hormone that is normally made by the body to

Table 22.2. Treatments for children with osteoporosis.

Agent	Class of drug	Advantages	Disadvantages
Calcium Carbonate and Citrate	Calcium	Necessary to maintain calcium stores	Elevated calcium in the urine and kidney stones
Ergocalciferol	Vitamin D	Necessary to absorb calcium	Only with overdose: calcium levels too high, weakness, headache
Calcitriol	Vitamin D	Active form, necessary if there is renal and liver failure	Only with overdose: calcium levels too high, weakness, headache
Calcitonin	Hormone	Builds bone density, useful for bone pain from fracture, comes as a nasal spray	Stuffiness, runny nose, rare allergic reaction
Alendronate	Bisphosphonate	Prevents bone breakdown, can take weekly	Irritation of the esophagus with heartburn
Pamidronate	Bisphosphonate	Prevents bone breakdown	Given intravenously, low calcium levels; infusion reaction with first infusion—increased fluid, elevated temperature, nausea
Fluoride is not used in kids	Mineral	Increases bone density	Builds poor bone, which results in increased fracture rate

promote bone formation. It is often used to treat the pain that immediately follows a fracture, but it is generally not used long-term for building bone density.

Of all the new medicines, bisphosphonates seem to be the most promising. Bisphosphonates are antiresorptive agents that slow the loss of bone from osteoporosis and restore bone density. Until recently, the use of bisphosphonates in children has been limited because of the possibility of adverse effects on the growing skeleton and because the drug is stored in the bones for many years. More recently, bisphosphonates have been shown to be safe, at least in the short term (i.e., adults taking the medicine for ten years), even in paediatric patients. Examples of bisphosphonates include alendronate (Fosamax), which can be taken orally; pamidronate (Aredia), which is given intravenously; and newer agents such as zolendronic acid (Zometa), which are very long-acting and can be administered every few months and in some cases even just once a year. If swallowing is impaired or if there is gastroesophageal reflux, risedronate (Actonel) might be useful. Side effects of medicines taken by mouth include stomach upset and low calcium levels. Intravenous preparations can cause fever, bone pain, intestinal symptoms, and changes of calcium level and other chemicals in the body. These adverse effects have been reported equally frequently in children and adults. When considering bisphosphonate therapy for children with JDM, your child's doctor should consider the potential irritation to the esophagus, which could be worse in someone who cannot adequately swallow the pill, such as a child with active JDM. Although bisphosphonates are being used more widely, they are not yet approved for use in very young children. Thus, they should be considered only when treating severe osteoporosis or in a research study. If your child develops jaw pain, report this to the doctor immediately.

Occasionally, adults with myositis receive bisphosphonate therapy at the start of corticosteroid treatment to prevent the development of osteoporosis. This strategy is highly controversial, particularly in children, where the development of osteoporosis cannot be predicted, and some individuals could be exposed to this medication unnecessarily.

Key Points

- Porous bone, or osteoporosis, occurs in children with JM but usually can be slowed down and repaired.

- Children who are weak often do not walk around as much, which also contributes to the osteoporosis.

- The state of bone health can be measured by a bone density scan (DXA), which may not be available for children in all geographic areas.

- Controlling the inflammation of JM will help prevent a decrease in bone density.

- Making sure that your child takes in enough calcium and vitamin D helps the bones heal.

To Learn More

Mayo Clinic.

Osteoporosis. Available from: www.mayoclinic.com.
>   Facts about the disease, signs and symptoms, diagnosis and screening, treatment, and self-care.

National Institutes of Health.

Osteoporosis and Related Bone Diseases—National Resource Center. Available at: www.osteo.org.

Information on metabolic bone diseases such as osteoporosis and Paget's Disease.

National Institutes of Health.

Why Milk Matters Now for Children and Teens. Available at: www.nichd.nih.gov/milk/milk.htm.

Recommendations for calcium and milk consumption for children and adolescents.

National Library of Medicine (NLM).

Osteoporosis. Available at: www.nlm.nih.gov/medlineplus/osteoporosis.html.

Links to online information on osteoporosis, calcium, and bone density from NLM's MedlinePlus database.

Organizations:

National Osteoporosis Foundation. 1232 22nd Street NW, Washington DC 20037-1292; Phone: 202-223-2226; Internet: www.nof.org.

Information on osteoporosis and its treatments, including fast facts, bone basics, risks, and prevention.

International Osteoporosis Foundation. 73, cours Albert-Thomas 69447, Lyon Cedex 03 France; Phone: 33-472-91-41-77; Internet: www.osteofound.org; Email: info@osteofound.org.

Supports national osteoporosis societies to increase the awareness, understanding, and prevention of the disease worldwide.

Reports in the Medical Literature

American College of Rheumatology Task Force on Osteoporosis Guidelines. Recommendations for the prevention and treatment of glucocorticoid-induced osteoporosis. *Arthritis and Rheumatism.* 1996 Nov;39(11):1791–1801. Available online at: www.rheumatology.org/publications/guidelines/osteo/osteo.asp.

Cassidy JT, Langman CB, Allen SH, Hillman LS. Bone mineral metabolism in children with juvenile rheumatoid arthritis. *Pediatric Clinics of North America.* 1995 Oct;42(5):1017–33.

Cimaz R. Osteoporosis in childhood rheumatic diseases: prevention and therapy. *Best Practice and Research. Clinical Rheumatology.* 2002 Jul;16(3):397–409.

Stewart WA, Acott PD, Salisbury SR, Lang BA. Bone mineral density in juvenile dermatomyositis: assessment using dual X-ray absorptiometry. *Arthritis and Rheumatism.* 2003 Aug;48(8):2294–8.

CHAPTER 23

Tune to Your Voice

Beth Solomon, MS, CCC-SLP

In this chapter...

We discuss the voice problems that develop in some children with myositis, how they are detected, and how they can be treated.

From the family's point of view...

"I noticed my child's voice becoming more hoarse and raspy about a month before her diagnosis. It continued to sound rough off and on during her first two years of treatment, but now after three years these changes are less frequent. It doesn't seem to coincide with her blood test results but instead occurs more when she's tired."

What Are the Common Childhood Voice Problems?

Voice disorders can be caused by many different medical and psychological issues, which often affect a child's self-perception and mental and social well-being. It is estimated that about one million children in the United States have voice disorders.

Many children with juvenile myositis (JM) often have difficulties performing daily activities, such as getting dressed, eating, and participating in sports. Although vocal difficulties are not usually the first thing children, parents, or doctors focus on, they can be an important concern in children with myositis.

The medical term for symptoms involving voice problems is dysphonia. The actual number of children with myositis who have problems with their voices is not known. However, experts in this area suspect that vocal symptoms are more common than is generally recognized. Dysphonia often is associated with other symptoms, such as muscle weakness, shortness of breath, and difficulty swallowing. Voice alterations in children with JM include hoarseness, vocal straining, low and loud voices. Many parents report that the child's voice sounds "weak." The severity of voice symptoms seems to vary and can be influenced by an individual's overall endurance and performance level.

How Is Sound Produced?

To understand the mechanisms of voice production, you must first understand the underlying structural engine and its source of fuel. The parts of the body used in the process of speaking are shown in Figure 23.1. The engine is the voice box (larynx), which is the primary vibratory mechanism. Inhaled and exhaled air is the fuel that powers the larynx. The process begins with respiration, that is, inhalation (breath in) and exhalation (breath out). Sound is produced by air exhaled from the lungs. This air travels from the lungs through the windpipe (trachea) and causes the vocal cords, which are muscular elastic membranes housed within the voice box (larynx), to vibrate like a rubber band or guitar string that has been plucked. The vocal cords are always open at least a little bit during breathing, but they can be partially closed to change the voice. The quality and strength of an individual's voice is determined by how hard you breathe out combined with how much the vocal cords vibrate.

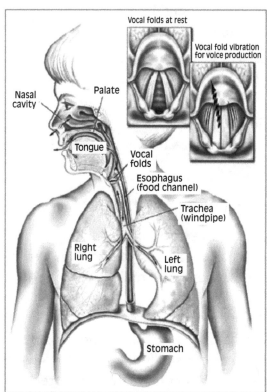

■ **Figure 23.1. Parts of the upper respiratory tract and larynx.**

How Do I Know Whether My Child Has Voice Problems?

The most common finding in children with active myositis is a nasal quality to their speech; however, in a large study of children with myositis, parents and caregivers reported a variety of vocal symptoms (Table 23.1). Often, children with myositis who have trouble speaking talk less frequently. They might use short phrases rather than complete complex sentences. Tiredness can also reduce a child's desire to talk.

Table 23.1. Voice problems that parents notice in children with myositis.

- Loud voice
- Hoarse voice
- Soft voice
- Low pitch
- Strained voice

- Breathy voice
- Whispered voice
- Harsh voice
- Wet, gurgly voice
- Nasal speech

How Do Healthcare Providers Recognize Voice Problems?

Usually a parent or teacher is the first person to notice a change in a child's voice. When a teacher notifies the parents, they often then contact their child's doctor. Sometimes your doctor will need to work with specialists to evaluate and treat a child's voice problems. These specialists might include otolaryngologists (ear, nose, and throat doctors), pulmonologists (lung doctors), gastroenterologists (intestinal tract doctors), and speech-language pathologists (specialists in voice and language problems). If your child's doctor doesn't know any specialists in your local community, then you can contact professional organizations, such as those listed at the end of the chapter.

Vocal changes lasting longer than two weeks should be assessed by a doctor to determine if there is a voice disorder. Typically, the assessment is geared toward providing the maximal amount of information while minimizing anxiety and fear. A number of approaches are frequently used in evaluating voice problems:

- *Comprehensive history:* A complete assessment of the possible contributors (medical, environmental, behavioral) affecting voice production, including the timing and severity of the symptoms and other factors that might maintain the dysphonia, is done.

- *Examination:* Examination of the head and neck are critical elements to the diagnosis of a voice disorder. Looking at the larynx is frequently the most useful portion of the assessment and is done by an ear, nose, and throat doctor. This can be done by using a tiny mirror inserted into the child's mouth or by using a procedure called flexible nasendoscopy. For this procedure a small flexible tube with a scope at the end is inserted through the nose after it has been numbed with an anesthetic. Children will frequently have mild complaints with both the mirror examination and the nasendoscopy. These are short tests usually lasting only ten to fifteen minutes. With the mirror assessment, children might feel a gagging sensation occasionally. Children occasionally will complain of a bitter taste when the topical anesthetic is applied for the nasendoscopy. When the doctor can see the larynx and true vocal fold structures clearly, he or she can determine the specific problem in the vocal cords that is causing the voice to change. These can include inflammation, vocal nodules, polyps (two different types of growth on the vocal cords that can result in hoarseness), or possible reflux.

- *Voice evaluation:* The speech-language pathologist routinely evaluates the nature and quality of the voice and how it changes over time. The comprehensive assessment includes a day-to-day history of vocal function, evaluation of voice use and misuse, perceptual voice ratings, and sophisticated assessments of a child's habitual vocal pitch and hoarseness. Other vocal qualities, including breathiness, loudness levels, and nasality, are also assessed.

- *Swallowing assessment:* The esophagus (see Figure 23.1) is examined to determine whether reflux (spilling of stomach contents into the esophagus), which might irritate the vocal cords, is causing the hoarseness or other dysphonic symptoms. This assessment is done with a barium swallow or other tests (see *Chapter 18, Swallowing and Other Digestive Problems*).

- *Respiratory assessment:* Pulmonary function testing and chest X-rays are often done to assess respiratory function and problems (see *Chapter 24, When Children Have Difficulty Breathing*).

What Laryngeal Problems Are Associated with Myositis?

Structural problems of the larynx are often found in children with myositis. The following are common laryngeal problems found in children with myositis, which can require evaluation by a speech pathologist:

Laryngitis is inflammation (swelling) of the laryngeal muscles and cartilages. Laryngitis is most frequently caused by respiratory infections from bacteria or viruses. The major symptom of laryngitis is a hoarse voice, which sounds raspy or deeper than normal, but this is usually temporary and improves in a few days to weeks. Often a child is only able to whisper and may be without a voice entirely. Other causes of laryngitis include straining and overuse of the voice from prolonged periods of talking or shouting.

Vocal fold nodules and *polyps* are different kinds of bumps on the vocal cords mainly caused by vocal abuse or misuse. Vocal nodules are callous-like formations that typically occur on the front third of the true vocal folds and are responsible for most long-term hoarseness in children. Polyps are similar to, but softer than, nodules. They can develop on one or both vocal folds and often persist.

Laryngopharyngeal reflux is caused by the backwash of stomach contents (typically a combination of food and acid) into the throat. In this condition direct exposure of the laryngeal tissue to the reflux causes redness and swelling in the larynx. Many adults have gastroesophageal reflux disease (GERD) also known as acid reflux disease; however, laryngopharyngeal reflux disease differs from GERD in that it lacks the heartburn symptoms (burning sensation and discomfort in the mid-esophageal region). The most common symptoms of laryngopharyngeal reflux disease are intermittent hoarseness, chronic throat clearing, and bad breath.

This condition can occur at the beginning of the illness as well as with JM flares and can be more severe in families with a history of GERD.

How Are Voice Problems Treated?

Treatment of voice problems in children with JM typically falls into two major categories: medical treatment and voice therapy. Medical treatment is usually used when acid reflux is present. The most common medicines used to decrease acid and help the reflux are ranitidine (Zantac) and omeprazole (Prilosec). In addition to these medicines, doctors recommend dietary changes, such as eating fewer acidic foods (for example, chocolate, tomatoes, and oranges) and fatty foods. People with acid reflux are also advised to eat a larger meal in the middle of the day and a lighter meal in the evening. It is also helpful to raise the head of the bed to decrease the possible reflux while children are sleeping. Occasionally, medications such as mucous-thinning agents are given to decrease the thickness and ease the flow of oral and nasal secretions.

Vocal cord nodules and polyps are often treated with voice therapy offered by a speech-language pathologist. Surgery to remove the nodules or polyps is rarely recommended in children for two reasons: 1) when the polyp is removed, it usually comes back because of persistent vocal behaviors; and 2) often the problem can be treated with voice therapy. Furthermore, surgery can cause subtle scarring of the true vocal folds, which can alter the voice quality permanently.

Voice therapy is often recommended for children with voice problems. Although speech-language pathologists try voice therapy in many children, its success can be variable, as children might not consider the voice problem serious. Usually adults, such as parents, caregivers, or teachers, are most bothered by the child's voice problems and are the ones who want to treat it.

Speech pathologists try to design an appropriate individual program to meet the specific needs of the child and the family. First, they identify factors that contribute to the dysphonia. These typically include patterns of vocal abuse and misuse. To ensure vocal change, the program incorporates improved vocal behaviors into a child's daily activities (see Table 23.2). For example, the child is told not to yell or shout and is complimented when she does not. The success of voice therapy often involves the use of a behavior modification program (that is, a behavior charting system with rewards given if the desired behavior is achieved).

Voice therapy should also teach the correct use and coordination of breath support during voice production. Strategies for integrating continuous breath and voice production are easily taught and established as daily routines with children. These strategies also help reduce the vocal strain and demands to the larynx resulting from trying to speak without using enough exhaled air.

Children should begin therapy by themselves, without the parent or guardian, so the therapist can work one-on-one with the child and address her specific needs.

Table 23.2. Example of a chart that can be used by parents or teachers to monitor desired vocal activities in a child with voice problems.

Vocal behavior	Days of the week with number of times behavior occurred						
	SUN	MON	TUES	WED	THUR	FRI	SAT
No yelling or shouting							
No throat clearing							
Avoid character voices							
No talking over television or electronic devices							
Increase hydration (Water intake: 8 glasses per day)							

Parents and guardians should be involved in their child's voice therapy at home to help with the treatments. Once the therapeutic goals are met, a child should have occasional checkups to make sure she continues the behaviors learned in therapy. Voice therapy usually lasts six to eight weeks, with reevaluation of a child's and family's progress at that time. Additional therapy and/or monitoring may be needed depending on the seriousness of the problem and associated factors.

In summary, hoarseness, soft speech, a scratchy voice, and other voice problems develop in some children with myositis, but in most cases they can be resolved with proper evaluation and treatment.

Key Points

- Voice is produced in a well-organized and highly sophisticated coordination of breathing and laryngeal (vocal cord) movements that are often affected by inflammation and tiredness.

- A team of professionals, including a speech-language pathologist and otolaryngologist, should evaluate voice disorders in a child with JM if voice problems last longer than two weeks.

- Evaluation of voice problems may include looking at the larynx along with assessment of voice production, respiration, and swallowing.

- Treatment of voice problems includes medicines in combination with voice therapy.

- Parents and other caregivers should be active participants in a child's voice therapy program to ensure incorporation of behavior modification techniques and vocal strategies into day-to-day activities.

- Most voice problems in children with myositis are resolved with proper evaluation and treatment.

To Learn More

To find a specialist, see *Finding a Specialist for Other Complications (Voice)* in the *Finding a Doctor or Specialist* section of the *Resource Appendix*, specifically:

American Academy of Otolaryngology and Head and Neck Surgery

American Speech-Language-Hearing Association (ASHA)

Voice Foundation

Additional Information:

Voice Foundation. 1721 Pine Street, Philadelphia PA 19103; Phone: 215-735-7999; Internet: www.voicefoundation.org; Email: office@voicefoundation.org.

Dedicated to solving voice problems. Funds research, promotes public education, and raises the professional level of voice care. Provides information on the different types of voice issues, various specialists, resources, fundraisers, and events.

Reports in the Medical Literature

Boone DR. *Is your voice telling on you?: how to find and use your natural voice.* San Diego: Singular Publishing, 1991:1–17.

McMurray JS. Disorders of phonation in children. *Pediatric Clinics of North America.* 2003 April;50(2):363–80.

McMurray JS. Medical and surgical treatment of pediatric dysphonia. *Otolaryngologic Clinics of North America.* 2000 Oct;33(5):1111–26.

Sonies BC. Evaluation and treatment of speech and swallowing disorders associated with myopathies. *Current Opinion in Rheumatology.* 1997 Nov;9(6):486–95.

CHAPTER 24

When Children Have Difficulty Breathing

Fernanda Falcini, MD; Susanna A. McColley, MD; and Rolando Cimaz, MD

In this chapter...

We discuss the reasons why children with myositis sometimes develop breathing problems, how we diagnose them, and what can be done to treat them.

From the family's point of view...

"Our daughter started having trouble breathing when running, especially up and down stairs. It could have been her extra weight from steroids, but we decided to see a pulmonary specialist. The specialist thought her breathing problems were due to weakness of her rib cage muscles, and we were relieved to know he thought they would improve as her myositis responded to treatment."

Why Do Children with Myositis Develop Breathing Problems?

Difficulty breathing or shortness of breath in children with myositis can occur for different reasons and is potentially serious. It can be caused by weakness of the muscles that move air into and out of the lungs or by problems inside the lungs that can block air from getting to the bloodstream. Breathing problems have been carefully studied in adults with myositis but are not as well researched in children with myositis. Almost half the adults with myositis develop short- or long-term lung problems during the first few years of their illness. Recent studies in children suggest that the problem may be more common than previously thought. Children with breathing difficulty are often referred to a specialist in lung problems called a pulmonologist; a pediatric pulmonologist is a lung specialist for children.

Difficulty breathing or shortness of breath in children with myositis can be due to different causes. Shortness of breath after physical activity is a potentially serious finding. It can be due to lung impairment, to involvement of the heart, which is rarely affected in juvenile myositis, or even to deconditioning of the muscles. Sometimes, lung problems may be found by chest X-rays or breathing tests in persons with myositis who are not aware that they have any lung problems.

Chest Wall Weakness

The respiratory muscles, which include muscles of the diaphragm (the muscle just below the lungs, which separates them from the digestive system) and muscles between the ribs, are important for breathing. These muscles can become weak because of the myositis itself, as a result of the use of corticosteroids to treat the myositis or from lack of exercise of these muscles. It can be difficult to determine the cause of respiratory muscle weakness, but evaluating the general level of myositis disease activity can sometimes help (see *Chapter 10, Charting Your Child's Progress*). Because respiratory muscle weakness can prevent secretions in the lungs from being coughed up, these secretions can sometimes remain in the lungs too long, become infected, and require treatment with antibiotics.

Problems in the Lungs Themselves

Another cause of breathing problems in children with myositis is inflammation in the lungs. In interstitial lung disease the lung tissue becomes inflamed, which can lead to a scarring of the lungs, called pulmonary fibrosis. The lungs can become scarred after the inflammation is reduced, just like in other body tissues. For example, in the skin, after inflammation has gone down, the skin that was affected can scar and remain rougher and less flexible than unaffected skin. This same process can happen in the lungs. These processes of lung inflammation and scarring can affect the gas-exchanging areas of the lung where oxygen from the air enters the bloodstream.

Symptoms of interstitial lung disease include shortness of breath (even at rest) and cough, which is lasting and may worsen over time. Interstitial pulmonary fibrosis is often associated with the presence of particular autoantibodies called anti-PM/Scl autoantibodies and antisynthetase autoantibodies.

Other Causes of Breathing Problems

When the swallowing muscles of the throat and swallowing tube (esophagus) become weak and lose their coordination, it causes a complication called pharyngeal dysmotility or dysphagia. Weakness of the swallowing muscles can cause food or liquid to enter the lungs during swallowing (i.e., go down the wrong throat), causing choking or aspiration pneumonia.

How Do Doctors Identify Lung Problems?

First, the doctor will listen to your child's lungs and see how short of breath she is. Then your doctor might order some tests to determine whether lung problems are present. These tests will not be done on all children, and your child's doctor will decide whether and when they should be done. It can be difficult to know whether your child has lung problems because not all children with lung problems complain of problems breathing. In a small group of children that was carefully studied, about half of the children with myositis had lung problems that were detected by changes in some lung function tests but were not noticed by the children, their families, or their doctors. Children who have difficulty breathing should have a thorough evaluation with several of the tests described below.

Breathing tests, also called pulmonary function tests, are useful for evaluating children who have persistent breathing problems. The most common reasons to have a pulmonary function test are persistent or worsening shortness of breath. These tests are done by asking your child to breathe as hard as possible in and out of a tube connected to a machine. The machine can measure many things, including the volume of air in the chest (lung volume measurement), the maximum volume of gas that can be exhaled from the lungs during a relaxed breath (slow vital capacity) or during a forced breath (forced vital capacity), the ability of the blood vessels in the lung to put the oxygen and other gases in the air you breathe into the blood within the lungs (diffusing capacity for carbon monoxide or transfer factor), and other aspects of lung function. Breathing tests might not be done in children younger than six to eight years old because they require a lot of effort and attention. When children are in the early stage of the illness, they may be too weak to have the test done properly.

A person with normal breathing tests will have lung volumes and air flow rates within the normal range for people their age, ethnicity, gender, and height. If the results are below normal, it is likely that your child has a restrictive disorder. A restrictive disorder is one caused by stiffness of the lung tissue (for example, from scarring) or by weakness of the chest muscles, both of which cause the lungs to be smaller. Restrictive pulmonary defects are common abnormalities in adult and juvenile myositis (JM).

The chest X-ray is useful in the diagnosis of pneumonia. In an X-ray, which is a picture of your child's lungs and rib cage, the lungs are not visible unless there is interstitial lung disease, aspiration, or pneumonia from another cause. To tell whether a patient has interstitial lung disease, more advanced X-ray techniques, such as computed tomography (CT) scans, are needed. CT scans can detect inflammation scarring in lung tissue so that interstitial lung disease can be recognized and appropriate treatment can be instituted.

How Can We Treat the Breathing Problems of Children with Myositis?

Breathing problems can be treated by exercises that can help strengthen the breathing muscles and by medicines to block the inflammation, which can be causing some of the problems in the lungs. Your child's healthcare team, including the pulmonologist, can advise you and your child on the types of breathing exercises and when they should be done. Many of the medicines used for the other symptoms of JM are also useful for treating the lung problems. In case of severe, short-term shortness of breath caused by underlying myositis activity (as in a flare), pulses (boluses) of intravenous corticosteroids (methylprednisolone), sometimes at very high doses, can be life saving. Other medications might be used (such as cyclosporine and/or methotrexate) in addition to treatment with corticosteroids.

Interstitial lung disease is often treated with cyclophosphamide (Cytoxan), cyclosporine (also called cyclosporine A, Sandimmune, Neoral, SangCya, GenGraf), or other potent immunosuppressants. More information, including the side effects of the different drugs used to treat myositis, can be found in *Chapter 12, Possible Medicines During the Course.*

If your child has swallowing problems, your doctors should be sure that your child is not at risk of swallowing food the wrong way so that it ends up in the airways. If that happens and causes pneumonia, then oxygen, respiratory care, and antibiotic treatment should be administered promptly.

What Will Happen in the Long Term?

Most children with chest wall muscle weakness recover full breathing function as they recover from the myositis. However, lung involvement that leads to progressive shortness of breath can be severe. Interstitial lung disease has a variable outcome but is generally serious. It should be treated aggressively and followed closely under the care not only of your child's JM doctor but also a lung specialist or pulmonologist.

Key Points

- Shortness of breath in children with myositis can be caused by weakness of the respiratory muscles from myositis or corticosteroids or from inflammation or infection of the lungs.

- For children with unexplained shortness of breath or coughing, a thorough evaluation is needed and includes tests such as chest X-rays, breathing tests (pulmonary function tests), and computed tomography (CT) scans, which can help determine the cause of the breathing problem.

- If a child is choking on food, she should immediately seek medical attention. There is a risk that the food can be swallowed incorrectly and end up in the lungs, causing pneumonia.

- Treatment for breathing problems in children with myositis depends on the cause, but many problems will respond to breathing exercises designed to strengthen the breathing muscles and corticosteroids and other medicines used to treat the myositis.

To Learn More

COPD International.

Living with Dyspnea—Four Ways to Breathe Easier. Available at: www.copd-international.com/Library/dyspnea.htm.

A patient information publication.

American Lung Association. 61 Broadway, 6th Floor, New York NY 10006; Phone: 800-LUNGUSA; Internet: www.lungusa.org.

The oldest voluntary health organization in the United States, with a national office and constituent and affiliate associations around the country. Aims to prevent lung disease and promote lung health through research, educational, professional, advocacy, and outreach programs. Its web site contains information on the anatomy of the lung, various lung diseases and how to cope; current stories regarding lung health; and more.

Reports in the Medical Literature

Cerveri I, Bruschi C, Ravelli A, Zoia MC, Fanfulla F, Zonta L, Pellegrini G, Martini A. Pulmonary function in childhood connective tissue diseases. *European Respiratory Journal.* 1992 Jun; 5(6):733–8.

Kobayashi I, Yamada M, Takahashi Y, Kawamura N, Okano M, Sakiyama Y, Kobayashi K. Interstitial lung disease associated with juvenile dermatomyositis: clinical features and efficacy of cyclosporin A. *Rheumatology (Oxford).* 2003 Feb;42(2):371–4.

Trapani S, Camicittoli G, Vierucci A, Pistolesi M, Falcini F. Pulmonary involvement in juvenile dermatomyositis: a two-year longitudinal study. *Rheumatology (Oxford).* 2001 Feb;40(2):216–20.

CHAPTER 25

Attention to Sugar and Fat Metabolism

Jean-Pierre Chanoine, MD, PhD, and Barbara S. Adams, MD

In this chapter...

We describe how your child with myositis might develop elevated blood levels of sugar (glucose), insulin (a hormone that helps process blood sugar), or lipids. In some children, these problems are mild and get better as the inflammation quiets down. In other children with myositis, who have symptoms such as intense hunger or thirst or greater abnormalities on the blood testing, specific treatments under the care of an endocrinologist may be needed.

From the family's point of view...

"Members on both sides of our family have been told to watch our diet and our weight and to try to lower our cholesterol. When a couple of our family members did in fact develop diabetes, I really began to worry because I thought the prednisone that our daughter had to take for her JM might increase her chances of developing diabetes herself. With this in mind, the doctors continued to monitor her blood tests for any signs of a problem, and all of us more diligently stuck to a healthier diet."

In order for your body to work, it needs energy. You get different forms of energy from food, which your body stores in fat cells. In juvenile myositis (JM) problems sometimes develop in the way your child's body processes or metabolizes the energy from food and stored energy.

When you eat foods high in complex sugars (such as bread, pasta, or potatoes) or more simple sugars (such as candy, soft drinks, or juice), they are broken down in your stomach and intestine and turned into glucose. If you eat a big meal, afterward you will have a high blood glucose level. Your body uses glucose as fuel for muscles and brain function. This fuel is transported from your intestines to your muscles through the bloodstream.

In order for the glucose to get inside your muscles to be used as fuel, it needs insulin. Insulin is a hormone produced by the pancreas, which facilitates the transfer of glucose into the muscles. Your pancreas makes more insulin if your blood glucose levels are high. Insulin has another function: It protects your stored energy, i.e. your fat cells. It stops the fat cells from breaking down and releasing their contents, called lipids, into your bloodstream. Two well-known lipids are cholesterol and triglycerides (Figure 25.1).

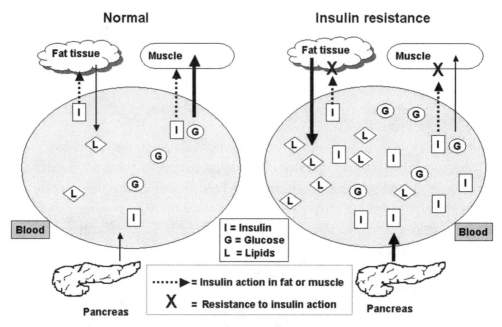

■ Figure 25.1. Blood insulin, glucose, and lipid levels in normal individuals (left panel) and in patients with juvenile myositis who have insulin resistance (right panel).

Dashed arrows reflect the *action* of insulin on fat or muscle. Plain arrows reflect the *transfer* of insulin from pancreas to blood, of glucose from blood to muscle, or of lipids from fat tissue to blood.

Insulin is made by the pancreas. In normal individuals insulin action stimulates glucose entry in muscle where it can be used as fuel. Insulin action also prevents breakdown of the lipids stored in fat tissue. In patients with juvenile myositis and insulin resistance, insulin action is impaired and despite the production of more insulin by the pancreas, less glucose enters the muscle and more fat is broken down. This can lead to diabetes and high blood lipids.

Some children with myositis develop problems with their glucose levels, lipid levels, or insulin levels. For example, in some children with myositis, the muscle and fat cells become less sensitive to the effects of insulin. This means that more insulin is needed to move glucose from the blood into muscle cells, and more insulin is also needed to keep the fat stores from breaking down. This condition is called insulin resistance. When a child with myositis becomes insulin resistant, the pancreas pumps more insulin into the blood to try to keep the blood levels of glucose and lipids normal and steady.

When insulin resistance is severe, the pancreas cannot make enough insulin to keep moving glucose into muscle cells or to protect the fat stores from breaking down. As a result, the blood glucose level rises, which can cause increased urination or thirst. These are the major symptoms of diabetes, or glucose intolerance. Other symptoms of diabetes include tiredness, weight loss, changes in vision, or general feelings of illness (malaise).

Some children with myositis have high levels of lipids in the blood, called hyperlipidemia. At first, high levels of lipids in the blood do not cause any symptoms, but if lipid levels stay high for a long time, health problems, such as high blood pressure, heart problems due to high blood pressure, and atherosclerosis (partial clogging of the arteries with material containing lipids, sometimes known as "hardening of the arteries") can develop.

Why Do Some Children with Myositis Have Insulin Resistance and Hyperlipidemia?

Children who have a longer course of active myositis or more calcinosis are more likely to have insulin resistance. However, no one knows exactly why high insulin levels (insulin resistance) and high levels of lipids in the blood (hyperlipidemia) are more common in children with myositis, even before their myositis has been treated with medication. It is possible that inflammation in the muscle changes the way insulin works with the muscle cells, so that more insulin is needed to move the glucose into the muscle. In addition, some medicines that are used to reduce the muscle inflammation, especially prednisone or cyclosporine, can bring on insulin resistance and high blood lipids or make these problems worse. If your family has a history of diabetes, this could make your child more likely to develop insulin resistance. You can see that your child's doctor must balance all these issues when deciding which medicines will best treat your child's myositis.

How Can Your Child's Doctor Tell Whether Your Child Has Insulin Resistance or Hyperlipidemia?

Your child's myositis doctor might ask whether members of your close family have diabetes or heart disease (including atherosclerosis). If so, your child could be more prone to high levels of glucose or lipids in the blood. Your child's myositis doctor might also look for signs of insulin resistance, such as extra dark areas of skin that may also be thickened, especially around the neck and in the armpits. These skin changes are called acanthosis nigricans (Figure 25.2). There is no treatment for the skin changes alone, but treating the insulin resistance will cause acanthosis nigricans to lessen or disappear. Insulin resistance can also cause high blood pressure or, very rarely, growth of coarse, dark body hair, especially noticeable in girls.

■ **Figure 25.2. (Color plate 15 on page 230.) Acanthosis nigricans.**
Note the pigmentation and the thickening of the skin at the back of the neck. In young individuals, acanthosis nigricans mostly reflects the existence of elevated blood levels of insulin and of insulin resistance. *Photo courtesy of Dr. H. Tildesley, Vancouver Canada.*

No matter what symptoms or signs your child may have, blood tests are the only way to tell whether insulin resistance, diabetes, or hyperlipidemia is present. Your child's doctor will have your child's blood tested in the morning after not having eaten for eight to twelve hours, in order to check fasting levels of glucose and lipids, including cholesterol and triglycerides. Testing the blood after your child has not eaten for a while allows the glucose, insulin, and lipid levels to be checked when they are not fluctuating from food intake. If you eat or drink anything other than water before they are checked, the levels may be artificially high and will be inaccurate. Fasting blood glucose and lipid levels have been well studied in children, so we know what is normal for children of different ages.

If your child's blood glucose levels are too high, the doctor may keep track of these levels on a regular basis. If the levels are much higher than in healthy children of the same age, your child's doctor may order a special test called a glucose tolerance test. In this test, blood glucose levels are measured just before and two hours after drinking a glass of very sweet sugar solution. This test measures how well your body processes glucose and how quickly it can make enough insulin. It helps your child's doctor determine whether your child has diabetes.

Some doctors think that JM patients with a family history of diabetes, hyperlipidemia, or significant heart disease (including high blood pressure) should have their blood tested regularly because they could have a greater chance of developing these problems. However, we do not yet have any scientific studies that prove this to be true. Doctors generally agree that children with myositis who have symptoms that could be the result of insulin resistance or hyperglycemia, (especially high blood pressure, frequent urination and thirst, or acanthosis nigricans) should have special testing of their blood to look for high levels of insulin, glucose, and lipids.

Children with insulin resistance and other problems related to how the body deals with sugars and fats should be seen and treated by an endocrinologist or a diabetologist. These are doctors who have special training in caring for diseases of the organs that make hormones. These doctors know a great deal about how the body handles sugars and fats. Some even specialize in the care of children with these problems. Your child's myositis doctor may be able to refer your child to a pediatric or adult endocrinologist/diabetologist. You can choose a specialist doctor from listings of members of groups like the American Association of Clinical Endocrinologists, The Hormone Foundation, the Lawson Wilkins Pediatric Endocrine Society, or the National Committee for Quality Assurance. Information to patients is also available on the web sites of the Endocrine Society and the American Diabetes Association. See *To Learn More* at the end of this chapter.

How Is Insulin Resistance Treated?

Children with myositis and insulin resistance rarely get full-blown diabetes. Diabetes is usually mild in children with JM, and it goes away on its own over time. When insulin resistance is not severe or lasts only for a short time (weeks to months), treatment might not be required. However, your child's doctor might re-check the level of blood glucose during follow-up visits. The first step in treating insulin resistance is to have your child increase her physical activity and eat a healthy diet similar to a diabetic diet, which contains more complex sugars (pasta, bread) and more fibers (vegetables, cereals). Your child's doctor and nutritionist will give you diet and exercise advice that best fits your child's needs. It can be difficult for children and teenagers with active myositis to increase their level of activity because their muscles are not strong enough for the amount of exercise needed to decrease insulin resistance.

When insulin resistance is caused by a medication, such as prednisone or cyclosporine, your child's myositis doctor may try to decrease the dose of that medicine if possible. When insulin resistance is caused by a medicine, it is usually reversible. However, it is not always possible to discontinue a medication such as prednisone if the myositis is active. In addition, prednisone should never be stopped abruptly. Therefore, another approach is to add a different medicine—one that does not cause insulin resistance—to control the muscle inflammation, so that the prednisone or cyclosporine can be reduced more quickly. Insulin resistance increases when the dose of prednisone increases. The amount of corticosteroid medication (such as prednisone) in the body is highest when these medications are given by mouth or intravenously. If your child uses corticosteroid skin cream alone, that is not likely to reach the high levels of high-dose oral or intravenous corticosteroids and is unlikely to affect insulin resistance.

If diabetes develops, then medicines can be prescribed along with diet and exercise to improve the action of insulin and decrease insulin resistance. These medicines include metformin (Glucophage, Glucovance) and a family of drugs called thiazolidinediones. Although these medications are often prescribed, many of these types of medicines are not specifically approved for use in children. Occasionally, insulin injections are needed to treat diabetes that is not controlled by changes in diet or by these other medicines.

How Is Hyperlipidemia Treated?

In many children blood lipid levels will improve as their medicine doses are lowered or as the muscle inflammation becomes less active. If your child exercises more (if the myositis is well-controlled) and eats a low-fat diet, the blood lipid levels might also decrease. Your child's doctor may feel that using medicines to treat hyperlipidemia in children with JM does not have clear, demonstrated long-term advantages. Furthermore, the medicines used to lower the blood lipid levels frequently injure muscle cells. For these reasons your child's doctor may decide not to prescribe any medication, except when the lipid levels are very high.

Several medications developed recently are helpful for treating hyperlipidemia. Some of the more effective drugs are members of the statin family, which by themselves can damage muscle, even in patients without myositis, and in general are not recommended for patients with myositis. Other lipid-lowering drugs do not damage muscle, but they are generally not as good at improving hyperlipidemia, and most of them have other side effects. Currently, there is very active research to develop new lipid-lowering medications with few side effects.

Key Points

- Insulin resistance occurs in some myositis patients, when more insulin is needed to move glucose from the blood into muscle cells or to keep fat stores from breaking down.

- The only way to tell whether your child has insulin resistance, diabetes (high blood glucose levels), or hyperlipidemia (high blood lipid levels) is to check fasting levels of insulin, blood glucose, and lipids.

- Myositis patients should have their blood tested if they have a family history of diabetes or high blood lipids or symptoms of insulin resistance, especially high blood pressure, frequent urination and thirst, or acanthosis nigricans.

- Treatment for insulin resistance includes a healthy diet, increased exercise, and, if possible, reducing the doses of medicines that can worsen insulin resistance. In many children with myositis, insulin resistance is mild and goes away with time. Myositis patients with severe insulin resistance or full-blown diabetes may need medication or even insulin injections.

- High blood levels of lipids (hyperlipidemia) can be treated with a low-fat diet, exercise, and, if needed, lipid-lowering medicines. Some of these medicines can cause muscle damage, even in patients without myositis.

To Learn More

To find a specialist, see *Finding an Endocrinologist* in the *Finding a Doctor or Specialist* section of the *Resource Appendix*, specifically:

American Association of Clinical Endocrinologists

The Hormone Foundation

Lawson Wilkins Pediatric Endocrine Society

National Committee for Quality Assurance

Additional Information:

American Diabetes Association. National Call Center, 1701 North Beauregard Street, Alexandria VA 22311; Phone: 800-342-2383; Internet: www.diabetes.org; Email: AskADA@diabetes.org.

Information and other services to people with diabetes, their families, health professionals and the public.

Resources for parents and children. Available from: www.diabetes.org/for-parents-and-kids/resources.jsp.

Information and resources for managing diabetes, with nutrition information, recipes, and exercises (much of it kid-friendly).

American Heart Association. National Center, 7272 Greenville Avenue, Dallas TX 75231; Phone: 800-242-8721; Internet: www.americanheart.org.

Cholesterol and Atherosclerosis in Children. Available at: www.americanheart.org/presenter.jhtml?identifier=4499.

Information on keeping children healthy to prevent heart disease as an adult.

Dietary Guidelines for Healthy Children. Available at: www.amhrt.org/presenter.jhtml?identifier=4575.

Recommendations for calorie and fat intake, with links to other relevant web sites.

Cincinnati Children's Hospital Medical Center.

Hyperlipidemia/Cholesterol Problems in Children. Available at: www.cincinnati childrens.org/health/heart-encyclopedia/disease/hyperlipidemia.htm.

Issue of high cholesterol in children, including how to prevent or control it.

Reports in the Medical Literature

Bhatnagar D. Should pediatric patients with hyperlipidemia receive drug therapy? *Paediatric Drugs.* 2002;4(4):223–30.

Huemer C, Kitson H, Malleson PN, Sanderson S, Huemer M, Cabral DA, Chanoine JP, Petty RE. Lipodystrophy in patients with juvenile dermatomyositis: evaluation of clinical and metabolic abnormalities. *Journal of Rheumatology.* 2001 Mar;28(3):610–5.

Valente AM, Newburger JW, Lauer RM. Hyperlipidemia in children and adolescents. *American Heart Journal.* 2001 Sep;142(3):433–9.

CHAPTER 26

Too Much Body Fat Loss

Barbara S. Adams, MD, and Elif Arioglu Oral, MD

In this chapter...

We describe how loss of body fat, called lipodystrophy, affects some patients with juvenile dermatomyositis (JDM) and tell you how to recognize it. We will also explain how the accompanying complications of high blood levels of insulin, glucose, and lipids can be treated. Children with lipodystrophy benefit from care by an endocrinologist experienced in metabolic problems. If you have not already done so, please read *Chapter 25, Attention to Sugar and Fat Metabolism*, before you read this chapter.

> ### From the family's point of view...
>
> *"During the fall, our daughter, a cute and somewhat chunky eleven-year-old, started to lose that baby fat she had carried for so long and to grow into puberty. Or so we thought. During the ski season, she had lost considerable body fat and felt the cold easily. She was slimming down, but her weight loss (almost twenty pounds) was starting to be a concern. I was watching what she ate, which wasn't very much. She didn't know why she wasn't hungry or why she couldn't eat as much as she used to."*

What Is Lipodystrophy?

In normal weight loss, fat cells shrink but they stay healthy. In areas affected by lipodystrophy, fat cells are partly or completely damaged or lost. Lipodystrophy, the loss of fat tissue from areas of the body, is a problem that occurs in some children and adults with myositis. Lipodystrophy also occurs in other autoimmune diseases, including scleroderma, systemic lupus erythematosus (also called lupus), thyroid disease, insulin-requiring diabetes, and juvenile rheumatoid arthritis. There are many other causes of lipodystrophy that are not linked to autoimmune diseases, including some purely genetic causes.

Partial lipodystrophy, or loss of body fat from one or more parts of the body but not the whole body, is the pattern found most often in children with JDM (Figure 26.1). Although the fat loss tends to be similar on both sides of the body, it can sometimes affect one side of the body more than the other. In some patients fat deposits in certain areas of the body increase while fat is lost from other areas. How much fat is lost and the location(s) from which it is lost varies a lot from patient to patient, and there is no way to predict the pattern.

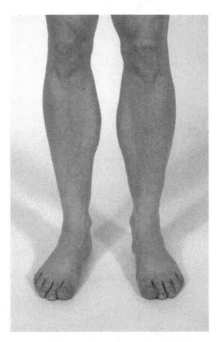

■ **Figure 26.1. Partial lipodystrophy affecting the legs of a patient with juvenile dermatomyositis.**
Notice that her calf muscles appear especially prominent, in part because of the loss of body fat in this area.

Generalized lipodystrophy, or widespread fat loss from most of the body, is not as common as partial lipodystrophy. Loss of most or all fat tissue happens more often in children whose JDM is severe and has been active for a long time. We also know that children with lipodystrophy are more likely to have calcinosis than most patients with JDM. Children with generalized lipodystrophy often have problems related to the way that their body uses sugars and fats as sources of energy. These problems are described below (see also *Chapter 25, Attention to Sugar and Fat Metabolism*).

In addition to storing energy, body fat serves as a cushion over bones and inner organs and supports blood vessels, nerves, and other body structures under the skin. When lipodystrophy decreases this protective cushion, some children feel discomfort over bony areas when they are in certain positions or when they are doing certain activities, depending on which areas are affected with loss of fat. Lipodystrophy also decreases the support for body structures such as blood vessels and nerves, so that muscles and veins are often seen through the skin more easily, and the arms or legs may appear very thin.

The fat loss in JDM, which is noticeable in 5% to 20% of patients, can show up when the illness is active, when it is being treated, or even after the myositis has gone into remission. It can develop slowly or rapidly. If fat loss started before remission, it can get worse even during remission. Most patients with lipodystrophy also have some insulin resistance (higher-than-normal levels of insulin in the blood). (See *Chapter 25, Attention to Sugar and Fat Metabolism.*) Researchers are working to find blood tests and other types of tests that can predict which JDM patients will get lipodystrophy, but there are no tests that can give us that information right now.

Why Do Some Children with Dermatomyositis Have Lipodystrophy?

In JDM, immune cells cause inflammation of the skin (producing the rash) and inflammation in the muscle tissue (producing muscle weakness). The immune cells also cause inflammation in the deeper fat tissue under the skin, which can damage or destroy fat cells. Although no one knows exactly why only some children with JDM have lipodystrophy, almost all JDM patients with a lot of fat tissue damage have problems with their body's ability to use sugars and fat for energy. People with lipodystrophy from many different causes all develop similar problems with sugars and fats, which suggests that the loss or damage of fat tissue itself leads to the metabolic problems of insulin resistance, extra fat in the liver, and high blood lipid levels.

Recent research shows that insulin resistance can be caused by damage to fat cells and is also likely to be made worse by the loss of fat cells. Research using laboratory animals has shown that the presence of normal fat tissue is very important for the body's regular metabolism of sugar and fats. Why are fat cells so important in keeping metabolism normal? One possibility is that fat-cell hormones give signals that control the body's response to insulin and control blood lipid levels. In addition, when fat cells are lost, the energy usually stored in fat tissue gets stored instead in other tissues, such as the liver and the muscles. The presence of fat in the liver and in the muscle decreases these tissues' sensitivity to insulin.

Recent research has shown that fat cells make hormones, including a hormone called leptin. Leptin controls the appetite and also controls how the body uses stored energy. Children who have lost a lot of fat (especially those with generalized lipodystrophy) have low levels of leptin in the blood, which causes them to feel very hungry and to seek food more than other children. Patients who have lost a lot of body fat also describe feeling hot, mainly after meals, for reasons we do not understand.

What Problems Occur in JDM Patients with Lipodystrophy?

Lipodystrophy causes problems with the body's ability to use sugars and fats as sources of energy, otherwise known as metabolic problems. In general, these problems occur when a large amount of fat is lost. Partial lipodystrophy usually does not cause metabolic problems. The specific changes in the body's ability to use sugars and fats include insulin resistance (higher-than-normal levels of insulin in the blood needed due to decreased sensitivity to the effects of insulin, see next paragraph) and hyperlipidemia (higher-than-normal levels of lipids in the blood) (see *Chapter 25, Attention to Sugar and Fat Metabolism*).

Insulin Resistance

Muscle tissue is the most important factor controlling the body's sensitivity to insulin. Because JDM involves inflammation and loss of muscle, all patients with a lot of muscle involvement have some amount of insulin resistance. Insulin resistance causes the pancreas (the body's insulin factory) to put more insulin into the blood, resulting in higher-than-normal insulin levels (Figure 26.2). That is the body's way of trying to keep blood levels of glucose and lipids normal and steady. However, this extra insulin cannot get into muscle and liver cells in the usual way, so it is free to act on other cells, such as the skin and the ovaries (in girls). High insulin levels cause coarsening and darkening of the skin, especially at skin folds around the neck, in the armpits, and in the groin (see Figure 25.2, Acanthosis nigricans, [color plate 15 on page 230] from *Chapter 25, Attention to Sugar and Fat Metabo-*

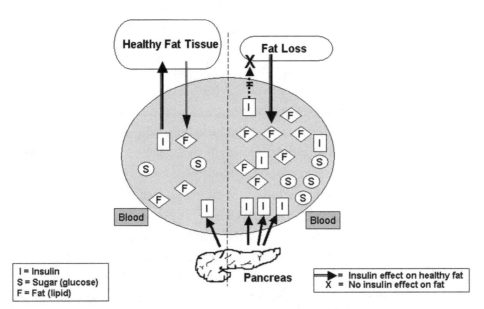

I = Insulin
S = Sugar (glucose)
F = Fat (lipid)

= Insulin effect on healthy fat
X = No insulin effect on fat

■ Figure 26.2. Blood insulin, glucose, and lipid levels in normal individuals (left panel) and in patients with lipodystrophy (right panel).

In healthy individuals the body's extra energy is stored in healthy fat tissue. Insulin keeps fat tissue healthy so that very little fat is broken down into lipids. In patients with lipodystrophy (right side of figure), there is a loss of fat tissue. With the loss of fat tissue, there is a loss of insulin action on fat tissue. Fat (lipid) rises in the blood and builds up in muscle and liver. Fat build-up in the liver and muscle decreases the ability of insulin to move sugar into the muscle and liver (insulin resistance). The pancreas tries to keep insulin and sugar balanced by pumping more insulin into the blood. The extra insulin can affect skin, ovaries, and other organs.

lism). Levels of insulin in the blood that remain high over a long period of time can also cause the ovaries to get bigger, to develop cysts, and to change so that they make male hormones instead of female hormones. These hormone changes can cause menstrual periods to become irregular or even stop, and they very often cause more hair growth over most of the body, especially in children with generalized lipodystrophy. Hair growth on the face is often a major problem for girls.

JDM patients with insulin resistance need higher-than-normal levels of insulin to move blood glucose into muscle cells and to prevent fat cells from breaking down. Insulin resistance can lead to glucose intolerance (high levels of glucose in the blood for an unusually long time after eating) and to diabetes mellitus (also called diabetes). In lipodystrophy these problems develop mainly because the body's fat tissue does not properly dispose of the glucose and lipids in the blood. The fat loss of lipodystrophy can also cause insulin resistance. When that happens, the insulin resistance is usually more severe and more difficult to treat.

Hyperlipidemia and Pancreatitis

In patients who have lipodystrophy, blood lipid levels increase because fat cells break down, spilling their contents (including cholesterol and triglycerides) into the blood, causing a condition known as hyperlipidemia (see *Chapter 25, Attention to Sugar and Fat Metabolism*) (Figure 26.2). In addition to increasing the risk of heart disease, high levels of triglycerides can cause painful inflammation of the pancreas (pancreatitis). Severe stomach or abdominal pain, bloating, and vomiting are all symptoms of pancreatitis. If your child's blood lipid levels are abnormally high, she should be evaluated by an endocrinologist.

Other Problems

Another metabolic problem linked to lipodystrophy is the buildup of fat in other parts of the body, especially in muscles and the liver (Figure 26.2). Extra fat in muscle tissue makes it less sensitive to insulin, which causes insulin and glucose in the blood to go out of balance. Extra fat in the liver, known as steatosis, also results in insulin resistance, which can make high blood glucose levels even worse. Buildup of fat can damage the liver, too, sometimes to the point of causing scarring and decreased liver function. If blood tests show signs of liver damage, your child's doctors may want to do a liver biopsy to find out how much damage has occurred.

How Can Your Child's Doctor Tell Whether Your Child Has Lipodystrophy?

It is not easy to be aware of lipodystrophy when it starts because changes in body fat can happen very slowly and can be hard to detect. Your child's doctor might be able to tell whether your child has lipodystrophy just by looking closely at her face, arms, and chest/stomach areas to see if there appears to be a loss of the fat tissue under the skin. Sometimes, there are firm, painful lumps under the skin resulting from inflammation of the fat tissue (called panniculitis), which can be seen or felt before lipodystrophy appears. Some patients also notice swelling in certain areas of the skin before fat loss is noticed. Loss of fat in the face often shows up first in the cheeks. Looking at old photographs from before your child's illness can help you and your doctor determine whether your child has lost body fat recently. Symptoms of insulin resistance, such as high blood pressure, acanthosis nigricans (see Figure 25.2 [color plate 15 on page 230], from *Chapter 25, Attention to Sugar and Fat Metabolism*), or new growth of coarse body hair, can also alert your doctor to look for the symptoms of lipodystrophy sooner. Fasting blood tests to measure blood glucose, insulin, and lipid levels (discussed in *Chapter 25, Attention to Sugar and Fat Metabolism*) can help your doctor tell whether your child has insulin resistance, hyperlipidemia, or diabetes.

Other ways to detect lipodystrophy include using an instrument called skin calipers to measure skin folds and the thickness of body fat tissue. Changes in tiny electric currents across the skin (skin impedence) can also be measured with a special instrument. Other ways that researchers measure fat loss include special X-ray studies, such as dual X-ray absorptiometry (DXA). This is the same instrument and the same method used to measure the thickness and strength of bones; consequently, body fat and the strength of the bones are often studied at the same time. In magnetic resonance imaging (MRI) fat appears white; researchers can measure the thickness and the shapes of white areas to find out whether important fat loss has occurred.

How Is Lipodystrophy Treated?

Children with lipodystrophy who have metabolic problems related to the body's use of sugars and fats should be examined and treated by an endocrinologist. Lipodystrophy is treated by controlling the underlying insulin resistance and problems with glucose and lipid levels in the blood (see also Chapter 25). Many of the same treatments for insulin resistance are used to treat lipodystrophy, including diet, decreasing the corticosteroid dosage, and adding second-line medicines that control the inflammation without causing insulin resistance.

Insulin resistance can also be treated with medicines that help the body use glucose better. Some of these medicines work by increasing the body's sensitivity to insulin; examples include pioglitazone (Actos) and rosiglitazone (Avandia). Other medicines, such as metformin (Glucophage or Glucovance), treat insulin resistance by decreasing extra glucose produced by the liver. Although these medicines have not been studied in children with JM, they have been helpful in treating other symptoms of insulin resistance, such as excessive body hair and irregular menstrual periods.

Children who develop severe diabetes are usually treated with insulin injections. They often need very large doses of insulin to bring their blood glucose level down and keep their diabetes under control.

Children who have high blood lipid levels are usually placed on a diet that reduces the amount of fat they eat. Drugs that lower blood lipid levels might be prescribed if diet alone does not bring the levels to normal. Blood lipid levels, especially triglyceride levels, are often high in patients with lipodystrophy. Medicines that lower the levels of those lipids are fenofibrate (Tricor) and gemfibrozil (Lopid). Another group of medicines that lowers blood lipid levels by blocking the body's production of cholesterol are called statins. Statins such as atorvastatin (Lipitor) and simvastatin (Zocor) are often used to treat adults with high cholesterol levels. Statins are generally not recommended for use in children with myositis, because statins cause breakdown of muscle tissue and worsening of myositis. If your child must take these medicines, your child's myositis doctor should follow her progress very closely to make sure that the medicines themselves are not causing extra muscle damage. At the present time, however, no medicines have been proven to be effective in treating lipodystrophy.

Key Points

- Lipodystrophy is the loss of fat tissue under the skin as well as deeper fat tissue around bones and organs.

- No one knows exactly why lipodystrophy occurs in JDM. Recent research suggests that fat loss can cause insulin resistance. Patients who have a lot of fat loss tend to have greater problems with insulin resistance.

- Onset of lipodystrophy may be gradual or sudden. Fat loss can occur during active JDM or after it has gone into remission.

- All patients with large areas of lipodystrophy have insulin resistance (problems with the body's ability to use glucose [sugar] as a source of energy), with or without diabetes (high blood glucose levels). Blood lipid levels may also be higher than normal.

- Treatment of lipodystrophy involves treating the underlying insulin resistance, high blood glucose, and high blood lipid levels. Increasing physical activity and eating a healthy low-fat diet similar to a diabetic diet are important lifestyle changes that can reduce blood glucose and lipid levels. There are effective medicines that can decrease insulin resistance, although they have not been tested in children.

To Learn More

To find a specialist, see *Finding an Endocrinologist* in the *Finding a Doctor or Specialist* section of the *Resource Appendix*, specifically:

American Association of Clinical Endocrinologists

The Hormone Foundation

Lawson Wilkins Pediatric Endocrine Society

National Committee for Quality Assurance

Additional Information:

American Dietetic Association. 120 South Riverside Plaza, Suite 2000, Chicago IL 60606-6995; Phone: 800-877-1600; Internet: www.eatright.org.

Information on healthy eating habits, dieting, and finding a nutrition specialist.

The Hormone Foundation, an affiliate of The Endocrine Society. 8401 Connecticut Avenue, Suite 900, Chevy Chase MD 20815-5817; Phone: 800-HORMONE; Internet: www.hormone.org.

Resource for the public by promoting the prevention, treatment, and cure of hormone-related conditions through public outreach and education.

University of Texas Southwestern Medical Center.

Welcome to Lipodystrophy.Info at UT Southwestern. Available at: www.utsouthwestern.edu/utsw/cda/dept105803/files/106777.html.

Current research into rare body fat disorders, types of lipodystrophy, therapies (management of metabolic problems, diet, surgical management, treatment of diabetes, treatment of high blood lipids, others), and enrollment in studies.

Reports in the Medical Literature

Garg A. Acquired and inherited lipodystrophies. *New England Journal of Medicine.* 2004 Mar 18;350(12):1220–34.

Huemer C, Kitson H, Malleson PN, Sanderson S, Huemer M, Cabral DA, Chanoine JP, Petty RE. Lipodystrophy in patients with juvenile dermatomyositis: evaluation of clinical and metabolic abnormalities. *Journal of Rheumatology.* 2001 Mar;28(3):610–5.

Misra A, Peethambaram A, Garg A. Clinical features and metabolic and autoimmune derangements in acquired partial lipodystrophy: report of 35 cases and review of the literature. *Medicine.* 2004 Jan;83(1):18–34.

Oral EA. Lipoatrophic diabetes and other related syndromes. *Reviews in Endocrine and Metabolic Disorders.* 2003 Mar;4(1):61–77.

CHAPTER 27

Eye Health

Janine A. Smith, MD, and Manuel B. Datiles, III, MD

In this chapter...

We describe the eye problems that may be associated with juvenile myositis (JM) and their treatment. We also discuss side effects of medication that can occur in the eye.

From the family's point of view...

"Even though she was on every-other-day prednisone to lessen the possible side effects, she started to have problems with her eyes. We went to an ophthalmologist and found she had slight glaucoma and cataracts in both eyes. We have to monitor the cataracts every six months, and she wears sunglasses because her eyes are more sensitive to the light. Fortunately, the doctors said the cataracts would stop growing once she stopped taking prednisone."

How Does My Child Get to See an Eye Doctor?

Your child's myositis doctor can refer your child to see a physician who is trained in the care of eye problems, called an ophthalmologist (or a pediatric ophthalmologist who cares for children only). The ophthalmologist will perform a dilated eye examination, which is part of your child's medical care and should be covered by your medical insurance. Children with juvenile myositis (JM) should see their ophthalmologist at least twice yearly; sometimes the eye doctor will request more frequent visits.

What to Expect in the Eye Exam

Eye exams involve measuring the vision, testing for the need for glasses, measuring the pressure within the eye, and examining the structures in the front of the eye with an instrument called a slit lamp biomicroscope to look for cataracts. The eye doctor puts drops in the eye to make the pupil bigger (called dilation) so that he can examine the back of the eye, including the retina and optic nerve. These drops may sting for one or two minutes. Your child will place her chin on a chin rest, and the doctor will use a special microscope with high magnification and light to examine the structures of the eye. This is not painful. A bright light and magnifying lens will be used to examine the retina, and afterward your child's vision may be blurry for one or two minutes, like after having your photograph taken with a flash camera. The pupil dilation lasts for one to two hours and makes near vision blurry and reading difficult. Your child will need to wear sunglasses for a few hours after the appointment because dilation of the pupils makes your eyes more sensitive to light.

What Eye Problems Occur in JM?

Eye problems associated with JM are rare. Typically, in juvenile dermatomyositis (JDM) patients have a rash on the face, which is characterized by redness around the eyes, but this rash is not associated with any problems inside the eyes. One of the early eye findings in children with JDM is dilation, or enlargement, of the small blood vessels along the eyelids, which may make the eyelids appear more red than normal. Another finding in some children with JDM and severe vasculitis is damage to the tissue at the corner of the eyes near the nose, which may leave small areas that are below the surface of the rest of the skin when healed (healed infarcts). Very rarely, children with JM have inflammation of the blood vessels in the back of the eye.

Inflammation and Eye Problems

In JM, inflammation is the main abnormality. Inflammation can cause abnormalities of the blood vessels of the retina; however, this is very rare. The retina is the thin tissue in the back of the eye, which is similar to the film in a camera. Rarely, blood vessels in the retina can become narrowed in small areas, resulting in loss of oxygen to the retina. This may give rise to a white spot called a cotton-wool spot, which can be seen by an eye doctor during an eye examination. When the inflammation is controlled by medications, these white spots go away. These spots do not result in permanent loss of vision. Even more rarely, the inflammation in the retina may result in abnormal new blood vessels (neovascularization), which can sometimes leak and bleed into the eye. The leaky blood vessels can often be treated safely and effectively with lasers.

Effects of Treatment on Your Child's Eyes

Side effects from some medications used to treat JM can also cause eye problems. Children with JM who are taking corticosteroids should visit their eye doctor for a thorough eye examination twice yearly to be certain that cataracts are not developing. Children receiving hydroxychloroquine (Plaquenil) should visit their eye doctor once yearly for special eye tests, discussed below. Sometimes the eye doctor will request more frequent visits.

Cataracts Related to Corticosteroids

A cataract is a clouding of the lens of the eye (see Figure 27.1). The lens is a disk-like transparent tissue suspended inside the eye, which focuses light on the retina, allowing a person to see objects clearly. This lens is like the lens of a camera, which focuses light on the film.

■ **Figure 27.1. (See color plate 16 on page 230.) Posterior subcapsular cataract in a twelve-year-old girl with JM treated with prednisone, as seen through a dilated pupil with a slit lamp biomicroscope.** Note the central location of the cataract (cloudy spot in the center of the lens) with characteristic "bubbles." The background is reddish because of the reflection of light from the retina behind.

Treatment using large doses of oral corticosteroids, such as prednisone or methylprednisolone (Solumedrol), is often required to control the myositis. Long-term steroid treatment can cause cataracts, and the main goal of having frequent eye checkups is to detect a cataract early in order to change the amount of steroid being given and to prevent the cataract from expanding. If your child is taking corticosteroids, she should have an eye exam at least two or three times a year or more frequently if she notices a change in vision.

Cataracts caused by steroids are located on the back of the lens and look like a snowflake or bubbles (see Figure 27.1). They are easily detected by an ophthalmologist using a device called a slit lamp biomicroscope. Cataracts can grow or enlarge slowly or quickly, depending on the dose of the steroids. They are related to dose and duration of steroid treatment. For steroids to cause cataracts, they must be used for a long time. Some people are also more likely to develop steroid-related cataracts than others. The cataracts stop growing when the steroid treatment is stopped, and in some children cataracts can even get smaller. If a cataract is detected, your child's myositis doctor may suggest new medicines for the JM to reduce the steroid dose quickly and to prevent the cataract from becoming larger.

The cataract may cause glare and light sensitivity, which is most noticeable in bright sunlight or when looking at the headlights of oncoming cars. The headlights look like a starburst is coming from them. When the light hits the cloudy part of the lens, it is scattered in such a way that it is dispersed onto the retina, creating the sensation of glare, sometime called photophobia, or light sensitivity.

Frequently Asked Questions

How do I know whether my child has any signs of early cataract?

Ask your child whether she has any trouble reading or seeing, such as blurred vision, double vision, or pain in or around the eyes. Ask your eye doctor whether your child's vision is normal and whether any abnormalities like a cataract have been detected.

If your child has a cataract, her eyes should be protected from sunlight. Wearing sun glasses designed to block ultraviolet (UVB) rays can make the eyes more comfortable in bright sunlight. Wearing a hat with a brim can also help protect the eyes.

If your child has a cataract, does it affect your child's daily activities, such as performance at school? When the cataract reduces a child's vision, as measured on an eye chart, and the child has difficulty performing her normal tasks (such as seeing the blackboard, studying, playing, watching TV, eating, bathing, etc.), then it is time to consider cataract surgery. Children need to have clear vision during their formative years for their eyes to develop normally. A cataract causes cloudy vision and, if it is not removed, could result in permanently worse vision in children less than seven years of age. Cataracts that develop after nine years of age do not cause this potential problem.

Treatment for cataracts is needed only when the cataract is so large that it gets in the line of sight and causes difficulty seeing. A temporary treatment involves dilating (enlarging) the pupils, which allows the child to see around the cataract. This may be done if your child's general condition temporarily will not allow cataract surgery under general anesthesia. This treatment will prevent the child from developing "lazy eyes" or amblyopia. Amblyopia can result in a permanent decrease in vision if the cataract is not removed and becomes large enough to block the light and prevent the eye from forming a sharp image on the retina.

How is cataract surgery done?

Cataract surgery has advanced recently and is now done with a small instrument that uses sound waves to break up the cataract. Once the cloudy lens is removed and after the eye has grown sufficiently, a plastic lens implant is inserted to replace the cloudy lens in order to help the eye focus. Otherwise, glasses or contact lenses are fitted later to aid the eye so that the child can see clearly. The surgery is relatively short, painless, and usually successful. A patch is placed over the eye after surgery, and the healing period ranges from one to four weeks. Sometimes an "after cataract" or clouding of the lens capsule, which holds the lens implant in place, can occur. This is readily treated with a laser procedure.

Research is being done to find a medical treatment using eye drops for cataracts, but currently the only effective treatment of cataracts is surgical removal.

What are the risks of cataract surgery?

Cataract surgery is usually done on children under general anesthesia. Therefore, your child's myositis doctor will have to give medical approval that it is safe for your child to have the surgery. Cataract surgery with intraocular lens implantation usually restores the child's sight back to normal, but she might need thin glasses, especially for reading. In young people, the lens power required may change with age, and in time she may need new glasses or contact lenses.

Steroid Side Effects: Glaucoma

Steroids can also promote the development of glaucoma, which is a painless eye condition associated with elevated pressure inside the eye. It results in damage to the optic nerve, which carries the visual image on the retina from the eye to the brain. Steroid-induced glaucoma occurs only after six weeks to several months of steroid treatment. Individuals differ in their susceptibility: only a small percentage of children will have a clinically significant elevation of eye pressure leading to glaucoma. Other factors related to susceptibility include the dose and frequency of steroid treatment. It is therefore important to monitor the eye pressure regularly during the entire time that oral steroids are being used, to make sure that no permanent damage to the optic nerve occurs.

Glaucoma is usually treated by special eye drops that lower the eye pressure and prevent damage to the optic nerve. Withdrawal of steroid treatment, if possible, can also help the eye pressure return to normal levels and avoid optic nerve damage. If steroid treatment needs to be continued, anti-glaucoma medications (usually eye drops) can be used to control the eye pressure. Glaucoma related to steroid use is usually reversible by stopping the steroids if the medicine has not been used for more than one year, but it may be irreversible if treatment is continued for eighteen months or more. If it is reversible, pressure usually returns to normal within two weeks. Because steroid treatment used in JM is frequently relatively short and episodic, loss of vision due to glaucoma rarely occurs.

Hydroxychloroquine and Effects on the Eye

Another medication commonly used to treat JM is hydroxychloroquine (Plaquenil). Hydroxychloroquine is very rarely associated with any eye problems because of the low dosage currently used for treating JM. Hydroxychloroquine rarely causes changes in the retina affecting color vision and field of vision. These retinal changes, which can be detected by an ophthalmologist, sometimes reverse when the medicine is discontinued. They occur mainly with long-term use in high doses that add up to more than one thousand grams. Hydroxychloroquine rarely has been associated with deposits on the cornea, which is the clear part of the front of the eye, like a crystal on a watch. An earlier form of the drug (chloroquine) was associated with this problem; however, in the doses of hydroxychloroquine used to treat JM, this is exceedingly rare. In the rare case that this would occur, it does not cause vision loss and goes away when the medication is stopped.

For children who need to take hydroxychloroquine, toxicity screening is done before starting the medicine to get baseline values for comparison to future tests. This evaluation involves color vision testing, a dilated retinal exam, and sometimes specialized visual field testing in older children. Color vision is tested by asking the child to read numbers printed in color on a dark or light background. This is especially important if there is a history of red-green color blindness in the family. The visual field test involves looking straight ahead and pushing a button when a small light is flashed on the side to test the peripheral vision.

Always ask the eye doctor how often your child needs to have an eye exam, and make sure you make the next appointment before you leave.

Frequently Asked Questions

Will my child become blind from myositis?

This is highly unlikely. The ophthalmic manifestations of JM in general do not result in blindness. Cataract, the most common abnormality, is a side effect of steroid treatment and not JM itself and can be treated surgically.

What should I look for to help determine whether I need to take my child to the eye doctor?

If your child is having problems with any one of the following:

- Bumping into things
- Complaining of seeing double
- Having blurred vision
- Complaining of headaches
- Complaining of light hurting her eyes

…you should have the eye doctor check your child. Your child should have at least yearly eye checkups, and you should ask the eye doctor whether he or she would like to see your child more often. Children receiving steroids should have eye checkups more often, for example every four to six months.

Does my child need to wear eye protection for sports?

There is no additional risk of eye injury from JM; therefore, there is no need for special eye protection other than what is usually recommended for particular games or sports. It is important for all children, not just those with JM, to wear appropriate eye protection when playing sports.

What are the side effects of chloroquine?

In the past, chloroquine, also known as Aralen, was used at high doses to treat many inflammatory diseases, including JM. This drug, however, can result in loss of central vision, loss of color vision, and a particular pattern of pigment deposits in the retina. Recently, a less toxic version of this medication, hydroxychloroquine, has been formulated and is currently being used. It has drastically reduced the risk of eye problems and is also used at a much lower dose than chloroquine.

Key Points

■ The child with JM should have a dilated eye examination by an eye doctor (ophthalmologist) to check for signs of active myositis and drug-related side effects affecting the eyes.

■ Corticosteroids can cause cataracts and glaucoma, both of which are treatable and easily detected on eye examination, which should be done every four to six months while a child is receiving steroids.

■ Hydroxychloroquine rarely can cause loss of vision or color vision. This can be prevented with frequent eye examinations and a relatively low dose of medication. Before starting hydroxycholoroquine and once yearly while receiving treatment, a color vision test should be done.

To Learn More

To find a physician, see *Finding an Eye Care Specialist* in the *Finding a Doctor or Specialist* section of the *Resource Appendix*, specifically:

American Academy of Ophthalmology

American Optometric Association

Additional Information:

National Eye Institute (NEI), U.S. National Institutes of Health (NIH). Information Office, 31 Center Drive MSC 2510, Bethesda MD 20892-2510; Phone: 301-496-5248; Internet: www.nei.nih.gov; Email: 2020@nei.nih.gov.

General information about various eye conditions, including photographs and images, publications list, and more.

National Eye Institute (NEI).

NEI Publications Catalog. Available from: http://catalog.nei.nih.gov/productcart/pc/viewCat_L.asp?idCategory=3 or call 301-496-5248.

Order or download pamphlets: *Don't Lose Sight of Cataract* (under "Cataract"); *Don't Lose Sight of Glaucoma* ("Glaucoma"); *See All You Can See: Activity Book for Ages 6 to 8* ("Activity Books"); and more.

The Medem Network.

Children's Health: Eye Care and Conditions. Available at: www.medem.com/medlb/articleslb.cfm?sub_cat=546.

Links to information on common eye problems and diseases, safety, and medical eye exams. Brochures available in Spanish.

Reports in the Medical Literature

Cohen BH, Sedwick LA, Burde RM. Retinopathy of dermatomyositis. *Journal of Clinical Neuro-ophthalmology.* 1985 Sep;5(3):177–9.

Marmor MF, Carr RE, Easterbrook M, Farjo AA, Mieler WF. American Academy of Ophthalmology. Recommendations on screening for chloroquine and hydroxychloroquine retinopathy: a report by the American Academy of Ophthalmology. *Ophthalmology*. 2002 Jul;109(7):1377–82.

McGhee CN, Dean S, Danesh-Meyer H. Locally administered ocular corticosteroids: benefits and risks. *Drug Safety*. 2002;25(1):33–55.

Spiera H. Rheumatic disease in children. *Journal of Pediatric Ophthalmology and Strabismus*. 1982 Mar-Apr;19(2):103–7.

When Your Child Has More Than One Autoimmune Disease

Clarissa M. Pilkington, MBBS, and Ann M. Reed, MD

In this chapter...

Here we discuss other disorders that commonly occur in children with myositis as overlapping illnesses and how they are identified.

From the family's point of view...

"A dermatomyositis patient read my post on an online bulletin board about my concerns and suggested that my daughter, who has juvenile dermatomyositis, might also have celiac disease. The dermatomyositis patient had celiac disease and had found that a number of other myositis patients also had this overlap condition."

What Are Overlapping Illnesses?

If your child has juvenile myositis (JM) as well as another connective tissue or autoimmune disease, such as arthritis, lupus, or scleroderma, then your child has a JM overlap condition. Most children with myositis, however, do not have another autoimmune disease. For those few children who have possible indications of another autoimmune condition, additional testing might be helpful. Your child's doctor will examine your child and order blood tests and sometimes other tests to determine whether your child meets the criteria for these other autoimmune conditions. Often children with overlapping illnesses have autoantibodies that are related to one or both of the illnesses. People with one autoimmune disease can be at more risk of developing a second autoimmune disease than people in the general population. This could be from having shared genetic and environmental influences for each of the diseases.

JM is considered one of a spectrum of systemic autoimmune diseases, in which many parts of the body can be involved. JM in this way is similar to other systemic autoimmune diseases such as lupus (systemic lupus erythematosus, SLE) and scleroderma. These diseases can occur alone, or features of these diseases can coexist with each other, in which case they are called overlap disorders (Figure 28.1).

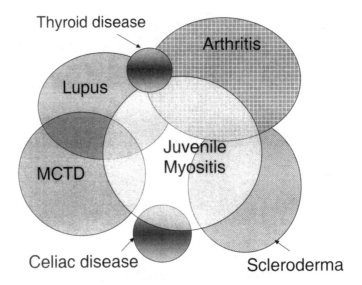

■ **Figure 28.1. Diagram showing how different autoimmune diseases can overlap with juvenile myositis and with each other.**
MCTD stands for mixed connective tissue disease.

Other autoimmune diseases that coexist with JM less commonly are the organ-specific autoimmune diseases, illnesses in which the immune system attacks one organ in particular. Examples of these organ-specific illnesses that overlap with JM include diabetes (the pancreas gland is the organ attacked by the immune system), thyroid disorders (in which the thyroid is attacked), and celiac disease (the small intestine is attacked). Some children initially have pure JM and later develop an overlap condition; some start with the other illness and later develop JM; and some children have both conditions from the beginning. Although in some cases it can be difficult to identify overlaps, several studies suggest that overall about 8% of children with myositis in the U.S. have overlapping illnesses. The frequency of different JM overlaps likely varies from location to location, however.

Juvenile Myositis/Scleroderma Overlap

Scleroderma causes thickening and tightness of the skin. Often the swallowing muscles, blood vessels, and other organs become stiff and do not work properly. Scleroderma is the most common overlap condition seen with JM in the United Kingdom. At a large children's hospital in London UK, about 15% of children with myositis also have scleroderma, which means they have JM/scleroderma overlap disorders. The frequency of JM/scleroderma overlap is lower in the U.S.

Some of the symptoms in children with scleroderma overlap include tightening of the skin and soft tissues of the fingers, which can cause difficulties with fully bending the fingers. In more severe cases children can lose tissue on the fingertips, resulting in tapering fingertips. Less commonly, there can be tightening of the skin around the mouth and nose. Both children with JM alone and children who have overlap with scleroderma can have changes in the nailfold capillaries with what is called "capillary drop-out," where fewer blood vessels than normal are seen in the skin around the edge of the fingernail. Children who have myositis overlapping with scleroderma tend to have milder myositis features: weakness is often mild to moderate, the muscle enzyme levels are only slightly increased in the blood, and the muscle involvement is usually short lived.

Some persons with myositis and scleroderma, especially adults, have an autoantibody called anti-PM-Scl (named after the overlap of polymyositis/scleroderma) and a strongly positive antinuclear autoantibody. Children with JM/scleroderma overlap frequently develop arthritis in the hands as well as calcinosis. They can also develop lung problems that are evident on lung function testing and might require a high-resolution computed tomography (CT) scan of the chest to monitor their illness.

Some children with JM/scleroderma overlap have a type of scleroderma called linear scleroderma, in which the skin thickening and tightening is confined to just one region of the body.

Juvenile Myositis/Lupus Overlap

Systemic lupus is a chronic, often lifelong, autoimmune disease that can affect many parts of the body, but it most often causes problems in the skin, joints, blood, and kidneys. The difficulty in defining JM/lupus overlap syndrome is that JM and lupus have many features in common. These features include myositis, rashes on the face, headaches, tiredness, joint pain, joint swelling, low white blood cell counts (low lymphocytes), and positive antinuclear autoantibodies (ANAs). In JM/lupus overlap syndrome, however, the myositis is often less severe, with only a moderate increase in the muscle enzymes, and it is often short lived.

The characteristic rash in lupus, called a malar rash, is in the shape of a butterfly on the cheeks. The malar rash can also occur in JM. The facial and finger rashes, however, can differ between children with JM and those with lupus. For example, the heliotrope rash and swelling around the eyes (called periorbital edema) in children with juvenile dermatomyositis (JDM) is not seen in persons who only have lupus. Also, the rashes on the hands in JDM, called Gottron's papules, occur over the knuckles, whereas in lupus the hand rashes usually occur between the knuckles (see *Chapter 16, Skin Rashes and Sun Protection*). Headaches and kidney involvement are often more of a problem in lupus than in JM. The autoantibodies can be the same, although a positive anti-double stranded DNA autoantibody is found only in lupus.

Another area of overlap between lupus and JM is the presence of anti-cardiolipin autoantibodies. These are characteristically found in lupus, but they can also be present in children with myositis, particularly JDM. Some children with myositis can develop high levels of these antibodies and have some of the same symptoms as in lupus (for example, a lacy skin appearance called livedo reticularis, blood clots, or recurrent miscarriages in young adults).

Juvenile Myositis/Mixed Connective Tissue Disease Overlap

Some children have features of several different autoimmune conditions and high levels of autoantibodies called anti-RNP (U1-ribonucleoprotein) autoantibodies, which together have been called mixed connective tissue disease (MCTD). There is controversy over this category of overlap syndrome because some doctors believe that MCTD is a separate illness and some do not. MCTD is a condition with clinical signs of two or more of the following: arthritis, lupus, myositis, or scleroderma. To have MCTD, your child must have high levels of anti-RNP autoantibodies in the blood, and she might also have specific genetic markers. However, it is often difficult to say whether a child has MCTD or JM/MCTD overlap because many children start off with myositis predominantly and then over time (as the myositis lessens) develop features characteristic of other autoimmune diseases, which can include Raynaud's phenomenon (a condition in which strong emotion or exposure to the cold causes the fingertips, toes, ears, or nose to undergo a series of color changes from white to blue to red), tightening of the skin, and problems with breathing and swallowing. Some physicians believe that children with MCTD are a subgroup of those whose illness evolves into lupus or scleroderma. However, many children with mild MCTD resolve their complaints over time, and the child might be left with only symptoms of Raynaud's phenomenon.

Juvenile Myositis/Celiac Disease Overlap

Celiac disease (also called gluten-sensitive enteropathy) is an autoimmune disease that occurs in genetically susceptible persons after eating gluten (a protein found in wheat, barley, oats, and rye). Celiac disease can be mild and almost undetectable, or it can cause severe problems, such as diarrhea, inability to absorb food in the intestine (called malabsorption), weight loss, problems with nerves and muscles, and iron-deficiency anemia. A few children are known to have both JM and celiac disease. In some of these cases the muscle weakness and elevation of muscle enzymes in the blood appear to respond to corticosteroids or other immunosuppressive agents. The symptoms of malabsorption, diarrhea, or gas continued and were worse than what could be explained by JM alone. The celiac disease was diagnosed by symptoms, biopsy, and in some cases autoantibody testing that is specific for celiac disease (called anti-gliadin and anti-transglutaminase autoantibodies).

Some children and adults with myositis/celiac disease overlap were started on gluten-free diets to treat their celiac disease, and they noticed weight gain and improvement in the other symptoms, including improvement in the muscle enzymes. The authors of one study thought that the elevation of muscle enzymes in the blood could be partially controlled with diet. It remains unknown why these two illnesses appear together and, more importantly, why the myositis in some individuals improves when they are placed on a gluten-free diet.

Juvenile Myositis/Diabetes Overlap

Type I diabetes is an autoimmune condition in which blood sugar levels are elevated because of a decreased amount of insulin (a hormone produced by the pancreas) as a result of an immune system attack on the pancreas. Insulin is a key regulator of the body's metabolism. It helps many tissues use sugar or glucose, which is needed, as an energy source. Although some children develop diabetes as a result of the corticosteroids used to treat their myositis (see *Chapter 25, Attention to Sugar and Fat Metabolism*), a few children have type 1 diabetes before they develop JM.

Corticosteroid treatments in diabetics can cause large swings in their blood sugar levels. For this reason, when high-dose intravenous or pulse corticosteroid therapy is given, it is usually done in a hospital, where the child and the sugar levels can be monitored carefully.

Juvenile Myositis/Psoriasis Overlap

Psoriasis is a condition in which thick red patches that look like scales form on the skin. Some children are misdiagnosed as having psoriasis when they first go to the doctor for their JDM rash. A few children with JM, however, have true psoriasis skin rashes in addition to rashes associated with JDM. A study in the U.S. showed that 3% of children with JDM also have psoriasis. Psoriasis can be treated by some of the same medicines used to treat JM. For example, methotrexate can be especially helpful for both conditions. But psoriasis often improves in sunlight, whereas JDM rashes usually worsen after excessive sun exposure. Psoriasis also tends to worsen as the prednisone used to treat JM is reduced.

Juvenile Myositis/Thyroid Disease Overlap

Both hypothyroidism (low levels of thyroid hormone) and hyperthyroidism (high levels of thyroid hormone) have been rarely reported as overlap disorders with JM. Anti-thyroid autoantibodies, including anti-microsomal and anti-thyroglobulin autoantibodies, are often used to screen for autoimmune or other thyroid disease. Thyroid disease can be an important cause of muscle disease unrelated to JM, and this problem usually is resolved with correction of the blood levels of thyroid hormone.

What Treatments Are Used for Overlap Disorders?

The treatment of overlap disorders is directed at controlling the child's specific symptoms at that time no matter which illness is causing them. Luckily, many of these conditions can be treated with the same or similar medicines used to treat

JM (see *Chapter 7, Treatment Possibilities in the Beginning* and *Chapter 12, Possible Medicines During the Course*).

Key Points

■ Other autoimmune conditions can occur with JM, and when this happens they are called myositis overlapping with another connective tissue disease or overlapping illnesses.

■ The most common autoimmune illnesses that overlap with JM are scleroderma and lupus, although others, including celiac disease, diabetes, psoriasis, and thyroid disease, occur less frequently in association with JM.

■ The treatment of overlap disorders is directed at controlling the child's specific symptoms at that time no matter which illness is causing them. Many of these overlapping conditions can be treated with the same or similar medicines used to treat JM.

To Learn More

The Myositis Association (TMA).

Overlap syndrome: when myositis isn't your only obstacle. Available from: www.myositis. org/jmbookresources.cfm or 800-821-7356.

American Autoimmune Related Disease Association (AARDA).

Patient Information. Available at: www.aarda.org/patient_information.php or 810-766-3900.

Information on more than sixty autoimmune diseases, including arthritis, thyroiditis, and lupus.

National Organization for Rare Disorders (NORD). Phone: 203-797-9590.

Index of Organizations. Available at: www.rarediseases.org/search/orglist.html.
Links to hundreds of rare disease support organizations around the world.

Index of Rare Diseases. Available at: www.rarediseases.org/search/rdbsearch.html.

Reports in the Medical Literature

Falcini F, Porfirio B, Lionetti P. Juvenile dermatomyositis and celiac disease. *Journal of Rheumatology.* 1999 Jun;26(6):1419–20.

Jury EC, D'Cruz D, Morrow WJ. Autoantibodies and overlap syndromes in autoimmune rheumatic disease. *Journal of Clinical Pathology.* 2001 May;54(5):340–7.

Rider LG, Targoff IN. *Single organ systems and autoimmunity: Muscle diseases.* In: Lahita RG, Chiorazzi N, Reeves WH, editors. *Textbook of Autoimmune Diseases.* Philadelphia: Lippincott-Raven; 2000. p. 429–74.

CHAPTER 29

Vaccines and Infection Protection

Laura J. Mirkinson, MD; Judy A. Beeler, MD; and Ildy M. Katona, MD

The statements in this chapter are those of the authors and do not necessarily reflect the official views, policies, or positions of the U.S. Food and Drug Administration or the U.S. Department of Health and Human Services.

In this chapter...

We provide information about immunization practices and ways to minimize infections in children with myositis.

From the family's point of view...

"When she caught any type of cold, it would linger about one week longer than normal. The nursery teachers and other parents we knew all took pains to let us know in advance whether there were any viruses or infections about."

"We stress hand washing and have been very fortunate that he has had very little problem with infections while his immune system is suppressed. We provide nice-smelling antibacterial soaps to the school, which has kept all of the kids interested in washing their hands often!"

What Information About My Child's Past Infections and Vaccinations Should I Give My Child's Doctors?

The therapy for myositis will include medications, such as corticosteroids and possibly other agents, that can lead to immunosuppression. This means that these treatments may interfere with your child's ability to fight infections or respond properly to vaccinations. Your child's healthcare providers will want to know whether your child has ever had problems with recurrent infections (such as multiple ear infections or sore throats) or serious infections (such as meningitis or pneumonia). They may want to check your child's blood for total or specific immunoglobulin (antibody) levels. When your child is first diagnosed with myositis or if your child sees a new doctor later on, it is important for your child's doctor to know several things about your child's history regarding vaccines and infections:

- First, does your child have all the recommended immunizations for her age? Your child's doctor will want to see a copy of your child's immunization record. The United States' recommended childhood immunization schedule is pub-

328 • Myositis and You

lished yearly and can be found on the web sites for the Centers for Disease Control and Prevention (www.cdc.gov/nip), the American Academy of Pediatrics (www.aap.org), or the American Academy of Family Physicians (www.aafp.org). Your local health department is another good source of information about vaccines. The Internet sites for immunization schedules used outside of the United States may be found at the end of this chapter.

- Second, has she ever had chicken pox (varicella)?

- Third, has she been exposed to someone with tuberculosis (TB)? If your child has not had a recent skin test for tuberculosis (called a PPD), then she may need to have one before starting treatment for myositis. If your child has a positive PPD skin test, then you should discuss with her doctor when to initiate therapy for myositis.

What Are the Different Types of Vaccines?

For this discussion, we divide vaccines into two main types:

- *Inactivated vaccines.* Inactivated vaccines have no live viral or bacterial parts. These vaccines include influenza vaccine (except Flumist), inactivated polio vaccine (IPV, given by injection, but not by mouth), pertussis, hepatitis A, hepatitis B, diphtheria, tetanus, pneumococcus, meningococcus, haemophilus influenza B (HIB), and rabies vaccines.

- *Live-attenuated vaccines.* Live-attenuated (weakened) vaccines have live viral or bacterial parts that produce a mild infection, which stimulates immunity to a virus or bacteria but rarely causes illness in healthy individuals. Live-attenuated vaccines include the nasal influenza vaccine called FluMist; varicella (chicken pox); smallpox; yellow fever; and measles, mumps, and rubella (MMR) vaccines. In some countries oral polio vaccine (OPV, given as drops by mouth) and a live-attenuated tuberculosis vaccination (called BCG) are used.

Many of these vaccines are routinely given to children between birth and four to five years of age. The meningococcal vaccine is recommended for young adolescents eleven to twelve years of age, adolescents entering high school or fifteen years of age who have not been previously vaccinated, and teenagers entering college who will be living in dormitories for the first time. Most schools require these vaccines before entry, so it is likely that many children will have received the recommended set of immunizations for their age before they have any symptoms of myositis. (See Table 29.1 for vaccines currently recommended in the U.S.)

What If My Child Has Not Received All the Recommended Vaccines?

For each child at each stage of the myositis illness, the benefit of a vaccine and the risk of an unexpected or unusual reaction to the vaccine should be weighed by you and your child's doctor. When vaccines are given to very ill children receiving

Table 29.1. Recommended immunizations for healthy children in the United States, 2006.*

Vaccine	Inactive or live virus in the vaccine
Diphtheria-tetanus (dT, DT)	Inactive
Diphtheria, Pertussis, Tetanus (DPT, DTaP, Tdap)	Inactive
Hemophilus influenza b (HIB)	Inactive
Hepatitis A	Inactive
Hepatitis B	Inactive
Influenza (intramuscular)	Inactive
Meningococcal (MCV4, MPSV4)	Inactive
Pneumococcal conjugate	Inactive
Polio (inactivated polio vaccine, IPV)	Inactive
Human papillomavirus (HPV)	Inactive
Varicella	Live
Influenza (nasal) (FluMist)	Live
Measles, Mumps, Rubella (MMRII)	Live
Measles, Mumps, Rubella, Varicella (ProQuad)	Live

*It is important that you discuss the risks and benefits of all vaccines with your child's doctor before immunization. For current updates in this rapidly changing field, see http://www.cdc.gov/mmwr/pdf/wk/mm5451-Immunization.pdf.

high doses of steroids or other immunosuppressive medicines, they might not work properly. The vaccine might not produce an immune response to protect your child from future infections because the immune system cannot develop a protective immune response when it is so suppressed by the different medicines. Also, for live viral vaccines, the child could become sick with the virus from the vaccine because the immune system is suppressed. Because each child with myositis is unique, it is important that your child's doctor decide with you how best to adjust your child's immunization schedule.

For children with myositis whose immunizations are currently due or overdue, catch-up immunizations are not generally recommended during the initial diagnosis and treatment phase. In general, the same childhood immunizations that are recommended for healthy children may be appropriate for children with myositis only when the myositis is well controlled and when doses of medicine are relatively low. Possibly the safest approach is to wait to administer immunizations after your child's myositis is fully controlled for several months and your child has discontinued all immunosuppressive therapy. Based on the experience of some juvenile myositis (JM) experts, there is also concern that some immunizations can cause JM to become worse in some patients. However, these reports are uncommon, and there is no current scientific evidence that vaccination will definitely make myositis worse. Your child's doctor may determine that it is more important to start therapy for myositis immediately and to provide catch-up immunizations later on, after medicine doses are lowered and the myositis is under good control, stable, and quiet for a period of time.

The decision to withhold immunizations may be based on several factors, such as the combined effects of several medications and the overall activity of your child's disease. A brief description of which vaccines can be given with which medications is provided in Table 29.2. Because each child with JM is different, your child's doctor will need to decide when the time is right to begin immunizations again. For more specific information about treatments for JM, see *Chapter 7, Treatment Possibilities in the Beginning* and *Chapter 12, Possible Medicines During the Course.*

Can the Other People in Our Household Still Be Vaccinated?

It is important that neither your child with myositis nor other household members receive live viral vaccines while your child is taking high doses of steroids or other immunosuppressive medicines. This includes live attenuated influenza vaccine (FluMist) because of a risk of transmitting the viral infection from the vaccinated person to your child with myositis. Oral polio vaccine may also be shed after vaccination and infect close contacts. Although this vaccine is not currently recommended for routine use in the U.S., it may be important to consider whether your child will have any risk of exposure to recently vaccinated individuals when traveling outside of the U.S. or when family and friends visit from regions that still use oral poliovirus vaccine. Only inactivated polio vaccine and inactivated influenza vaccines should be used in this situation. Varicella (chicken pox) vaccine virus can also be transmitted from immunized persons to immuno-suppressed children with myositis. It is generally recommended that individuals who have received the varicella vaccine avoid contact with immunosuppressed persons for six weeks after immunization. There may be new live viral vaccines in the future, and these recommendations would apply to any live viral vaccines.

However, whenever one person in a household is more susceptible to infection, it is very helpful for all the other members of the household to be up-to-date with their immunizations of inactivated vaccines. This is a good way of protecting your child who is being treated for myositis and decreases the chance of family members getting sick at home. This may include making sure everyone in the household has had a recent tuberculosis skin test and gets an inactivated influenza vaccine every year.

The MMRII vaccine, which contains three strains of live attenuated viruses (measles, mumps, and rubella), is not used to immunize immunosuppressed children but may be given safely to household members. The risk of transmitting the infection to other family members in the house who did not receive the vaccine is

Table 29.2. Medications, risks of infection, and vaccines that might be used in JM.

It is important that you discuss the risks and benefits of all vaccines with your child's doctor before immunization.

Medicine	Increased risk of severe infection while taking this medicine?	Vaccines your child might receive while taking this medicine	Vaccines your child and other household members *should not* receive while your child is taking this medication***
Corticosteroids* Prednisone, Prednisolone Medrol, SoluMedrol	Yes	Inactivated vaccines**	Live virus vaccines should not be given when on high doses of corticosteroids
Methotrexate* (Rheumatrex, Trexall)	Yes	Inactivated vaccines	Live virus vaccines
Hydroxychloroquine (Plaquenil)	No	Inactivated and live vaccines	No vaccines are prohibited
Intravenous immune globulin (IVIG)	No (However, IVIG is a pooled blood product and can potentially transmit a blood-borne infection.)	Inactivated vaccines	IVIG may interfere with normal responses to live vaccines. Patients should not receive live vaccines, such as MMR and varicella, for up to eleven months after IVIG is given.
Cyclosporine* (Sandimmune, Neoral)	Yes	Inactivated vaccines	Live virus vaccines
Cyclophosphamide* (Cytoxan)	Yes	Inactivated vaccines	Live virus vaccines
Azathioprine* (Imuran)	Yes	Inactivated vaccines	Live virus vaccines
Tacrolimus* (by mouth) (Prograf)	Yes	Inactivated vaccines	Live virus vaccines
Mycophenolate* (CellCept)	Yes	Inactivated vaccines	Live virus vaccines
TNF-alpha inhibitors* Etanercept (Enbrel) Infliximab (Remicade) Adalimumab (Humira)	Yes	Inactivated vaccines	Live virus vaccines

* Immunosuppressive medication. See *Chapter 12, Possible Medicines During the Course,* for more information about medicines used in the treatment of myositis.

** See Table 29.1 for which vaccines contain inactivated or live virus.

*** While receiving immunosuppressive medicines, your child may get sick with the virus in live virus vaccines and should not receive these vaccines. Likewise, live viral vaccines, such as oral polio vaccine, live-attenuated influenza vaccine, and varicella vaccine, should not be given to household members if your child is receiving these medicines because these vaccine viruses can be transmitted to those in close contact. However, measles, mumps, and rubella vaccine(s) can be administered to household members even if your child with JM is receiving immunosuppressive medicines.

quite low for rubella and is not known to occur for the measles or mumps vaccine viruses that are currently included in MMRII. In contrast, there is some evidence of symptomatic transmission of some mumps vaccine strains that are included in vaccines used in other countries.

What If My Child Has Never Had Chicken Pox (Varicella) and Never Received a Varicella Vaccine?

Sometimes a very mild chicken pox infection (varicella) goes unnoticed. However, these mild infections can be sufficient to provide protection against the chicken pox virus. Your child's doctor can check blood levels of antibodies to varicella virus. If varicella antibodies are present, your child should be immune to chicken pox and would not become sick with it if she had been in contact with someone with chicken pox. If your child does not show signs in the blood of adequate protection against chicken pox, it is important to avoid anyone with chicken pox while your child is receiving steroids or other immunosuppressive medicines to treat the myositis. In many cases it is not appropriate to delay the treatment of myositis so that your child can first receive the chicken pox vaccine.

If your child has been exposed to someone with chicken pox, let your child's doctor know immediately. If your child is exposed to chicken pox, she may be treated with varicella-zoster immune globulin to help lessen the severity of chicken pox that could develop. This medicine must be given by injection as early as possible and no more than four days after exposure to chicken pox. If this medicine is not available, the Advisory Committee on Immunization Practices is recommending the use of intravenous immune globulin (IVIG) as a substitute. An antiviral medication called acyclovir (Zovirax) is occasionally used in patients who have been exposed to chicken pox and develop symptoms. Later, when your child is no longer on high-dose corticosteroids or other immunosuppressive medicines and the myositis is under good control for a period of time, the varicella vaccine may be administered. Your child's specialist or doctor should plan the right timing for your child to receive the chicken pox vaccine.

A unique feature of chicken pox is the ability of the varicella virus to reactivate as herpes zoster or "shingles" years after the primary infection. This reactivation appears as a localized, often painful rash made up of groups of small, red, fluid-filled bumps. In immunosuppressed patients, such as in children with myositis taking high doses of prednisone or other medicines, herpes zoster can occasionally become a widespread and serious infection. Herpes zoster infection can occur after natural chicken pox infection and has been reported infrequently after vaccination. The appearance of that type of rash requires prompt evaluation by a healthcare provider.

Should Children with Myositis Receive an Influenza Vaccine Each Year?

Influenza is a highly contagious winter illness that can cause high fevers, chills, severe cold symptoms, and upset stomach. It is spread easily from one person to another. There are two types of influenza vaccine available, and each is administered in early autumn in the United States and Canada. The most commonly used one is inactivated influenza vaccine. It is given by a shot injected into the muscle and can be used in most individuals. As with other vaccines, it may be less effective in immunosuppressed individuals, and it may be prudent to delay immunization, if possible, until immunosuppressive medicines are discontinued. Recommendations for the use of influenza vaccine can be reviewed at www.cdc.gov/mmwr/preview/mmwrhtml/rr55e628a1.htm. It is worthwhile for children with myositis and their family members to consider being immunized with inactivated influenza vaccines each year, as early as possible, because it can help to decrease your child's possible exposure to influenza. Children receiving high-dose corticosteroids, cytotoxic drugs, and/or biologic agents that suppress the immune system are usually able to respond to inactivated influenza vaccine and often do not have any serious or unexpected reactions after vaccination. For some patients receiving high-dose or daily corticosteroids or multiple medicines, it may be best not to receive the inactivated influenza immunization until their illness is less active and medication doses are decreased.

The second type of influenza vaccine (FluMist) is a live-attenuated influenza vaccine given as a nasal spray. It may be used in healthy children five years old and older. *FluMist should not be used by individuals taking corticosteroids or other immunosuppressive therapies or by their household members or other close contacts because it contains live influenza virus.*

The influenza virus changes constantly, allowing it to cause illness even in people who have had influenza in the past. For this reason the virus strains used to make the vaccine are re-evaluated yearly to make certain that the vaccine will include new strains that are expected to cause influenza during the coming season. Annual immunization helps boost existing immunity against influenza virus and stimulates additional protection against new strains.

If your child is exposed to the flu or develops symptoms of a flu-like illness, you should contact your child's doctor immediately. It may be necessary for your child to take antiviral drugs shown to be effective against current strains of influenza viruses, such as oseltamivir (Tamiflu), to prevent or treat influenza infection. These types of antiviral drugs work best if administered within two days of the onset of symptoms. Oseltamivir may be used to treat influenza A and B infections in children one year old and older. Another medication, zanamivir (Relenza), is approved for use against A and B strains in children seven years old and older.

Are There Any Special Concerns About Using Vaccines in Children on Immunosuppressive Therapy?

How much the immune system is suppressed influences how well the vaccine will work. For example, children using only topical corticosteroids, like those used for skin rashes, can be effectively immunized on schedule with live or inactivated vaccines because they are only minimally immunosuppressed. However, live virus vaccines should not be administered to persons receiving high doses of corticosteroids by mouth or by vein. Live viral vaccines can make the child get sicker than usual with the infection from the vaccine. "High dose" may mean an individual dose of corticosteroid that is considered by your child's doctor to suppress the immune system. Alternatively, it may reflect the prolonged use of a corticosteroid or a combination of several medicines that when used together produce a strong suppression of the immune system.

The American Academy of Pediatrics recommends that children do not receive a live virus vaccine until they have stopped taking high-dose corticosteroids, or other such medicines that suppress the immune system, for about one to three months. Similar precautions are advised in children receiving cytotoxic and biologic agent therapy. In children receiving moderate doses of therapy that can potentially suppress the immune system, a risk-benefit ratio needs to be considered before vaccination. The potential risks are a side effect of the vaccine (including a potential worsening of the myositis) and/or an inadequate immune response to the vaccine. The benefits are partial or complete protection against infection. If the immune response to the vaccine was reduced, later re-immunization, when the child is off treatment for myositis, is an option. Again, these decisions about when the time is right to initiate or restart immunizations should be made in consultation with your child's myositis doctor or primary care provider.

How Does Immunosuppressive Therapy Affect the Signs and Symptoms of Infections?

Immunosuppressive therapy, such as corticosteroids, can decrease the typical signs and symptoms of infections. For example, you may see less redness and tenderness at the site of a skin infection. Any minor illness, such as an upper respiratory infection or "cold," fever, or symptoms of illness such as headache, ear pain, cough, sore throat, nausea, decreased appetite, vomiting or diarrhea, or a change in the level of activity should be carefully monitored and evaluated by your child's primary care provider. These same medicines also increase your child's chances of becoming sick with various infections, including bacterial and viral infections. Children with myositis who are receiving steroids or other immunosuppressive treatments require early and aggressive medical treatment for viral and bacterial infections.

What If Someone Else in Our Household Is III?

It is important to have the sick household member evaluated by his or her healthcare provider. If they have a treatable infectious illness, early treatment may prevent exposing your child with JM to the illness. Of course, standard precautions for avoiding infectious illnesses, such as regular and thorough hand washing, using disposable bathroom cups, and not sharing food, drinks, utensils or dishes, are always appropriate.

Will My Child Get More Infections While on Medicines for Myositis?

Once the medications for myositis are begun, your child might get more minor infections, such as ear or sinus infections. Common infections, such as strep throat and infections around the nails, are important to treat early. Sometimes your child may develop a cheesy white layer on the inside of the cheeks or in the vaginal area that becomes red and itchy; this may be a yeast infection. Let your doctors know when your child has these infections so they can be checked out and given the proper antibiotics or other treatment. Sinus infections need to be treated with antibiotics for three weeks.

A few children who develop myositis may have a lower level of factors (immunoglobulins, especially IgG and IgA) that protect against infection, even before the medications for myositis are started. If the infections persist, your child's doctor might want to check your child's IgG level to determine whether it is normal. If it is not in the normal range for your child's age, then your child may need to receive intravenous immune globulin (IVIG) to bring the amount in the blood up to normal levels. Because the body uses IgG to defend itself against infection, your child may need repeated infusions every three or four weeks until the doses of myositis medicines are lowered. It is helpful to check the IgG levels before the next dose of IVIG to see whether your child has recovered. Sometimes with medicines that cause a great amount of immunosuppression some doctors choose to start an antibiotic, such as trimethoprim/sulfamethoxazole (Bactrim or Septra), to help protect the lungs from infection, but there is no single approach to this problem. If your child receives cyclophosphamide, the white cells in the blood are usually at their lowest level nine to eleven days after each dose, and this too may lower your child's level of protection.

What Should I Tell My Child's Teacher or Day Care Provider About the Risks of Infection?

It is important that your child's teacher understand that medications used to treat myositis increase your child's chance of becoming sick with an infection. That doesn't mean your child shouldn't attend school. Your child's education is an essential part of her intellectual and social development. Teachers often notice the first signs and symptoms of illness in the classroom, such as tiredness and decreased activity. You should ask your child's teacher to tell you when your child's behavior in school does not seem normal. Also tell your child's teacher that it is important to alert you when one of your child's classmates develops an infection, such as chicken pox, influenza, or other serious infections so that you can be more alert to the signs of illness in your child or can seek the appropriate treatment early. Your child's teacher can help reduce the chances of infection by encouraging the same good infection control habits in school that you use at home, such as regular hand washing, and by teaching good hygiene.

What Can I Do to Reduce My Child's Risk of Infection?

Good, basic hygiene, such as regular hand washing and avoiding sharing food and utensils, is always important. Your child should avoid unpasteurized dairy products, undercooked beef or poultry, raw eggs, and raw shellfish. These foods have been associated with a number of different serious stomach bacterial and viral illnesses. Your child should not drink well water unless it is boiled, and fresh fruit and vegetables should be washed before being eaten. Your child should wear protective clothing (long sleeves and a hat when in wooded areas) to avoid tick bites and use insect repellent in the warm weather to decrease mosquito bites. These precautions decrease the risk of Lyme disease and infection with West Nile virus.

Children with JM sometimes develop specific skin problems, such as calcium deposits and skin ulcers. These areas may be especially prone to infection because the surface of the skin may be broken. In fact, any area where the skin is broken, such as cuts and abrasions, is more likely to become infected. It is a good practice to inspect the skin regularly for any signs of infection, especially if calcinosis or ulcers are present. If you notice redness or tenderness of the skin or if your child has a skin lesion that is not healing, your child's doctor should examine the skin and decide if antibiotics are needed. Exposure to lakes, oceans, and swimming pools should be avoided if the skin is broken.

In general, your child should avoid close contact with other children or individuals who have acute illness such as sore throats, stomach virus (vomiting and/or diarrhea), or pneumonia. There may be times when your doctor recommends that your child not attend school if there is a known outbreak of an acute infectious illness affecting many children in school. Special precautions, such as the use of face masks and avoidance of public spaces, may occasionally be considered.

Is It Okay for My Family and My Child to Travel?
Can Visitors Come to Our Home?

Before you travel, be sure that no one you are visiting has a serious infectious illness. The same is true for people visiting you. When your child is receiving intensive medical therapy, it makes good sense to avoid people whom you know are sick. Of course, this is not always possible. Everybody gets sick once in a while.

Most minor illnesses, such as colds and runny noses, will not likely affect the course of your child's illness or therapy. Alert your child's doctor if you know your child has been exposed to a serious infectious illness.

You should discuss any overseas travel with your child's doctor. In general, the routine immunizations that are recommended for U.S. citizens are adequate for most overseas travel. Information on immunization for travelers is updated regularly by the Centers for Disease Control (CDC) and can be found at www.cdc.gov/travel.

Key Points

- For each child at each stage of the myositis illness, you and your child's doctor should weigh the benefit of a vaccine and the risk of an unexpected or unusual reaction to the vaccine.

- Some immunizations may have to be delayed while the myositis is treated with medicines that suppress the immune system, but some can be given on schedule. "Catch-up" immunizations are generally not recommended during the initial diagnosis and treatment phase. Medicines that suppress the immune system interfere with your child's ability to fight infections.

- Live virus vaccines should not be given to patients receiving immunosuppressive therapy, and, in general, should not be given to their household members or other close contacts.

- Inactivated vaccines may be safe for patients whose myositis is stable or inactive and who are on low doses of immunosuppressive medicines. They may be given to household members and other close contacts, which help protect your child with myositis from developing these infections.

- Practice good infection control. Family members and your child with myositis should wash hands regularly, use disposable cups in the bathrooms, have tissues handy, and not share food, cups, or eating utensils.

- When your child is receiving treatments for myositis that suppress the immune system, seek medical evaluation quickly if you think she is ill. Be sure to have close household contacts examined if they are sick because they can pass infection on to a child with myositis.

To Learn More

Centers for Disease Control and Prevention (CDC). Phone: 800-232-2522 (English) or 800-232-2330 (Spanish).

Immunization Schedules. Available at: www.cdc.gov/nip/menus/vaccines.htm#Schedules.
    Updated immunization schedules.

Vaccine Information Statements. Available at: www.cdc.gov/nip/publications/VIS.
    Information sheets that explain both the benefits and risks of a vaccine. Federal law requires that VIS be handed out whenever certain vaccinations are given.

Contraindications To Childhood Immunization. Available at: www.cdc.gov/nip/recs/contraindications.htm.

Information Networks and Other Information Sources. Available at: www.cdc.gov/other.htm#states.

> Links to state and local health departments, public health partners, and other resources.

American Academy of Pediatrics.

Recommended Childhood and Adolescent Immunization Schedule. Available from: http://aapredbook.aappublications.org.

World Health Organization.

Vaccines, Immunization and Biologicals. Available at: www.who.int/vaccines/Global Summary/Immunization/ScheduleSelect.cfm.

> Information on international immunization programs.

Canadian Paediatric Society.

Routine Immunization Schedule for Infants and Children. Available at: www.caring forkids.cps.ca/immunization/vaccinationchild.htm#Table1 or 613-526-9397.

Immunization Action Coalition. 1573 Selby Avenue, Suite 234, St. Paul MN 55104; Phone: 651-647-9009; Internet: www.immunize.org; Email: admin@immunize.org.

A 501(c)3 nonprofit organization working to increase immunization rates and prevent disease by creating and distributing educational materials for health professionals and the public. Facilitates communication about the safety, efficacy, and use of vaccines within the broad immunization community of patients, parents, healthcare organizations, and government health agencies.

The National Advisory Committee on Immunization (Canada). Public Health Agency of Canada, 130 Colonnade Road, A.L. 6501H, Ottawa ON K1A 0K9; Phone: 604-666-2083; Internet: www.hc-sc.gc.ca/index_e.html.

Vaccine Adverse Event Reporting System (VAERS). P.O. Box 1100, Rockville MD 20849-1100; Phone: 800-822-7967; Internet: www.vaers.org.

Report adverse events or problems developing after immunizations to VAERS.

Reports in the Medical Literature

Centers for Disease Control and Prevention. Chapters 1, 18, and 19. In: Department of Health and Human Services. *Immunization Works: Everything you want to know about immunization in one CD.* Centers for Disease Control and Prevention National Immunization Program; 2003.

Hopes of Recovery

The Clinical Course and Outcome of Juvenile Myositis

Robert M. Rennebohm, MD; Brian M. Feldman, MD, MSc, FRCPC;
Adam M. Huber, MSc, MD; Charles H. Spencer, MD;
Robert P. Sundel, MD; and Lisa G. Rider, MD

In this chapter...

Juvenile myositis tends to follow one of three main clinical courses: a single cycle, several cycles, or chronic continuous course. With currently available treatments, the outcome appears very good. The mortality rate has been greatly reduced, and most children can carry on daily life functions and complete their schooling.

From the family's point of view...

"We didn't know what to expect, and from what we learned from other families, there were many different paths their children had followed in terms of responding to treatment and having flares of the disease. Luckily, our doctors were very honest with us, telling us they didn't know our daughter's exact prognosis and that we couldn't tell ahead of time what would treat her symptoms. They couldn't predict whether she'd go into remission, but we'd just have to keep trying."

When parents are first told that their child has a form of juvenile myositis (JM), they have many questions about the clinical course of the illness (how the illness behaves over time and what patients experience along the way) and the outcome (the final result after the illness is over). Common questions include:

- How long does this illness last?
- How severe can it get?
- How well can it be controlled?
- If it goes away, will it come back?
- Can permanent damage occur?
- What will most likely happen in my child's case?

Unfortunately, there is no single answer to these questions. The condition will be different for each child. In this chapter, we will talk about general patterns. Your child's illness might not follow one pattern exactly. Since juvenile dermatomyositis (JDM) is the most common form of JM, we will focus on it.

What Are the Possible Outcomes of JDM?

When children with JDM are treated with currently available medications of prednisone alone or in combination with other medicines (see *Chapter 12, Possible Medicines During the Course*), their illness tends to follow one of three main clinical courses:

- Monocyclic course
- Polycyclic course
- Chronic continuous course

Within each course there is a broad spectrum of illness severity and disease duration. Some children have a clinical course that does not fit neatly into any of these general patterns.

Monocyclic Course

The clinical course is defined as monocyclic (single cycle) if your child's illness goes into remission within twenty-four months after diagnosis and there is no relapse. Remission means there is no clinical or laboratory evidence of active JDM, and the child no longer needs to take medicine for JDM. Relapse (or recurrence) means a return of active JDM after a period of remission. Approximately 20% to 60% of children with JDM have a monocyclic course.

The illness in patients with a monocyclic course may start at a mild, moderate, or severe level of intensity. (A moderate example is shown in Figure 30.1.) This

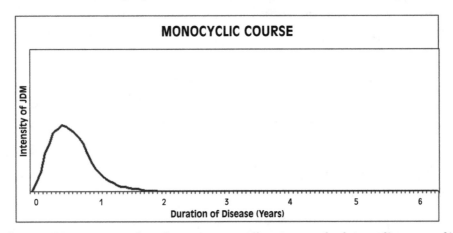

■ **Figure 30.1. Example of a monocyclic course in juvenile myositis.**
This child developed moderately severe juvenile dermatomyositis. Her illness went into remission (no clinical or laboratory evidence of active disease, off all medication) within two years after treatment and never returned.

results in mild, moderate, or severe muscle weakness and varying amounts of rash. Over the following months, while receiving medication to treat the JDM, the severity of illness decreases. Within two years the JDM becomes inactive, medication can be stopped, and the illness never returns. The monocyclic course is the least threatening and has the best outcome. A complete recovery, including a return to normal muscle strength, usually occurs. Calcinosis may occur, but it is usually mild.

Polycyclic Course

The clinical course is defined as polycyclic (many cycles) if your child's illness goes into definite remission but recurs at least once. Patients whose JDM follows a polycyclic course often initially appear to have a monocyclic course but then have one or more relapses (see Figure 30.2). Relapses usually occur after a period of remission that lasts for several months to a few years. It is less common for a relapse to occur after having been in remission for many years. Most patients have only one, two, or three recurrences. Usually, each relapse behaves much like a monocyclic episode, although the recurrences might be milder, particularly when appropriate treatment is started quickly.

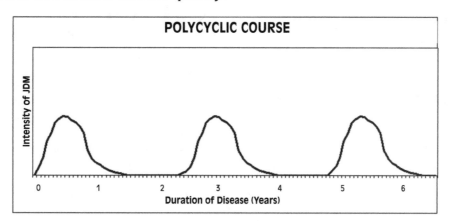

■ Figure 30.2. Example of a polycyclic course in juvenile myositis.
This child developed moderately severe juvenile dermatomyositis, which initially appeared to follow a monocyclic course but recurred (relapsed) twice, once at two years, five months and again at four years, nine months into the course of the disease. She was in remission (no clinical or laboratory evidence of active disease, off all medication) before each relapse.

We do not know why some children have a recurrence of illness after a remission. Often, recurrence seems to happen spontaneously. In some cases reducing the dose and number of medications too quickly can contribute to a recurrence. In other situations certain environmental factors, such as sun exposure without adequate use of sunscreen and protective clothing (see *Chapter 16, Skin Rashes and Sun Protection*) or an infectious illness or even exposure to other factors, can contribute to an illness flare or relapse, with recurrence of symptoms and active myositis. The exact percentage of JDM patients who experience a true polycyclic course is not known. Estimates range from 10% to 40%.

The long-term outcome of children with a polycyclic course is usually excellent or good. In one study 90% of such JDM patients recovered completely when followed up for an average of eight years, and in another study 40% recovered completely when followed up for an average of six years. This complete clinical recovery was achieved, on average, within four years after diagnosis but took eleven years in one case. Calcinosis occurs more frequently in polycyclic disease than in monocyclic disease, but less frequently in polycyclic disease than in chronic continuous disease. Several studies strongly suggest that the risk of calcinosis can be reduced in all three illness courses if JDM is treated aggressively and early at each recurrence.

Chronic Continuous Course

The course is defined as chronic continuous if your child has continuous clinically active disease for more than two years after diagnosis. Typically, the disease remains continuously active to some extent for several years, often for four to ten years, sometimes longer (Figure 30.3). Often, parents ask whether their child will "grow out of their myositis" or if the illness will "burn out on its own" when their child is a teenager or adult. With proper treatment JDM can be well controlled or cured by the time the child becomes older. For some people, however, the myositis remains active into adulthood. Approximately 10% to 50% of children with JDM have a chronic continuous course when treated with early, aggressive treatment.

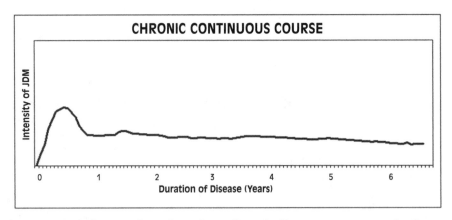

■ **Figure 30.3. Example of a chronic continuous course in juvenile myositis.**
This child initially developed moderately severe juvenile dermatomyositis, which improved after treatment was started but has remained continually active for more than six years. She is still on medication. Her disease will probably gradually become less and less active and finally go into remission over the next four years.

This course varies the most in terms of disease duration, disease severity, extent of fluctuation of illness intensity, and outcome. Some children have a chronic continuous course that fluctuates very little in intensity and continues for several years. The intensity of their illness throughout most of those years can be mild, moderate, or severe. The duration of their illness varies from a few years to more than a decade. Sometimes their illness remains slightly active into their adult years. The outcome for these children depends on whether their illness throughout the years has mostly been mild, moderate, or severe.

In other children with a chronic continuous course, the intensity of disease activity fluctuates widely. Their illness alternates between being very active and much less active, before finally going into remission. This course resembles a polycyclic course, except that true remission does not occur between recurrences. In fact, it is often difficult to know whether a child has a true polycyclic course or a widely fluctuating chronic continuous course because it is often hard to know whether the myositis has truly gone into remission between disease flares.

There is an important subgroup of patients with chronic continuous disease who have chronic continuous skin disease rather than chronic continuous muscle activity. Most of these children initially have at least some muscle disease (sometimes relatively mild), but the main concern becomes their considerable ongoing skin rashes. Their JDM rash is sometimes widespread, and it commonly continues (at varying degrees of severity) for several years, despite the presence of little or no disease activity in their muscles. Their skin rashes are often difficult to treat and can be very frustrating for the child and family. In addition to cosmetic concerns, these children may be at increased risk for calcinosis. More research is needed to determine how best to treat these children, but it is important to keep in mind that their skin rashes seem to require several different medicines (see *Chapter 16, Skin Rashes and Sun Protection*).

Why Do JDM Patients Follow Different Illness Courses? Can Early, More Aggressive Treatment Prevent a Severe or Chronic Course?

The three main clinical courses described above are the courses noted when children with JDM are treated with the currently available medicines, including high initial corticosteroid dosage (1–2 mg/kg/day, sometimes with several initial pulses of intravenous methylprednisolone), followed by gradual lowering of the corticosteroid dosage over many months and often with early addition of other medicines. Parents often ask, "Would even more aggressive treatment, particularly early after illness onset, prevent my child from having a polycyclic or chronic continuous course or reduce the severity of her illness?"

We do not have proven answers to that question. It seems that some children may be largely destined, perhaps because of differing genetic predispositions, to follow one course or another. When patients who seem to have the same symptoms at the onset of their illness receive similar medicines for their myositis, some follow a monocyclic course, others a polycyclic course, and others a chronic continuous course. Perhaps some children have a mild monocyclic course primarily because they are prone to develop only a mild version of JDM, which is able to be corrected fully within twenty-four months, after which time they are not prone to develop JDM again. Perhaps some children who have a severe, prolonged, difficult-to-treat course primarily do so because they are prone to develop a very intense version of JDM and have much less capacity for self-correction.

Other factors, such as exposure to certain viruses, sunlight, or other environmental conditions might also influence the course of your child's JDM. Such exposures could contribute to ongoing myositis or to relapses of myositis after achieving remission.

We currently do not know whether early, aggressive treatment with currently available medicines can prevent your child from having a chronic continuous course or a polycyclic course. We do know that aggressive treatment given early, soon after the first symptoms develop, is hugely beneficial and greatly improves outcome. Such treatment usually greatly reduces the severity of the illness so that your child has less severe muscle weakness and rash throughout the disease course and has a better outcome, including lower risk of developing calcinosis.

Pediatric rheumatologists and others who care for children with JDM are optimistic that there will be treatments that can break into the vicious cycles (or otherwise interfere with the disease process) so that the disease loses steam and grinds to a halt sooner than is the case with current therapies. The goal is to develop treatments that can safely convert all courses of JDM into mild, monocyclic courses of the shortest possible duration. Until such treatment becomes available, it is important to treat early and aggressively, and it is helpful to be aware of the monocyclic, polycyclic, and chronic continuous courses that have been observed.

Can Doctors Predict Which Clinical Course My Child Will Have?

Once a family understands the possible clinical courses of JDM, the next question usually is, "Which course do you think my child will have?" Unfortunately, it is difficult (if not impossible) for your child's doctors to predict which course your child will likely follow. Even children who show signs of very severe muscle weakness and extremely high muscle enzyme levels could follow a monocyclic course and enjoy an excellent outcome. On the other hand, some children who initially have only mild weakness could have a chronic continuous course.

There are some clues, however, that might indicate a greater likelihood of a chronic course and/or the presence of more severe illness. These factors include:

- Delay in diagnosis and delay of proper treatment may lead to a more prolonged illness or the development of calcinosis.

- Failure to respond adequately to the initial high doses of prednisone or other steroid medication suggests more intense disease and a need for more aggressive treatment.

- Failure to tolerate reduction of prednisone dosage suggests that the patient is at increased risk of a chronic continuous course.

- Extremely severe swallowing difficulty at the beginning of the illness suggests need for particularly aggressive treatment and can indicate greater likelihood of a chronic course.

- The clinical course of some JDM patients is complicated by the development of severe ulcers in the skin or digestive tract (esophagus, stomach, or intestines). These ulcers are holes in the skin or digestive tract tissue. Development of severe skin ulcers or gastrointestinal ulcers (including unusually severe abdominal pain) suggests that the patient has particularly severe illness and might have a more prolonged course. These conditions suggest the need for particularly aggressive therapy. Fortunately, only a small percentage of children with JDM develop severe ulcers. If ulcerative complications are recognized early and treated aggressively, a very good outcome can occur.

- Development of interstitial lung disease, i.e., inflammation of the lung tissue and air sacs (see *Chapter 24, When Children Have Difficulty Breathing*), suggests an increased risk for severe and/or chronic illness.

- Some studies indicate that results of the initial muscle biopsy related to the involvement of the muscle blood vessels might help predict whether the illness is likely to be chronic or severe.

- Genetic factors might play a role. Some JDM patients with a particular polymorphism (variation in the gene) of a cytokine called tumor necrosis factor alpha (TNF-α) are more likely to have a chronic course of JDM (see *Chapter 3, The Pathways to Juvenile Myositis*).

- Certain blood tests give clues to predict clinical course. Patients with the myositis-specific autoantibody Mi-2 (see *Chapter 1, What Is Juvenile Myositis?*) tend to have either a monocyclic or polycyclic course. Patients with anti-synthetase (Jo-1) autoantibodies tend to have a chronic continuous course. These autoantibody tests are not performed routinely and are available only in certain laboratories.

How Well Will My Child Function in the Long Term?

Although the clinical course influences the eventual outcome of JDM, most children have a remarkably good result. Several pediatric rheumatologists tracked the outcomes of their patients with JDM in the 1970s and 1980s. These patients, who at the time of the studies were teenagers or young adults, mostly had good outcomes and could participate in normal activities, although some of them had ongoing skin rash, weakness, or calcinosis.

A more recent study was done in Canada at four different hospitals. In this study, sixty-five children with JDM were contacted several years after the diagnosis of myositis was made. Half the children were contacted more than seven years after the time of their diagnosis. At the time they were contacted, almost all the children could take part in all normal life activities. Seventy percent had no measurable disability at all, and the rest had only minimal disability. The exception was one person who had many calcium deposits that limited her ability to walk and do other household activities. The 70%—those who had the most normal physical function—were least likely to have a chronic continuous course and least likely to have calcinosis.

Educationally, these children did extremely well. Three of the children had to stay behind a year in school because they had missed too much school at the beginning of the illness. Even so, all of the children were attending school or had finished, and all reported that they were doing well academically. All of the patients who had finished high school had gone on to university or college.

That study also looked at growth. Prednisone, one of the treatments for myositis, might stunt your child's growth if used for a very long time. Although most of the children were close to their predicted height, they were more frequently shorter than would be expected based on their parents' height. Those with a chronic continuous course were more likely to be shorter than expected.

Can Children Die from Juvenile Dermatomyositis?

With current treatments for JDM, children very rarely die of JDM (approximately 1% of patients or less). This is particularly true for those who do not have any of the high risk factors mentioned earlier (such as severe ulcerations or interstitial lung disease). Even when life-threatening factors are present, JDM can usually be brought under safe control if intensive, aggressive therapy is provided promptly, particularly if your child is in a hospital that is experienced with very sick children and if she is cared for by a specialist who has experience treating JDM. When death does occur, it is usually because of a hole developing in the digestive system (gastrointestinal perforation), lung disease, heart complications, or infection, in that order of probability.

The key to preventing death is early aggressive therapy and early recognition of and attention to high risk factors. Before 1960, JDM was not treated as aggressively or as early as it is treated today, and approximately one-third of patients died, one-third recovered, and one-third had chronic disabling disease; most patients had severe disability. During the past decade the importance of early aggressive treatment has been greatly emphasized, and the mortality rate has decreased markedly. The two most recently published articles on the long-term outcome of JDM reported death in only one of one hundred patients. The fact that even one patient died underscores the potential seriousness of the disease and the need for even more effective treatment.

No formal studies have been completed to determine whether JDM shortens life expectancy. It seems likely that, for most patients, life expectancy is normal. It also seems likely that the only patients who might be at risk of having a shortened lifespan are the infrequent patients with particularly severe, particularly prolonged, and particularly disabling disease. But even for those patients, life expectancy may be normal. Formal study of this issue is needed.

Some parents ask whether there is a link between JDM and cancer. They ask this because they have read or heard that there is a link between adult dermatomyositis and cancer. Fortunately, the link between JDM and cancer is very rare (see *Chapter 1, What Is Juvenile Myositis?*).

What Are the Outcomes of Juvenile Polymyositis and Other Forms of JM?

There are not much data on the clinical course and outcome of juvenile polymyositis (JPM) and other forms of JM, primarily because these forms of JM are much less common than JDM. Most, but not all, children with JPM have a chronic continuous course. In our experience the outcome of JPM is not appreciably different from that of JDM. JM overlapping with other connective tissue diseases (overlap myositis) frequently follows a polycyclic course. Myositis-specific autoantibodies can help determine the course (see *Chapter 1, What Is Juvenile Myositis?*). JPM or overlap myositis associated with Jo-1 and other anti-synthetase autoantibodies tends to follow a chronic continuous course. JPM associated with anti-signal recognition particle often follows a chronic continuous course. (These blood tests are not performed routinely in patients with JPM or myositis overlap syndromes.) Further careful study of more children with JPM and other forms of JM is greatly needed.

Key Points

- When children with JM are treated with currently available medicines, their illness tends to follow one of three main courses: monocyclic, polycyclic, or chronic continuous.

- There is a broad spectrum of illness severity and disease duration within each disease course pattern.

- It is difficult, if not impossible, to predict the course that your child's illness will follow.

- There are clues, however, that may indicate the presence of particularly severe disease activity and/or likelihood of a more chronic course.

- Early aggressive treatment gives children the best chance for a good outcome.

- Most children with JDM have a good outcome.

Reports in the Medical Literature

Bowyer SL, Blane CE, Sullivan DB, Cassidy JT. Childhood dermatomyositis: factors predicting functional outcome and development of dystrophic calcification. *Journal of Pediatrics.* 1983 Dec;103(6):882–8.

Fisler RE, Liang MG, Fuhlbrigge RC, Yalcindag A, Sundel RP. Aggressive management of juvenile dermatomyositis results in improved outcome and decreased incidence of calcinosis. *Journal of the American Academy of Dermatology.* 2002 Oct;47(4):505–11.

Huber AM, Lang B, LeBlanc CM, Birdi N, Bolaria RK, Malleson P, et al. Medium- and long-term functional outcomes in a multicenter cohort of children with juvenile dermatomyositis. *Arthritis and Rheumatism.* 2000 Mar;43(3):541–9.

Pachman LM, Liotta-Davis MR, Hong DK, Kinsella TR, Mendez EP, Kinder JM, Chen EH. TNFalpha-308A allele in juvenile dermatomyositis: association with increased production of tumor necrosis factor alpha, disease duration, and pathologic calcifications. *Arthritis and Rheumatism.* 2000 Oct;43(10):2368–77.

Ponyi A, Constantin T, Balogh Z, Szalai Z, Borgulya G, Molnar K, et al. Disease course, frequency of relapses and survival of 73 patients with juvenile or adult dermatomyositis. *Clinical and Experimental Rheumatology.* 2005 Jan-Feb;23(1):50–6.

Rennebohm R. Juvenile dermatomyositis. *Pediatric Annals.* 2002 Jul;31(7):426–33.

Spencer CH, Hanson V, Singsen BH, Bernstein BH, Kornreich HK, King KK. Course of treated juvenile dermatomyositis. *Journal of Pediatrics.* 1984 Sep;105(3):399–408.

CHAPTER 31

Planning for the Future

Patience H. White, MD, MA, and Patricia A. Rettig, RN, MSN, CRNP

In this chapter...

We define and discuss general principles concerning the transition from childhood to adulthood and provide a list of resources to assist you and your teenager with juvenile myositis (JM) to plan for a successful transition.

From the child's point of view...

"When I am older, I want to be a rheumatologist just like my doctor so that I can help kids who have to go through this terrible disease."

"My dermatomyositis definitely plays a role in deciding 'what I want to be when I grow up.' I want to ensure that the future I build for myself will allow me to have the healthy lifestyle that I know I need in order to maintain my well-being. Since my condition is constantly changing, I have to be able to adapt to new circumstances, no matter how challenging that may seem. Going to college has been one of the greatest challenges I have ever been faced with, but by going slowly, being realistic about my abilities, and seeking help when necessary, I am confident that I will be able to receive a well-rounded education for future success, even if it takes a little bit longer."

Teenagers face many changes and transitions as they prepare to leave high school, the home, and the pediatric healthcare setting. Therefore, it is important to learn about available resources to help the teen and family make these transitions successfully. Transition can be defined as the planned movement of youth with long-term illnesses and disabilities from childhood to adulthood. Transition includes:

- School to post-secondary education and/or work
- Home to independence
- Pediatric to adult healthcare systems

The optimal goal of transition is to provide services that are uninterrupted, coordinated, developmentally and age appropriate, psychologically sound, and comprehensive. No matter how transition care is organized, the following general principles apply:

Transition for children with myositis should be a process, not an event, and should involve the entire family. This process must be planned and must consider the young person's developmental stage and illness process. The lack of planning for transition was the most common reason given by service providers in the rehabilitative, educational, and medical areas for children's failure to move successfully into the adult world.

The transition process should begin on the day of diagnosis for both the doctors and the adolescents with myositis and their families. The plan should include goals for independence and self-management that are on a flexible schedule, designed to accommodate the young person's increasing capacity for choice and independence.

Different possibilities for moving into the adult medical system should be discussed with the adolescent, who should be an integral part of the decision-making process. The adolescent must learn to speak for herself, an important step in growing up. Parents need to understand that their roles will change as the focus moves toward fostering a confidential relationship between the young adult and the physician.

Pediatricians, other members of the healthcare team, and the family must also prepare for this transition and understand that letting go is in the best interests of their patient/child. Some of the major barriers to this process are fears of the unknown and difficulty recognizing the need for change when your child has a long-term illness. Many times, the philosophy of "Why change if there isn't a problem?" becomes the operating mode. Thus, when the transition isn't planned, it frequently occurs in a crisis situation when the young adult is forced by age, insurance, or life plans to change facility or provider. Choosing a new doctor when your child is doing well and is involved with the choosing usually results in a better psychological and medical outcome than a situation in which your child is forced to switch during illness or crisis.

Coordination between primary and specialty physicians is essential, as is the coordination between healthcare, educational, vocational, and social service systems.

What Does Your Child Want for Her Future and Transition?

Adolescents with special healthcare needs know what they are looking for regarding transition services. When they were asked what they wanted for their future, many studies found that they most wanted job training, with independent living skills and college or vocational guidance close behind. Of note, only 45% had had someone talk with them about how to make medical decisions, less than half had been asked about their work plans, and only 50% had heard of transition planning.

Recent studies in England confirmed that physicians and allied health professionals, along with youths with rheumatic diseases and their parents, considered the following to be the top "best practice" approaches for care during transition:

- Addressing education, career needs, and goals
- Developing an individualized transition plan
- Providing honest explanations of the adolescent's rheumatic condition and associated healthcare needs
- Giving adolescents the opportunity to express opinions and make informed decisions
- Giving adolescents the option of being seen by doctors and therapists without their parents

What Are Some of the Benefits of Transition Planning?

- Promotes continuity of rheumatology care
- Increases understanding of self-care expectations
- Promotes independence
- Addresses key developmental issues, such as insurance, finances, career planning, college education, and reproductive health issues
- Facilitates community and agency referrals
- Prevents gaps in service and unplanned transfer
- Offers reassurance, education, counseling, and support

From High School to Post-Secondary Education

Education is essential in today's knowledge-based economy. Studies by the U.S. Department of Labor showed that education level is directly related to lifetime earnings and to who is hired for a job. These relationships are true for people with chronic illnesses or disabilities as well. This means that in the United States, for example, in order for an individual with disabilities to have access to health insurance benefits, he or she must have a high-skill job requiring as much education as possible beyond high school. Thus, counseling to make post-secondary education a reality for young people with myositis is central to their success. A 2001 Harris poll found that 32% of persons with disabilities between ages eighteen and sixty-five work full- or part-time compared with 81% of the general population. Studies have shown that young people with chronic illnesses or disabilities have lower graduation rates and are less likely to attend a four-year college compared to those without chronic illnesses or disabilities. This is exemplified by the fact that 32% of individuals with chronic illnesses or disabilities say that their lack of skills, education, and training accounts for their lack of employment.

Post-secondary education can take many forms. Although most people think that it means college, it can actually be any type of education or training after high school, including trade or professional school, an on-the-job training program, apprenticeship, specialized course work, two-year community college, university, or even postgraduate study. The type of education or training your child will pursue after high school will vary according to her desired goals, abilities, and individual needs.

As with any life transition, planning is the key to success. Planning for the transition to higher education or training should start early. For example, your child should plan to take the appropriate courses in high school for what she wants to do later in life. Transition planning also includes gathering information about one's interests, skills, and abilities and applying that information to the formation of future goals; identifying the type of post-secondary education or training to be pursued; and assessing how the myositis will affect that education. Transition planning should identify the accommodations necessary for post-secondary education to be successful, as was done for elementary and high school (see *Chapter 36, School Issues*). It also means that your child must acquire the necessary knowledge and skills to make appropriate choices and access resources.

As a parent, one of the most important things you can do is to expect that your child with JM will participate, to the best of her ability, in activities that are developmentally appropriate. For many young adults who have graduated from high school, this could mean living independently, acquiring additional education or training in preparation for employment, and finally, getting a job. This expectation should be set early and revisited over the years as the young person matures. It is important for parents to incorporate this expectation into the many activities you do with and for your child. Parents can collaborate with schools to ensure that their children's needs are accommodated. Parents are an important partner in their child's post-secondary education and can be excellent partners in the development of their child's short- and long-range goals and transition plans. Partnering with your child's myositis doctor or primary healthcare provider is important in developing appropriate long-range plans.

For students attending post-secondary education, it is vital to understand how their disability affects them medically, environmentally, in activities of daily living, and educationally. Take the time to educate your child about her disability, discuss limitations and abilities, and have a dialogue about future goals as a first step in planning for her transition to another school or training program. This will help her acquire needed disability-related knowledge to succeed.

Transition services in an Individualized Education Plan (see *Chapter 36, School Issues*) are intended to prepare students to go from the world of school to the world of adult life. Transition services can include instruction, community experiences, setting goals regarding employment, and helping your child acquire daily living skills, as well as providing functional vocational assessment, if needed. The transition plan should include transition-related activities while children are in school. Community-based resources and support services should be identified and contacts made, as appropriate. Students who plan to pursue additional education or training after high school should identify course work needed to achieve those goals and list specific activities that will help them become an independent adult. After age twenty-one and at post-secondary education such as college, there is no law that guarantees your child rights to education as there is in high school. You can obtain free help regarding special education rights and preparing for transition at the Parent Training and Information Center in each state.

Transitioning from School to Work

Work skills start with taking on responsibilities in the family. The earliest working experience is in the home, with household chores. Long-term studies of children with chronic illnesses or disabilities report that giving your children household chores starting at a young age is essential for fostering competence and responsibility.

Early work experience is equally important. In 1996 *The New York Times* surveyed three hundred employers and found that the top three qualities that employers desired were a good attitude, communication skills, and previous work experience. Several American studies found that between 30% and 50% of healthy thirteen-year-olds are involved in a work experience once a week, such as babysitting or paper routes. Children with myositis also need to be exposed to the world of work at a similar age and to role models of working adults with chronic illnesses.

After age twenty-one few services are mandated for individuals with chronic illnesses or disabilities. However, there are three federal laws related to work and disability. Section 504 of the Rehabilitation Act of 1973 prohibits discrimination by employers receiving federal funds, mandates equal opportunities and programs for individuals with disabilities, and provides federal funds to agencies that develop programs for people with disabilities. The Rehabilitation Act Amendments of 1978 improved this initiative to guarantee access to programs for all individuals, even if gainful employment is not the outcome. The Rehabilitation Act Amendment of 1992 stated the role of vocational rehabilitation counselors in working with adolescents with disabilities.

Can My Child Receive Vocational Rehabilitation?

Frequently, contacts made through the individualized education planning process enable students and their families to use community-based providers of disability-related services, such as many kinds of training and educational, medical, and other services tailored to your child's needs. Although vocational rehabilitation counselors can provide services to the young adult, they frequently refer her to appropriate community-based organizations that offer services such as self-advocacy training, the development of employment readiness skills, and help finding and using assistive devices. Vocational rehabilitation services are intended to help individuals become or stay gainfully employed. Many programs prepare the individual for employment in specific occupations; others can provide a job coach to assist with job training at a community-based employment site.

A vocational rehabilitation counselor will work with your child to assess her disability level and help her develop an individualized program to achieve her goals. Together, the vocational rehabilitation counselor and young adult will develop an individualized plan for employment, which will identify an employment goal and how to attain it. The steps for achieving that might include some post-secondary education or training and will take into account any disability-related needs and accommodations that are necessary to achieve success.

Vocational rehabilitation traditionally has been viewed as an adult service agency; vocational rehabilitation routinely did not start until after graduation from high school. Today, with transition planning mandated under the Individuals with Disabilities Education Act, there is a movement for vocational rehabilitation counselors to participate in transition planning before the student graduates. Parents and students can request their participation, and it is highly desirable that they do.

Many students and their parents are surprised when the student leaves the school system and enters the adult service delivery system. While the student was in school, she was entitled by law to services, and school staff was responsible for identifying needs and providing appropriate services. Conversely, vocational rehabilitation is an eligibility-based system. The person must identify herself to the vocational rehabilitation center and must be found eligible for services before she can receive them. The services offered by vocational rehabilitation centers and the way in which they are provided may differ from services provided by the school. It is important that you and your child understand the differences in the systems at least one to two years before your child leaves high school. This will ensure that services will be coordinated and accessible immediately after leaving the school system. Contact your state vocational rehabilitation office to learn about the process, procedures, and timelines for establishing eligibility.

Vocational rehabilitation counselors can help individuals continuing their educations to learn about resources available through the college, such as the disability support services office. Most post-secondary institutions have disability support services on campus. To receive assistance or request accommodations for disability-related needs, a student must disclose the disability, provide documentation of disability, and identify needed accommodations. The documentation of disability must support the requested accommodations.

The disability support services office can assist students with disclosure, requesting accommodations, identifying supports and services, and assistive technology and can also address any other disability-related needs presented by the student. There is a lot of variability across schools as to what they do for students with disability as well as the types of accommodations provided. Public schools that receive federal funding must provide reasonable accommodations to qualified students with disabilities under Section 504 of the Rehabilitation Act of

1973 and Title II of the Americans with Disabilities Act (ADA). Private institutions and vocational schools must also provide reasonable accommodations as required by the amendments to the Rehabilitation Act and Title III (public accommodations) of the ADA. The young adult's physician will be asked to provide documentation of disability and justification for the requested accommodations and should work closely with the student to ensure that all disability-related needs and appropriate and reasonable accommodations are identified. Even if your child does not need any accommodations on entering post-secondary education, she should sign up with the disability support services office in case her myositis flares up and she requires accommodations, such as postponing an examination.

From Pediatric Medical Care to the Adult Medical System

Families need to make two major decisions about the medical care of the child with myositis as she becomes an adult, namely: 1) whom will she see for her care, and 2) how will she pay for her medical care? As the adolescent with JM prepares to leave her pediatric provider, the family and the pediatrician should plan this transfer of responsibility from the parent to the youth long before the date that the youth will go to a new physician or healthcare team, and her pediatrician may be able to refer her to an appropriate physician for her care as an adult. For example, your adolescent should:

- Understand who is needed as part of her healthcare team, such as physical therapists or occupational therapists
- See the physician alone and be prepared to tell her new providers about her illness and symptoms
- Make her own appointments
- Plan how to use transportation to get to her healthcare providers
- Understand her medications, their side effects, how to take them, and how to get them from the pharmacy
- Understand her health insurance and how to make claims and get reimbursed.

Planning how to pay for medical care is an important issue for youth moving into adulthood in the United States. Young adults are the largest group in the United States without health insurance. If the teenager is covered by her parents' insurance, then the parents must find out until what age and under what conditions their child can stay on their policy. If your child goes to work, essential questions include: does the job offer health insurance benefits; how much does it cost; are medications covered; and does the policy cover the doctors and hospitals the youth wants? If the youth meets the Medicaid income requirements and Medicaid is offered in your state, signing up for Medicaid coverage can be helpful because Medicaid covers medications. If a youth is already on Medicaid and also gets a job, it is important to find out how much she is allowed to earn and still stay on Medicaid.

How Do We Start Planning for Transition?

To prepare your adolescent for the adult world, check out the resources listed below. Moreover, participation in existing teen programs will help. Through camps, teen clubs, and family educational and support conferences, kids learn that they are not alone, that others have similar illnesses and need to take the same treatments, that there are older kids who have done very well in college, with their job, and with their new adult rheumatologist. Positive role modeling of others with the

Table 31.1. Transition to adult services for youth with chronic illnesses and disabilities.

How to "LEAVE"

L = Life	• Expect to have a full and productive life. • Your planning must include all aspects of your life: work, education, recreation, independent living, relationships, adult healthcare, etc. • Talk to your parents, friends, teachers, pediatric health provider, and other adults in your life about your goals and needs.
E = Education	• Get as much education as you can. This will help you obtain the job/career of your choice. • Learn about insurance (for example, co-pays, referral system for specialist or OBGYN, appeal process), power of attorney, living wills, guardianship, independent living places, colleges or technical schools, what is expected in the workplace, financing for your future plans.
A = Advocacy	• Speak up and ask questions if you do not understand your transition plan at school, medications, tests, your diagnosis and its effects on your future. • Contact local and national advocacy groups, hotlines, your doctor, your teachers, health agencies, and foundations if you need more information. • Go to the web—plug in at the library, home, or work to gather all the information you need.
V = Values	• What do you value in your medical and work relationships? Location, access, comfort, trust, support of a team? • What do you value in your insurance? Cost, access, speed, support? • Value and trust yourself to make good decisions. Consult with family and important adults in your life.
E = Empowerment	• Use your power to negotiate this transition. • Use your own power to find answers if those you ask do not know. • Establish a new independent relationship with your family, and begin the discussion on how to go out on your own.

Adaptation of Dr. Kathy A. Woodward's Adult Transition Nomogram (unpublished). Used with permission of Dr. Woodward.

same condition is one of the biggest benefits to the participants. Going to camp or a program offered by the youth's healthcare team might not sound like transition planning, but it really is (see *Chapter 37, Summer Camps*). Your child will learn useful strategies and resources to help her become a responsible participant in her own healthcare. She will learn ways to handle future situations or tap into resources. She will gain peer support and lasting friendships. Knowledge about what is going on with their bodies and their futures is very important to teens. Likewise, planning for that move to the adult rheumatologist is crucial. Take a moment to check out some of the great tools and resources to help make it all happen with success. Table 31.1 lists considerations as your child prepares to leave home, high school, and pediatric healthcare.

The section *To Learn More* at the end of this chapter lists some of the many resources available to families. In particular, the Institute for Child Health Policy has a comprehensive web site that has many of the resources listed as Internet links. The Illinois Chapter of the American Academy of Pediatrics offers some excellent timelines and checklists. Transition guides are also on the web sites listed under Adolescent Health Transition Project and Institute for Community Inclusion at Children's Hospital Boston.

Key Points

■ Start the transition process early, as soon as myositis is diagnosed. Know that your child will eventually have to leave her pediatric providers and handle her own healthcare.

■ Encourage your child to attend post-secondary education, and work with guidance counselors to help her choose the appropriate preparatory courses in high school.

■ After your child graduates from high school, take advantage of vocational rehabilitation services, which are based on eligibility. These can help her prepare for a job or for post-secondary education.

■ Work with your pediatric healthcare providers to make the switch to the adult healthcare system as smooth as possible. Don't wait for a crisis to force the change.

■ Use the many resources that are available to you and your teenager with myositis.

To Learn More

The Myositis Association (TMA).

Transition issues for teenagers and young adults. Available from: www.myositis.org/jmbookresources.cfm or 800-821-7356.

American Academy of Pediatrics.

AAP Medical Home, Transition Resources. Available at: www.medicalhomeinfo.org/tools/youthguides.html.

Institute for Community Inclusion/UCEDD. University of Massachusetts Boston, 100 Morrissey Blvd, Boston MA 02125; Phone: 617-287-4300; Internet: www.community inclusion.org (choose "Education & transition" under Browse ICI by topic).

Booklets and resources.

Institute for Child Health Policy. *Health Care Transitions.* University of Florida, P.O. Box 100147, Gainesville FL 32610-0147; Phone: 352-265-7220; Internet: http:// hctransitions.ichp.edu.

Training materials and resources for transitioning from pediatric to adult healthcare.

National Center on Secondary Education and Transition. Institute on Community Integration, University of Minnesota, 6 Pattee Hall, 150 Pillsbury Drive SE, Minneapolis MN 55455; Phone: 612-624-2097; Internet: www.ncset.org; Email: ncset@umn.edu.

National Dissemination Center for Children with Disabilities. P.O. Box 1492, Washington DC 20013; Phone: 800-695-0285; Internet: www.nichcy.org.

National Transition Network, University of Minnesota. Internet: http://ici2.umn.edu/ntn; Email: ntn@icimail.education.umn.edu.

University of Washington. *Adolescent Health Transition Project,* a project of the Washington State Department of Health and Center on Human Development and Disability, Box 357920, University of Washington, Seattle WA 98195; Phone: 206-685-1358; Internet: http://depts.washington.edu/healthtr.

Resources of the United States Federal Government:

Social Security Administration, Office of Public Inquiries. Windsor Park Building, 6401 Security Blvd, Baltimore MD 21235; Phone: 800-772-1213; Internet: www.ssa.gov.

U.S. Department of Labor, Office of Disability Employment Policy (ODEP). Frances Perkins Building, 200 Constitution Avenue NW, Washington DC 20210; Phone: 866-633-7365; Internet: www.dol.gov/odep.

Reports in the Medical Literature

American Academy of Pediatrics; American Academy of Family Physicians; American College of Physicians-American Society of Internal Medicine. A consensus statement on healthcare transitions for young adults with special healthcare needs. *Pediatrics.* 2002;110:1304–6.

Blum RW; Rosen D; Suris JC; Bowes G, Sinnema G, Suris JC, Buhlmann U, Kelly A. Proceedings of the working conference, "Moving On: Transition from Pediatric to Adult Health Care." *Journal of Adolescent Health.* 1995;17(1):3–36.

Blum RW, Garell D, Hodgman CH, Jorissen TW, Okinow NA, Orr DP, Slap GB. Transition from child-centered to adult health-care systems for adolescents with chronic conditions. A position paper of the Society for Adolescent Medicine. *Journal of Adolescent Health.* 1993 Nov;14(7):570–6.

Rettig P, Athreya BH. *Leaving home: preparing the adolescent with arthritis for coping with independence and the adult rheumatology world.* In: Isenberg DA, Miller JJ, editors. *Adolescent Rheumatology.* London: Martin Dunitz Publishers; 1999.

CHAPTER 32

Approaching Adolescence

Cynthia J. Mears, DO

In this chapter...

We discuss issues that arise in adolescence, such as sexuality and risky behavior, and give parents and teens with juvenile myositis (JM) guidance for dealing with them. Teens taking immunosuppressants are at much greater risk of sexually transmitted infection than their healthy peers and should take extra precautions, for infection itself can cause the JM to flare. JM and many of the medications used for treatment impair liver function so that recreational drugs and alcohol are not handled normally and can reach dangerous blood levels.

From the family's point of view...

"We are used to thinking about our daughter as a child, and now she's trying out a lot of things—makeup, piercing, who knows what! We're not comfortable talking with her about adult behavior, but we're afraid of what will happen if we don't 'communicate.'"

During the teenage years your child will develop in many different ways. She'll gain the capacity for abstract thought and reasoning; she might have a growth spurt; and potent hormones are released that foster sexual development. Girls will have their first period, and boys will grow facial hair. When your teen has myositis, she will go through the same physical and developmental changes, but many of the medications, such as steroids and immunosuppressive agents, can cause physical side effects that make growth and development more challenging, both physically and psychologically. As adolescents struggle to understand their emerging bodies and sexualities within the framework of a complex social environment and the demands of a chronic illness, parents, teens, and their doctors need to talk openly and honestly.

Facts About Teens and Sexuality

- Approximately 50% of U.S. high school students report having sex.[1]
- Each year, three million teens contract a sexually transmitted infection.[1,2]
- Nearly fourteen thousand sexual references and behaviors are shown each year on television.
- Among U.S. adolescents, young women reach puberty and sexual maturity younger than ever before, so their bodies are more mature, but their minds are not![3]

1. Centers for Disease Control and Prevention. Youth Risk Behavior Survey. *MMWR CDC Surveillance Summaries.* 2000;49(27):1–104.

2. Institute of Medicine, Committee on Prevention and Control of Sexually Transmitted Diseases. *Hidden epidemic: confronting sexually transmitted diseases.* Eng TR, Butler WT, eds. Washington DC: National Academy Press, 1997.

3. Herman-Giddens, ME, Slora, EJ, Wasserman, RC, et al. Secondary sexual characteristics and menses in young girls seen in office practice: A study from the Pediatric Research in Office Settings Network. *Pediatrics.* 1997;99(4):505–512.

If you have a hard time talking about sex with your teens, admit it! If you're uncomfortable, they will be too. Practicing with your spouse or partner can help reduce the anxiety, and it will ensure that you both know each other's thoughts about the subject before you talk to your teen. If you really can't imagine having this discussion yourself, make an appointment with a pediatrician, adolescent medicine specialist, or an organization like Planned Parenthood, or give her this chapter to read, but don't avoid the topic; otherwise, someone else may misinform your teen. Remember that talking about sex does not necessarily encourage her to have sex; in fact, it could even discourage her.

Whenever an opportunity presents itself to share your wisdom with your teen, use it. She might appear not to be listening, but teens do hear it. Opportunities present themselves every day. TV commercials are often a way to start the discussion. "How do you think they are trying to sell that product?" is a great way to open the subject with teens. That first pubic hair or pimple is a teachable moment. Now you can talk about hormones and puberty. Read up if you need to know more about development. There are many web sites, including www.youngwomens health.org, or booklets from the American Academy of Pediatrics. It can be less threatening to both of you to have several short talks, for instance, when you see a tattoo, a body piercing, a drunk, revealing clothing, or an open display of affection, rather than one long "sex talk." These opportunities are your chance to bring up the subjects in an open, nonjudgmental way. Ask open-ended questions, such as, "What do you think about that?" You will be amazed at what your teen already knows.

For Teens: Protecting Yourself

As you grow from childhood to adulthood, your sexuality will awaken. If your myositis is still active, there are two main areas of concern for you—birth control

> ### Tips for Talking with Teens
>
> - Respect your teen's privacy, and don't embarrass her, especially in front of other teens.
>
> - Validate that it's okay to have sexual feelings and dreams and sensitive spots on your body. We all do.
>
> - Be sensitive to your teen's feelings. To say "Help me understand your concerns" shows that you are trying to be sensitive, rather than critical or judgmental.
>
> - Make sure you both are talking about the same thing. A young doctor asked a teen if she was sexually active. The teen bent her head in a questioning manner and said to the resident, "No, I lie still. Don't you?" Teens might not consider oral or anal sex to be "real sex" and might engage in these activities to "keep their virginity." Parents need to let their teens know that these forms of sex are just as risky for getting sexually transmitted infections.
>
> - Take your teen seriously. If she says she is in love, don't laugh or make fun of it. If she says she wants to kill herself, you should get help *immediately*.
>
> - Tell your teens you love them, often. Teens really need that safety net of unconditional love.
>
> - Let teens blame things on you when they're challenged to do something that's not right. For example, curfews will give kids an "out" for getting away from a difficult situation.

and sexually transmitted infection. Either is much more risky for a teen with JM than for a healthy teen. It is important to know what those risks are and how to decrease them.

Birth Control

If you are abstaining from sex when you're a teenager, you have made a great decision! Abstinence is the safest action: you can be sure you won't get pregnant or get sexually transmitted infections, such as HIV. If you're not abstaining from sex, we advise you to use birth control because it's easy to get pregnant, and you can get pregnant the first time you have sex and at any time during the month. Pregnancy complicates myositis in many ways (see *Chapter 33, Pregnancy and Fertility*). If you are considering having sex, here are some things you need to consider because you are also dealing with myositis:

- Practice the 100% rule. Sex is the responsibility of each participant. You must fully protect yourself against sexually transmitted infections whether your partner does or not. You must also take full responsibility for birth control whether your partner does or not.

- Know that you can get birth control in all fifty states, confidentially, and without parental notification or consent.

- Pelvic exams using a speculum to see internally are not needed to start birth control but external exams are a good idea so your doctor can make sure that you are developing normally and check you for problems. Request routine urine tests for sexually transmitted infections, like gonorrhea and chlamydia. Some other sexually transmitted infections are not routinely tested for, so if you might have been exposed to them, you should tell your doctor. Pap smears for cervical cancer screening should be done three years after starting sex or yearly after 21 years.

- Some medicines that treat myositis can be harmful to an unborn baby, causing deformities and even death (see *Chapter 33, Pregnancy and Fertility*).

There are many methods of contraception, most of which can be classified into barrier methods (such as male and female condoms, diaphragms, cervical caps, sponges, and spermicides) or hormonal methods (such as the pill, the ring, injections, and the patch). You should discuss with your doctor which one is best for you. If you choose a hormonal method, you should be checked for anti-cardiolipin antibodies in the blood, and you should tell your rheumatologist.

If one of these primary methods of contraception is not used correctly or fails, you can get "emergency" contraception from a clinic or your doctor. You must call within 72 hours of intercourse. Emergency contraception contains high doses of hormones and should not be substituted for your primary form of birth control. Check with your myositis doctor to see whether these hormonal birth control methods might interact with any of the medicines that you take.

The hormonal methods of birth control do not protect against sexually transmitted infections. Condoms provide some protection against HIV. Remember that there is no way of telling whether people have a sexually transmitted infection just by looking at them.

Sexually Transmitted Infections

Teens who are taking medications for JM have suppressed immune systems and are therefore at higher risk of getting sexually transmitted infections because of their weakened immune defenses against infection. Sex and drug use lead to risks of infection with HIV (Human Immunodeficiency Virus) and other sexually transmitted infections. The medicines that are given for myositis knock down your body's defenses against these infections, making you more susceptible to them— and these infections can in turn make the myositis worse. If your immune system has been compromised by the medications you're taking and you get a sexually transmitted disease, such as HIV or gonorrhea, it could make you very, very ill. If you thought that recovering from myositis was rough, you could have many more complications from sexually transmitted infections, not only because of the illness but also because the medicines that treat them do the opposite of what the medicines for JM do (i.e., they strengthen the immune system).

What kind of sexually transmitted infection could you get? Approximately twelve to fifteen million sexually transmitted infections occur each year in the United States, and adolescents have the highest age-specific infection rate. Human papillomavirus (HPV*) is the most common of these in adolescents, with chlamydia a close second. In addition, it is estimated that 22% of the U.S. population age twelve or over is infected with the herpes simplex virus type 2 (HSV-2). In addition, forty to eighty thousand new HIV infections occur each year in the U.S., and about half occur in people younger than twenty-five years old.

Sexually transmitted infections cause a variety of symptoms, ranging in severity from uncomplicated inflammation of the urinary tract to more serious conditions, including pelvic inflammatory disease, pregnancy problems, cervical cancer, and AIDS. One of the major consequences of sexually transmitted infections in young women is pelvic inflammatory disease. Adolescents with pelvic inflammatory disease can have long-term problems, including chronic pelvic pain or the inability to get pregnant or have a baby.

Many teens have sexually transmitted infections and don't even know it. The most common symptom of a sexually transmitted infection is no symptom at all. That being said, these infections can be divided into those that cause changes in mucous and those that cause bumps or sores on your private parts. The best way to find out whether you have a sexually transmitted infection is to go to your doctor immediately when you notice any sores around your privates, changes in the discharge from your vagina or penis, or changes in your ability to urinate. If you notice any change in your mucous, such as a change in color, consistency, or smell, it could be associated with a sexually transmitted infection or an infection related to steroids or other medicines. For more information, see www.teenshealth.org.

Finally, there is HIV (Human Immunodeficiency Virus), the virus that causes AIDS. You can get HIV through sexual contact, including anal sex, by sharing needles (e.g., body piercing or if you are shooting drugs), and by sharing blood (don't even think about being "blood brothers or sisters" with anyone). HIV can also be sexually transmitted between same-sex partners. You can't tell whether someone has the HIV virus by looking at them. You might never know if you have HIV unless you get tested. Some people may have symptoms that seem like a severe flu, but the symptoms get better after a short time. Others may lose a lot of weight or get lots of unexplained rashes that itch, like yeast or fungus infections. But most commonly, people have no symptoms when they first get the HIV virus. So be sure to get tested if you are uncertain; if the result is negative, you will have peace of mind, and if the result is positive, the earlier you can receive treatment, the better.

Confidential testing is when you get pre- and post-test counseling where you learn about HIV and what the testing means. You have a blood test and then you come back to talk about the results. Laws regarding patient confidentiality still protect a teen's privacy. This type of testing is recommended because teens who

---

*To prevent HPV and cervical cancer, teenagers may now receive the HPV vaccine. Discuss this with your doctor.

have positive results are then easily connected to care. Although there is no cure for HIV, there are effective treatments.

Alcohol and Drug Use and JM

You and your friends already know that drinking and driving are a lethal combination. Every year at holidays or graduation, reports of accidents bring grief to families. When you have JM, you are even more susceptible to the effects of alcohol because your liver, which breaks down the alcohol, might not function normally. This is because of the myositis-related inflammation or some of the treatments for the myositis itself. In particular, prednisone, methotrexate, azathioprine, and other JM medicines can impair your liver function and your ability to break down the alcohol, which can also cause more side effects of your myositis medicines. An impaired liver will make your body less able to handle alcohol and recreational drugs, so that a small amount has a big impact. If your judgment is clouded from drugs or alcohol, you are placing yourself at risk—a risk you do not need to take!

Key Points

- Adolescence is a critical period in the development of sexual identity as well as in the development of sexual behaviors that can lead to unintended pregnancies or sexually transmitted infections, including HIV.

- Having juvenile myositis doesn't change a teen's desire to fit in and experiment, but the risks associated with sexual activity are greater and include increased susceptibility to disease and complications from pregnancy.

- If you want to use hormonal contraception, check with your myositis doctor, and be sure to protect yourself against sexually transmitted infection, too.

- Transition to adulthood can be achieved with honest, clear discussions between parents, teens, and healthcare providers.

- Recreational drugs and alcohol do not mix with JM and the medicines used to treat it.

To Learn More

KidsHealth/The Nemours Foundation.
Teens Health, Answers and Advice. Available at: www.teenshealth.org.
Age-appropriate answers to many questions teens have about themselves, including healthy dieting, feelings and emotions, and sexuality.

Children's Hospital Boston.
The Center for Young Women's Health. Available at: www.youngwomenshealth.org.
Facts on teen issues geared toward girls and young women (ages 12–22), including nutrition, fitness, sexual health, general health and development, gynecology and reproduction, and emotional health.

Greydanus DE, Bashe P. *Caring for Your Teenager.* IL: American Academy of Pediatrics; 2003. [Visit www.aap.org and click on "Bookstore & Publications" to order a copy.]

CHAPTER 33

Pregnancy and Fertility

Ann M. Reed, MD, and Chester V. Oddis, MD

In this chapter...

In this chapter you will learn about how myositis can influence pregnancy and fertility, and how pregnancy can affect myositis. You will also learn how the medicines used to treat juvenile myositis (JM) can affect fertility and breastfeeding.

From the family's point of view...

"I had no problem getting pregnant. Although I had a high-risk pregnancy, I promised myself that I was not going to worry for the next nine months. After failing the glucose test, I was referred to a specialist who was concerned with the results but assured me that being on prednisone for a long time must have affected the test. I was on prednisone every other day for the entire nine months of my pregnancy. Since I have severe calcinosis throughout my entire body, it amazes me how much room the human body has inside for my baby to grow. I delivered a healthy, eight-pound baby girl. I have so much love for my daughter that I cannot even imagine my life without her."

Although about twice as many females are affected by myositis as males, only about 15% of all persons with myositis are women who develop the illness during their childbearing years (ages fifteen to thirty years). Girls with JM, however, need to consider the issue of pregnancy when they reach their childbearing years. Not all women with myositis will necessarily have high-risk pregnancies or develop complications during pregnancy. However, very little is known about the effect of pregnancy on myositis or whether women with myositis have more difficulty having babies. In addition, many women who have been diagnosed with JM might have to be treated during their pregnancy with medications that could affect the health of their infant. Information on the side effects of different types of drugs is very important to mothers because they should know whether the medications could harm them or their babies or affect their ability to breastfeed their newborn infants.

Can Women with Juvenile Myositis Become Pregnant and Deliver a Healthy Baby?

The first part of this question deals with the effect of the myositis on fertility (the ability to become pregnant), and the second part has to do with the outcome of pregnancy in women with JM. Researchers at the University of Pittsburgh recently mailed questionnaires across the country to almost 300 women with myositis and received responses from most of them. One of the questions concerned their pregnancies before and after they developed myositis. As you might expect, there were many fewer pregnancies after the onset of myositis; nevertheless, there were 35 pregnancies in 24 women, and 20 pregnancies resulted in full-term normal babies. Some of those pregnancies were discontinued at the request of the mother, and some resulted in miscarriages. Some of the women (7 of the 24) were pregnant at the time the myositis was diagnosed, and some of the pregnancies (28 of 35) occurred after the diagnosis was made. Some of these same mothers, however, were still able to deliver healthy babies after they developed myositis. About two-thirds of the pregnancies that occurred after the women were diagnosed with myositis were successful. In the group of 17 women who had babies after they received a diagnosis of myositis, three had developed myositis as children (all had juvenile dermatomyositis [JDM]). These three women delivered four full-term babies, but they also had had one miscarriage and one stillbirth, where the baby was not alive when it was born.

In a separate study of 22 women with JDM from Duke University Medical Center and the University of North Carolina, all six women who tried to become pregnant were successful, resulting in nine pregnancies and nine healthy babies. None of these women had reactivation of their JDM or a flare of their illness with or after pregnancy. Two of the women went on to have four additional pregnancies. They had no problems with high blood pressure, swelling of their legs or body, or protein in the urine (together known as toxemia). Three of the infants were small for their gestational age (smaller than expected based on their birth age) but otherwise healthy.

In summary, although some experts have suggested that fertility rates are different before and after the onset of myositis, it remains difficult to evaluate accurately the influence of myositis on the ability to become pregnant and deliver a healthy infant. Many different factors, such as age, the use of contraception (birth control) and other drugs, and the effect of the myositis severity, may play a role in a woman's ability or choice to become pregnant after developing myositis. However, there is certainly enough evidence for women to be optimistic about future pregnancies leading to the delivery of healthy babies based on the information that we have now.

Will a Pregnancy Cause Worsening Muscle Weakness, Rash, or Other Problems in the Mother with Myositis?

A small study done in England showed no increase in the activity of myositis in four women who became pregnant some time after the onset of myositis. In fact, two of the women, in whom myositis was under good control during pregnancy, were able to decrease the medicines they were taking for myositis. Others have reported similar findings. In the Pittsburgh study mentioned above, in 28 pregnancies in women with an established diagnosis of myositis, their muscle weakness improved in five pregnancies, remained unchanged in 20, and became worse in only three of the pregnancies. These are encouraging results.

However, of the seven women who developed myositis during pregnancy, five had significant muscle weakness, and two had a rash of dermatomyositis. These two women later developed muscle weakness after they delivered their babies. Thus, the onset of myositis during pregnancy might be associated with more severe illness, and there is evidence from some studies that the outcome of the newborn infant might not be as good when myositis develops during pregnancy.

What Other Factors Might Affect the Pregnancy Outcome of a Woman Who Has a History of Myositis?

In general, women whose myositis is inactive when they become pregnant have good pregnancy outcomes. Mothers may even be able to lower their dose of prednisone and other immunosuppressive medicines during pregnancy, possibly because the body increases its own immunosuppression so that the fetus will not be rejected. Conversely, it is our experience that women who become pregnant when their myositis is active or flaring generally require higher doses of prednisone and have poorer pregnancy outcomes. The outcome of the newborn infant tends to go hand in hand with the degree of myositis activity in the mother.

Can a Woman with Myositis Who Is Pregnant Take Prednisone?

A woman with myositis who is pregnant can take prednisone if it is necessary. The risk to the developing baby from corticosteroid (prednisone) treatments is very low. Therefore, the need to start, stop, or taper prednisone should be the same whether or not a woman with myositis is pregnant. It is safe to take prednisone during pregnancy because the placenta cannot convert prednisone to its effective, active form, and so the fetus is not exposed to the active drug. However, pregnancy does not change the effect of prednisone on the mother, and the same side effects that occur in women who are not pregnant will occur in pregnant women. In addition, the use of prednisone or other corticosteroids before pregnancy does not have a later adverse effect on a woman's ability to become pregnant.

What Other Past or Current Medicines Might Cause Problems with the Ability to Become Pregnant or Affect the Pregnancy Itself?

This can be a very complicated question because many different medicines are used to treat people with myositis. We will discuss this question based on the different types of medicines that are used to treat persons with myositis. This information is summarized in Table 33.1.

Table 33.1. Summary of drugs and their possible effects on male and female fertility and pregnancy.

Drug	Male fertility	Female fertility	Use in pregnancy
Corticosteroids (Prednisone, Medrol)	No effect	No effect	Acceptable (in lowest possible dose)
Methotrexate (Rheumatrex, Trexall)	Causes reversible sterility; discontinue three to six months prior to attempted pregnancy	No effect	• Toxic to developing baby • Discontinue drug three to six months prior to attempted pregnancy in women to prevent damage to the developing baby
Hydroxychloroquine (Plaquenil)	No effect	No effect	Can be continued safely throughout pregnancy
Cyclosporine (Sandimmune, Neoral)	Limited information	Limited information	Avoid. May affect the baby's developing immune system
Azathioprine (Imuran)	No major effects	No major effects	• Minimal chance of serious birth defects • Use only with severe or life-threatening disease
Cyclophosphamide (Cytoxan)	Decreased (worse with daily oral use compared to intermittent monthly intravenous use)	Decreased • Daily oral dosing for one year results in ovarian failure in > 70% women • Less chance of ovarian failure with monthly intravenous use	Do not use. Discontinue at least three months before trying to become pregnant in both males and females

Nonsteroidal Anti-Inflammatory Drugs (NSAIDs)

NSAIDs consist of aspirin (trade names include Bufferin, Aluprin, Ecotrin, Empirin), ibuprofen (Motrin, Advil, Excedrin), naproxen (Aleve, Naprosyn), and many other similar drugs. In general, these drugs do not cause birth defects, but women who are trying to become pregnant should avoid them because they can interfere with conception. They can be used in the lowest effective dose during pregnancy and only intermittently, but NSAIDs should be avoided for at least six weeks before the expected delivery date.

Methotrexate (Rheumatrex, Trexall)

This drug does not seem to affect female fertility adversely, but it can cause reversible sterility in men. Men may have trouble fathering children while taking methotrexate, but after stopping this drug, men can usually father children later. Women of childbearing age *must* use adequate contraception with methotrexate, as this drug is toxic to a developing infant. Women must discontinue methotrexate at least three months before attempting to become pregnant because it causes serious birth defects.

Hydroxychloroquine (Plaquenil)

There are no reports that this drug causes problems with fertility. Even though it crosses the placenta and enters the developing infant, there is no evidence that it causes birth defects. In general, it can be continued safely throughout pregnancy and does not pose a significant risk to the baby. Some doctors feel it is better to stop the drug during pregnancy and instead prescribe low doses of prednisone to treat the symptoms for which hydroxychloroquine is given. Each woman and her doctor should make this decision jointly.

Cyclosporine (Sandimmune, Neoral)

In general, this drug should not be used during pregnancy, and a woman with myositis who can possibly become pregnant should take measures (contraception) to prevent pregnancy. Although there are no reports of increased birth defects, this is based on limited experience. There is the potential for cyclosporine to suppress or alter the immune system of the developing baby. Thus, it is wise to avoid this drug during pregnancy.

Azathioprine (Imuran)

This drug has much less risk for infertility than other cytotoxic agents, such as cyclophosphamide (discussed below). Many girls and women with myositis have received azathioprine and later become pregnant. In addition, the drug is associated with few birth defects because, similar to prednisone, the fetus is relatively protected from its effects. Nonetheless, this drug should be avoided during pregnancy or used only by women with severe problems.

Cyclophosphamide (Cytoxan)

This drug has been associated with ovarian failure when used in adults with lupus and vasculitis. Ovarian failure is a condition in which the ovaries no longer work properly, and a woman's menstrual periods stop and pregnancy cannot occur. Although there have not been any studies of these problems in children with myositis, in adult women with lupus who received seven intermittent doses of cyclophosphamide by vein, there was about a 12% chance of their periods stopping. This problem is likely to be higher in adult women who take this drug by mouth every day for a year or so. It seems that many factors can determine which problems develop with cyclophosphamide, and it is likely that the age of the person, how the drug is given (by mouth or by vein), as well as how long it is taken all influence the side effects of this drug. The other thing to remember is that these are estimates. It is very difficult to predict an outcome in an individual person.

Cyclophosphamide can also cause problems with sperm production when it is used to treat myositis in boys and men, and in some cases it can result in infertility. Because of the risk of infertility in males and females, however, cyclophosphamide is generally used for only the most severe JM cases involving certain serious problems, such as lung disease, skin ulcerations, and other serious illnesses that do not respond to other treatments. This drug should generally not be given during pregnancy because it might cause birth defects, and it should be withdrawn at least three months before a woman tries to become pregnant. For life-threatening complications, it can be given after the first trimester. Because of the risk of infertility with cyclophosphamide, you may want to discuss with your child's doctor the possibility of banking sperm or eggs before the treatment of your older children.

Other Medicines

Less is known about the effects on pregnancy and fertility of other, less commonly used medicines prescribed for JM, such as tacrolimus (Prograf) and anti-tumor necrosis factor-alpha (TNF-α) therapy (infliximab, etanercept). But these drugs should be avoided whenever possible during pregnancy. Because mycophenolate mofetil (CellCept) is known to cause birth defects, it should not be used during pregnancy, and women should be tested for pregnancy before using it.

What Restrictions Are There for Mothers Who Want to Breastfeed Their Babies?

Table 33.2 summarizes the medications that can be used or should not be used by mothers who wish to breastfeed their babies. Some drugs should be discontinued if the mother is nursing because they can enter the breast milk and potentially cause side effects to the newborn infant. This is an individual decision, and many women will not even take an acetaminophen (Tylenol) or aspirin if they breastfeed, for fear of harming their infants. If the mother needs to take the medicine to treat myositis or other problems, then a decision can also be made to discontinue breastfeeding.

Table 33.2. Medicines and breastfeeding.

Medicine	Breastfeeding
Aspirin (Bufferin, Aluprin, Ecotrin, Empirin)	Compatible
Other NSAIDs (Motrin, Advil, Naprosyn, others)	Compatible
Corticosteroids (Prednisone)	Compatible
Cyclophosphamide (Cytoxan)	Contraindicated
Azathioprine (Imuran)	Contraindicated
Methotrexate (Rheumatrex, Trexall)	Contraindicated
Cyclosporine (Sandimmune, Neoral)	Contraindicated
Hydroxychloroquine (Plaquenil)	With caution *

Abbreviation: NSAIDs = nonsteroidal anti-inflammatory drugs

Compatible = acceptable to use during breastfeeding, no current evidence that it harms the baby

Contraindicated = do not use, evidence suggests that this drug harms the baby

* Low amounts are found in breast milk of women who take hydroxychloroquine, but the American Academy of Pediatrics classifies this drug as compatible with breastfeeding

Summary

In summary, although there have only been a few small studies in this area, the current information we have suggests that most boys and girls with JM can look forward to having healthy children later in their lives. In general, the more active the myositis is, the more likely a woman will have problems during her pregnancy, so it is important that the myositis be controlled as much as possible before becoming pregnant. Some drugs used to treat myositis do not cause problems with fertility or pregnancy, but others can. You should carefully discuss these issues with your child's doctor.

Key Points

- Most boys and girls with JM can have healthy babies later in their lives.
- In general, the more active the myositis is, the more likely a woman will have problems during her pregnancy.
- Certain drugs used to treat myositis can cause problems with fertility or pregnancy, and all women should consult their doctor about these issues before becoming pregnant.
- Certain drugs used to treat myositis can be passed to babies during breastfeeding and cause problems. All women should consult their doctors about these issues before breastfeeding.

To Learn More

The Myositis Association (TMA).

How Will Pregnancy And Nursing Affect And Be Affected By Myositis? Available from: www.myositis.org/jmbookresources.cfm or 800-821-7356.

Reports in the Medical Literature

American Academy of Pediatrics Committee on Drugs. The transfer of drugs and other chemicals into human milk. *Pediatrics.* 2001 Sep;108(3):776–89.

Gutierrez G, Dagnino R, Mintz G. Polymyositis/dermatomyositis and pregnancy. *Arthritis and Rheumatism.* 1984 Mar;27(3):291–4.

Janssen NM, Genta MS. The effects of immunosuppressive and anti-inflammatory medications on fertility, pregnancy, and lactation. *Archives of Internal Medicine.* 2000 Mar 13;160(5):610–9.

Silva CA, Sultan SM, Isenberg DA. Pregnancy outcome in adult-onset idiopathic inflammatory myopathy. *Rheumatology.* 2003 Oct;42(10):1168–72.

Resources and Opportunities

CHAPTER 34

Protecting Your Child's Rights

Ann Kunkel, BS; Susan J. Wright, OT; Carol B. Lindsley, MD;
and Jane G. Schaller, MD

In this chapter...

Federal laws protect your child's rights and allow for special services for children with disabilities. These laws provide equal opportunity to receive services and education and protection from discrimination. We describe those laws and direct you to where you can find more information.

From the family's point of view...

"You are your child's best advocate. I have acted as my child's voice and tried to find as much information and help as I can for all of us. There are programs run by the state that can help with financial burdens. Sometimes they are not readily known. Contact your local health department or child services. The hospital social workers are a good source, too. But the best thing that I ever did was join a support group. We share so much information about where to get help in our community, as well as emotional support for one another. It has been a real blessing for me."

How Are My Child's Rights Protected?

Understanding laws and regulations at federal, state, and local levels is necessary to equip yourself to address your child's rights to receive adequate and comprehensive healthcare in the United States.

On the national level several statutes and laws relate to medical and educational services for children with disabilities, including arthritis and other connective tissue diseases such as juvenile myositis (JM). Children who have chronic illnesses often have fragmented medical care, in part because of the need for many specialists and long-term coordinated medical care. This challenge has become more difficult in our current managed-care environment.

In countries outside the United States children with disabilities are entitled to special care as defined in an international treaty called *The Convention on the Rights of the Child*, adopted by the General Assembly of the United Nations, November 20, 1989. This Convention can be an important advocacy tool for attention to children with dermatomyositis and any other condition. The rights of the child become enforceable only when they are encoded into the domestic laws of individual countries. A Committee of the Rights of the Child in Geneva reviews the status of child rights in various member countries and can comment on violations.

The following federal laws protect and provide services for children with disabilities and their families and ensure the confidentiality of medical information.

Which Law Protects the Confidentiality of My Child's Medical Records?

The Health Insurance Portability and Accountability Act of 1998 (HIPAA) protects your child's rights regarding shared medical information. It regulates how medical information about your child may be used and disclosed and how you can get access to this information. Each medical professional and medical facility has developed privacy practices. Each time your child sees a new healthcare professional, uses a new pharmacy, or requires her medical information to be shared, an HIPAA Notice of Privacy Practices form must be signed by the parent or guardian. Each facility might have a slightly different interpretation of HIPAA policy. Generally, health information about your child can be shared among healthcare professionals if they assist in taking care of your child. Your pediatric rheumatologist's team can communicate with your primary doctor's office and usually with the school nurse. You might need to sign a release of information form before they communicate any information. You can also sign the form to release either all medical information or only specific information. To communicate with anyone at your child's school other than the nurse, this form must be signed. Each school district has developed its own forms, and it is easiest to ask the school to fax the form to the doctors' offices. This Act ensures that medical information is shared only among healthcare professionals treating your child, but it can also cause frustration because some healthcare professionals interpret it to mean that they cannot communicate anything without a release and cannot share laboratory results and medication changes without your signed consent. You will need to check on the practices in each office to make sure each healthcare professional has access to the information needed to care for your child.

Which Law Protects My Employment If I Must Take Off Work to Care for My Child?

The Family and Medical Leave Act of 1993 (FMLA) requires covered employers to provide up to twelve weeks of unpaid, job-protected leave to eligible employees for certain family and medical reasons. When children with chronic illness like JM need additional care, such as when your child is first diagnosed or when the illness flares or relapses, this Act requires your employer to give you time off without risk of losing your job. Employees are covered if they have worked for a covered employer for at least one year and for 1,250 hours during the previous twelve months, and if the company has at least fifty employees within seventy-five miles.

Unpaid FMLA leave must be granted for any of the following reasons:

- To care for the employee's spouse, son, daughter, or parent with a serious health condition

- To care for the employee's child after birth or placement for adoption or foster care

- For a serious health condition that makes the employee unable to work

At the employee's or employer's option, certain kinds of paid leave may be substituted for unpaid leave. The employee may be required to provide advance leave notice and medical certification. Taking of leave can be denied if requirements are not met. The employee ordinarily must provide thirty days advance notice when the leave is "foreseeable," as for a scheduled surgery. If the employee is unable to work because of a serious health condition, an employer may require medical certification to support a request for leave and may require second or third opinions (at the employer's expense) and a fitness-for-duty report to return to work.

For the duration of FMLA leave the employer must maintain the employee's health coverage under any group health plan. Upon return from FMLA leave most employees must be restored to their original or equivalent positions with equivalent pay, benefits, and other employment terms. The use of FMLA leave cannot result in the loss of any employment benefit that accrued before the start of an employee's leave.

For additional information about the FMLA leave, contact the nearest office of the Wage and Hour Division, listed in most telephone directories under U.S. Government, Department of Labor.

Which Laws Protect My Child's Rights to Education and Special Services at School?

Beginning in the 1970s, several federal laws guaranteed children with disability the right to special services from schools. These laws include Section 504 of the Rehabilitation Act of 1973 and the more inclusive PL 94–142, the Education of All Handicapped Act.

Section 504 of the Rehabilitation Act of 1973 mandates that services and programs receiving federal funds must provide equal opportunity to all, including children with chronic illness. Schools are included in this mandate. The Education for All Handicapped Children Act outlines a special referral process and provides for parental participation in decisions regarding their child's education.

The Individuals with Disabilities Education Act Amendments of 1990 (IDEA) improved services for students with disabilities as provided in the Education for All Handicapped Children Act and changed the name to IDEA. For more information, see *Chapter 36, School Issues.*

The regulations to implement the Individuals with Disabilities Education Improvement Act of 2004 (IDEA) are in the process of being drafted at the time of the writing of this book. You can find current information about the status of this Act at the U.S. Department of Education web site, listed in the resource section (*To Learn More*) at the end of this chapter.

Which Laws Protect My Child's Rights to Rehabilitative Services and Access to Public Facilities?

Children with myositis need access to comprehensive medical and educational services, as well as social and rehabilitative services and physical access to public facilities. The Vocational Rehabilitation Act requires that state and federal agencies provide transitional services, including those that address independent living and vocational preparation (see *Chapter 32, Approaching Adolescence*). The Americans with Disabilities Act of 1990 (ADA) guarantees access to transportation and public facilities and programs for any child who has or has had a physical or mental impairment that substantially limits a major life activity.

Where Can I Find Help?

Understanding everything these laws provide and using them to help your child may seem overwhelming. Contacting parents of other children with JM through organizations that support myositis, such as The Myositis Association, the Arthritis Foundation, and the Cure JM Foundation (see *Resource Appendix*), can give you firsthand information about how they succeeded in getting their children the help they need. When confronted with a rare illness, networking with others who have had similar experiences can save you time and frustration and can be a good way of receiving moral support.

Your child's physician, nurse, therapist, social worker, or teacher might also have helpful information. Some hospitals have parent advocates who volunteer to assist parents by providing information and answering questions about which services are available. You are your child's voice and can make a difference in the quality of care and services she receives throughout her illness. It will require persistence. You need to ask questions until you get the answers and services your child is entitled to.

Key Points

- Understanding federal, state, and local laws and regulations can equip parents to be the best advocates for their child's healthcare needs.

- The following laws guarantee children with disabilities the right to special services:

  — Rehabilitation Act of 1973, Section 504

  — The Individuals with Disability Education Act (IDEA)

  — The Vocational Rehabilitation Act (www.firstgov.gov; toll free: 800-FED-INFO or 800-333-4636)

  — The Family and Medical Leave Act of 1993 (contact your local office of Wage and Hour Division, listed in most telephone directories under U.S. Government, Department of Labor)

- Networking with parents of other children with JM, through organizations such as The Myositis Association, the Arthritis Foundation, and the Cure JM Foundation, can provide firsthand information about how they have successfully obtained the services their children are entitled to.

To Learn More

National Council on Disability, 1331 F Street NW, Suite 850, Washington DC 20004; Phone: 202-272-2004; Internet: www.ncd.gov.

Detailed information on the federal laws and acts regarding disabilities, and valuable links to various government web sites.

National Dissemination Center for Children with Disabilities (NICHCY), P.O. Box 1492, Washington DC 20013; Phone: 800-695-0285; Internet: www.nichcy.org; Email: nichcy@aed.org.

Central source of information on disabilities in infants, toddlers, children, and youth; IDEA; No Child Left Behind, as it relates to children with disabilities; and effective educational practices.

U.S. Department of Education.

IDEA 2004 Resources. Available at: www.ed.gov/policy/speced/guid/idea/idea2004.html. Information on the Individuals with Disabilities Education Improvement Act of 2004 (IDEA).

CHAPTER 35

Insurance and Medical Expenses

Carolyn L. Yancey, MD; Donna LaRue, RN, BSN;
and Marisa S. Klein-Gitelman, MD, MPH

In this chapter...

We will define types of insurance and suggest methods for successful communication and navigation of the managed care system in order to receive quality healthcare. We will also discuss the appeal process for the insurance decision, should it be needed, and an approach to getting help for medication-related expenses.

From the family's point of view...

"It was hard enough having a sick child to take care of, especially while we both were working. But the bills were overwhelming. We didn't know where to turn but knew there had to be options out there."

Where Should I Start?

Access to medical care is one of the most significant issues faced by our nation. When a child suddenly becomes ill, it is unfortunate that one of the great difficulties you may face is how to access appropriate care and how to get your child's medical needs taken care of promptly and appropriately. As soon as you know that your child will require medical attention for juvenile myositis (JM), it will be helpful to you to learn specifics about how *your healthcare system* works and how to manage medical expenses.

What Types of Medical Insurance Are the Most Common?

There are several types of health insurance, a number of which are defined below. These descriptions are general; each specific plan may be different. The first step toward understanding how to advocate for your child is to understand what kind of insurance you have for your child, what services are covered, and what options are available if your child's needs are not met.

1. *Indemnity or Fee for Service* insurance allows the purchaser to choose any physician for medical care. There is a split between the insurer and the insured for

costs of care covered by the insurance plan until the out-of-pocket maximum cost of care is reached. After the out-of-pocket maximum cost has been reached, the provider (the insurance company) pays for all covered benefits.

2. *Preferred Provider Organization (PPO)* or Discounted Fee for Service is similar to Indemnity insurance; however, costs are lower within the specified network for care covered by the plan. Outside the network, co-pays are based on higher charges or are based on the difference between the charges for in-network and out-of-network care.

3. *Point of Service (POS)* can be a more expensive insurance plan, especially for individuals who require specialized care. In this plan each covered individual has a primary care physician (PCP) who will choose to refer an individual to the needed care provider within the plan or outside the plan. If you need care that can only be achieved outside of the plan, all or most of the cost will be covered by the Point of Service if the primary care physician makes the referral. If the primary care physician does not make the referral, you will have to pay a significant coinsurance cost.

4. *Health Maintenance Organizations (HMO)* were developed to try to manage medical costs for patients with the idea of reducing costs while assuring that those who need care can receive it. Although this is the least expensive type of plan, it is also the most restrictive for access to healthcare. Each insured member pays a monthly fee. A primary care provider or physician (PCP) coordinates medical care. There is focus on preventive care, which is valuable. Some plans charge co-pays for care of injuries or illness. Care by any physician outside the plan must be paid by the individual and will not be covered by the plan. Some plans will make exceptions in extraordinary situations for external physician evaluations.

5. *Medicaid* is a federal program developed to provide care to low-income families, especially the disabled, blind, aged, or selected families with dependent children. Although Medicaid is a federal program, each state deploys Medicaid independently, creating some discrepancies concerning who receives Medicaid and how. Most services are covered; however, home healthcare is usually not included. The requisites for coverage include:
   a. Ability to qualify for Aid to Families with Dependent Children (AFDC)
   b. Fewer than six years without family income or an income at or very much below the federal poverty level, which is periodically redefined
   c. Pregnant women with an income at or below the federal poverty level
   d. People who have supplemental security income (Kidcare) as allowed by the state in which they live
   e. Recipients of adoptive or foster care services
   f. Independent children, nineteen years of age or younger, with an income below the federal poverty level

6. *State Supported Supplemental Insurance (SSI)* or *Kidcare* is available in some but not all states, and the requirements for each state's plan vary by state. Kidcare programs like the Medicaid State Child Health Insurance Programs (SCHIP) can help cover costs not met by other insurance for those who qualify (individuals younger than age eighteen years and pregnant women), including covering more benefits, "outside" providers, day hospital or home healthcare, and medications. There are several excellent web sites that detail what each state does and does not provide and to whom in the reference section.

How Can We Cope with Insurance Issues and with Managing Medical Expenses?

Parenting a child with a chronic illness can be quite stressful. Coping with a denial for payment of a medical consultation or procedure can be overwhelming and often seem impossible to resolve until parents understand how to work with the system. We hope that the following guidelines will help patients and families understand the insurance claim process.

There are two important issues in managing medical expenses and in receiving quality healthcare: successful communication with a managed care organization (MCO), health maintenance organization (HMO), "point of service" (POS), or other type of integrated healthcare system (IHS) and understanding the appeal process should an adverse decision ever be received.

Public and legislative support for consumer protection and education continues to expand from employer groups and healthcare delivery systems. You can check your health plan rating with the National Committee for Quality Assurance (NCQA), which evaluates and certifies health plans, to better understand what you should expect from your plan's overall care delivery and member satisfaction.

People with chronic disease, such as juvenile myositis, and their families are often concerned about receiving doctor-recommended treatments within a health maintenance organization or integrated healthcare delivery system as individual doctor-recommended treatments may not be approved. A consumer's faith in his or her healthcare system is critical for persons with an acute or chronic disease requiring varying resources over time. Historically, we had complete trust in healthcare systems; however, in the climate of managing quality care and costs within an integrated healthcare delivery system, individuals and families are often uneducated about the best way to maximize their coverage or how to best manage the potential appeal of a perceived adverse decision. The patient-doctor relationship is the foundation for receiving quality care. Your physician is your strongest advocate should an appeal ever need to be challenged.

Integrated delivery systems have reinvented their in-house processes to review medical requests and utilization management decisions (i.e., for or against a doctor's recommendation). More decisions are now made in accordance with national accredited clinical care guidelines, there is enhanced documentation of final decisions, and there is expanded information sharing with consumers. Managed care organizations use customer service 800-telephone numbers and online tracking by membership identification to document telephone conversations for the benefit of consumers, claim issues under dispute resolution, and formalize each step in the review process for timely review and quality care.

Suggestions to Handle Issues with Your Managed Care Health Insurance

Know the telephone number of your member services department or customer service department, and call them *first* when you have a question or concern. Be willing to give them a chance to solve what seems to be a problem.

Select a primary care provider in the physician/provider network when you are initially enrolled in your insurance plan. Inquire about where your child will receive subspecialty care and which physician will provide this care.

Identify which pediatric subspecialty facility or hospital is contracted with your insurance plan so that your claims can be correctly processed.

Support your health plan by encouraging your subspecialty provider to join the insurance company's network if they are not currently a member. Supporting network membership for pediatric rheumatologists or pediatric neurologists and other subspecialists your child may see is a win-win situation for you and your family as much as it is for the health plan.

Notify the utilization review department when you join a new health plan, via the member services or customer service department, of your family member's existing diagnosis and past medical management. Also, request continued care by the physician you have seen previously. Recommend your physician for the network if they are not members. Your suggestion will be forwarded to the provider relations department for follow-up. Remember: the best network physician is often the one that patients recommend to the health plan.

Transfer records to ensure that your primary care and subspecialty care physician have all your medical records and full information, so that they can clearly present their treatment plans to your health plan. You have an important role in helping your physician serve your needs within the health plan.

Understand your options. As a member of an insurance plan, your affected family member may have a right as a "special needs" enrollee based on certain criteria. You may be able to have "open referrals" to a subspecialist. Please check with your health plan for these options.

Understand your coverage. Before you receive care, understand what is covered and what is not covered by your employer and health insurance plan. For example, some plans may not cover injectable medications that your physician may be considering to treat your child. Some insurance plans require pre-authorization or approval for certain treatments. Failure to receive this pre-authorization will result in the treatment being denied. Some plans will allow visits for subspecialty care but will only pay for laboratory or radiology tests at specific locations. Having tests performed at the wrong facility could incur a large bill that your insurer will not cover. If you are not certain, call your insurance plan member services or customer service department for the answer to your questions. If you are still unclear about your insurance benefit coverage, contact your employer's healthcare benefit representative for clarification.

You can request: Once you are enrolled in a healthcare plan, you can request to have your child assigned to a case manager. A case manager in the health plan's utilization management department will facilitate seamless submission and review of your physician's requests and ensure use of preferred in-network contracted resources, such as physical therapy or occupational therapy, for your child's management.

Case manager: If you need to speak with a nurse, ask to speak with a case manager in the utilization management department who is familiar with chronic diseases and even your individual issues.

Customer service might be helpful. The next step is to contact the customer service number listed on your insurance card. Keep a notebook with the date, time, and name of the person with whom you spoke, and take notes about your conversation. Find out the reason a claim is being denied. Many times the reason is a simple clerical error such as the wrong CPT code (an insurance code for your child's diagnosis or treatments) for the procedure that was used. These errors can easily be corrected most of the time.

Keep meticulous records. Make copies of everything you send to the insurance company. If there was no billing error, then you may need to proceed to a formal appeal. Often these requests need to be in writing, and additional documentation from your doctor might be necessary. Sending your request by certified mail helps to ensure that it is dealt with appropriately and gives you documentation that it was received. Some companies have a time limit within which the appeal process can be started, such as within sixty days of receipt of the denial.

Consider complaining. If you continue to have a problem with your healthcare plan, call your health plan again and explain that you want to file a formal complaint or formal grievance. Most health plans will assign your file to an individual manager, who will "shepherd" it through the final appeal process.

A formal grievance is indicated if the health plan denies a covered service or treatment or denies a claim for a covered service or treatment on the basis that the service was not medically necessary. Examples of grievances:

- Your primary care physician refuses to give you a referral to see a specialist on the basis that it is not medically necessary and that the condition can be treated by him or her.

- Your emergency claim was denied as the basis that it was not a true emergency.

If your issue relates to any other issue with your health plan, you need to inquire about filing a formal complaint. Examples of formal complaints:

- You have a hard time obtaining an appointment with your physician even for sick visits.

- Your health plan refuses to provide treatment on the basis that the procedure is cosmetic or experimental and is not a covered benefit.

- You disagree with the treatment you received from your physician.

At this point you should seek help from your child's physician. Most appeal processes require a letter stating the medical necessity for the procedure or treatment and any relevant information from the medical record. Your doctor may include articles from peer-reviewed medical journals or even chapters from this book that support the medical effectiveness of the proposed plan. Support from your doctor is critical if the claim is being denied because the procedure or treatment was not "medically necessary." Most physicians are very willing to provide these documents in order for their patients to receive the most appropriate care. It is valuable to speak with your provider/physician to find out what needs to be addressed in this letter in order to overturn the denial. You might even find that there is more support for your situation than you imagined. The written document should include the following information:

- Child's name and insurance identification number

- Child's medical diagnosis

- Current situation—a clear explanation of the condition

- Request for services—a clear explanation of what is needed to support medical care. For example, if the request is for pediatric rheumatology care, poll the available physicians in your network for their experience with your child's diagnosis. You might be able to demonstrate a lack of experience within the physician network that supports your request to see a non-participating physician. You might also be able to have the physicians designated by the provider sign your letter of request in support of your needs. If the request is for a new medication, your physician must be able to document why this medication is necessary.

- If you are able to, estimate the cost of not providing appropriate care, such as the need for long-term care, surgery, or devices that might surpass the cost of the requested care.

The health plans have several levels of internal review of all complaints and grievances. An initial review is made by a first-level complaint or grievance committee. If you are dissatisfied with the decision of the *first-level committee*, you can appeal that decision to the *second-level committee*. You have a right to appear before the second-level complaint or grievance committee and explain why you believe your disputed service or claim should be paid by the health plan.

Some states will allow your physician the option to file a grievance on your behalf with your written consent. Please note that separate processes of appeals for complaints and for grievances exist in many states and health plans. It is important to note that in some states, appeals must be made within fifteen days of notice of the health plan's second-level review decision. Check with your health plan for the regulated timeframe within which a member must appeal an adverse decision.

In some states, if you are dissatisfied with the decision of the health plan's internal *second-level grievance review committee*, you can notify the health plan that you want an appeal. The health plan, in turn, will contact the Department of Health, which will assign an independent certified utilization review entity to review your case. In some states there may be a charge for this step in the appeal.

In some states, if you are dissatisfied with the decision of the health plan's internal *second-level complaint appeal committee*, you can appeal that decision to either the Department of Health or the state insurance commissioner. Sometimes, just the idea of involving state regulators is enough to turn things around with the insurance company. Forty-one out of the fifty states, plus the District of Columbia, offer the option of appeal and review by an outside panel of physicians, nurses, and lawyers who are not connected to the insurance company in any way. According to a recent study by the Kaiser Family Foundation, the insurers are overruled in about 50% of the cases, with rate of patient victory ranging from a high of 72% in Connecticut to a low of 21% in Arizona and Minnesota.

Your best advocates are your primary and subspecialty care physicians who know you and your child's medical history and management. A good doctor-patient relationship lies at the heart of patient satisfaction. Please remember to be willing to work with your health plan and your employer group. The overarching goals of health plans and employer purchasers are to deliver quality care to each member and to retain a healthy, comfortable, and satisfied health plan member.

A final thought—know your rights, and understand your insurance plan thoroughly. Complete information coordinated by a well-informed physician advocate is the key to a favorable outcome for better healthcare. Document all communications with the health plan and your physician. Try to obtain and keep copies of diagnostic test reports and consultant letters.

How Can We Afford All the Medications?

For many parents, one of the biggest worries that accompanies the diagnosis of a serious autoimmune disease is how they will be able to afford the numerous medications needed to treat the disease. Even when medications are covered by insurance, the co-pays can really add up, especially for children taking several medications. Many of the new medications used to treat autoimmune diseases are extremely expensive, making it very hard to pay a 10%–20% co-pay for each prescription.

What Can Parents or Caregivers Do to Make Sure Their Children Receive the Medications They Need?

Is a less expensive but equally effective drug available? Determine whether you can switch to a less expensive but pharmacologically equal version of the medication, called a generic. Generic drugs are required to be equivalent to the brand-name drug, they are just as effective, and may be 30%–50% less expensive than the brand-name drug. There are a few generic drugs that may have slightly different benefits or side effects. Be sure to check with your physician to determine whether a generic substitution is an appropriate choice.

Can your child's medicine be ordered from a legal and reliable mail-order pharmacy? A second step would be to obtain prescriptions from a mail-order pharmacy. Instead of paying prescription co-pay every month, the co-pay is paid only every three months, cutting the cost to the family by two-thirds. Some states require a co-pay for each month's medication supply. It does require work on the part of the family in that they must request a three-month prescription from the physician, fill out the mail order forms, and mail both in.

Can a Family Receive Medication Directly from a Pharmaceutical Company?

Many pharmaceutical companies have drug assistance programs, which significantly reduce or eliminate costs. Drug assistance programs work in cooperation with your doctor. In most cases there are patient income requirements. The family's income cannot exceed a specified amount, and proof of income must be provided. Forms are generally required to be filled out and signed by both the doctor and the patient's family.

What Is Available Through State-Funded Programs?

Some states have their own state drug-assistance programs to help cover the cost of prescription drugs. The requirements vary from state to state. Some are only designed to help people over sixty-five. Programs are currently available in CT, DE, IL, MA, ME, MI, MD, NJ, NY, PA, RI, and VT. Many hospitals have social workers or patient-financial planning assistants who can help determine whether you qualify. State supported supplemental insurance or Kidcare/CHIPS is described in the previous section. Not all states have this opportunity, and requirements vary between states. Please see one of the resources for details about Kidcare in your state.

Can I Apply for Medicaid?

Medicaid is jointly funded by the federal government and individual states to provide insurance and prescription drug coverage for low-income and needy families. Each state has different income requirements and criteria for acceptance into the program. Again, most social workers or patient financial planning personnel would be familiar with their own state's requirements and can assist families with this process.

What About Purchasing Medications from Canada or Other Countries?

Families sometimes wonder about the possibility of purchasing prescription drugs in Canada. Some medications can be up to 50% less expensive in Canada than they are in the United States. A few drugs may cost as much or more in Canada than in the United States. Anyone who has medical insurance in the United States that covers prescriptions under a co-pay system would not be likely to save money by purchasing the prescription in Canada. There may be serious safety concerns relative in the drug you thought you ordered: 1) it might not be the correct drug, or the drug might have other unknown additives, 2) it might not be at the proper strength, and 3) you might not save money after all.

Currently, the United States Food and Drug Administration (FDA) does not regulate or approve prescription drugs that are purchased in Canada. This creates a safety concern, related to both the type of drug that you obtain and the strength and purity of the medication itself. There are currently several bills under consideration in Congress, which would allow the importation of drugs from Canada into the United States. We strongly advise patients to wait for the outcome of this legislation. Quality and safety of prescription drugs is most important for your child's successful care.

Key Points

- When you choose an insurance plan, it is helpful to understand the differences in types of insurance, including costs, benefits, and limitations.

- Once you have selected a health plan, successful communication and navigation of the managed care system includes:
  - Understanding your benefits
  - Maintaining excellent communication between your child's primary care provider or physician and sub-specialist
  - Obtaining support through a case manager if you confront complex care issues
  - Knowing how to initiate the appeal process, if indicated

- Medications used to treat a chronic illness can be very expensive. Families have several ways to reduce costs.
  - Within the insurance plan, generic medications and mail-order pharmacies can reduce costs significantly.
  - Many pharmaceutical companies have drug assistance programs to help patients who cannot otherwise afford a medication.
  - State programs for drug assistance and supplemental insurance are available, but there is considerable variability in what is offered in each individual state.

- Some families are eligible for Medicaid, which provides families with insurance and medication coverage that they could not otherwise afford.

To Learn More

The Myositis Association (TMA).

Help paying for prescription drugs. Available from: www.myositis.org/jmbook resources.cfm or 800-821-7356.

> Links to various web sites listing organizations that can help pay for your prescription medicines.

United States Department of Health and Human Services.

Insure Kids Now. Available at: www.insurekidsnow.gov or 877-543-7669.

> Links to every state, in English and Spanish, with contact numbers and requirements for KidCare/CHIPS coverage.

American Academy of Pediatrics (AAP).

State Children's Health Insurance Program. Available at: www.aap.org/advocacy/schip.htm or 847-434-4000.

> Information and links similar to the U.S. government web site, but with contacts within AAP, a physician-run organization.

Henry J. Kaiser Family Foundation.

Your Source for State Health Data. Available at: www.statehealthfacts.kff.org or 650-854-9400.

> State-level data on health policy, health coverage, demographics, access, financing, and state legislation.

The National Association of Boards of Pharmacy.

List of Pharmacies. Available from: www.nabp.net/vipps/consumer/faq.asp.

> Lists of approved online pharmacies. The Verified Internet Pharmacy Practice Sites™ (VIPPS) program and its accompanying VIPPS seal of approval identify to the public those online pharmacy practice sites that are appropriately licensed, are legitimately operating via the Internet, and have successfully completed a rigorous criteria review and inspection.

The Muscular Dystrophy Association (MDA).

Eligibility and Payment. Available at: www.mdausa.org/publications/mdasvcs/eligpmt.html or 800-572-1717.

> Resource for families who have no insurance but don't qualify for Medicaid or Medicare; provides free medical care to those who have been diagnosed with myositis.

The Medicine Program.

Medicine Information Form. Available from: www.themedicineprogram.com or 866-694-3893.

> Organization established by volunteers dedicated to alleviating the plight of an ever-increasing number of patients who cannot afford their prescription medication.

FFF Enterprises, 41093 County Center Drive, Temecula CA 92591; Phone: 800-843-7477 (Reimbursement Advisor Line); Internet: www.fffenterprises.com.

Major supplier of IVIG, working with the FDA to track the blood supply in the United States. Patient advocates work with families to obtain IVIG coverage when insurance companies deny it, having successfully helped many myositis patients.

Reports in the Medical Literature

AAHP Report. *Early Evidence Shows Independent Review Working for Consumers.* December 1999. Washington DC: American Association of Health Plans.

Jesitus J. Staking Their Claims—Health Plans Hope a Willingness to Offer Appeal of Denials Restores Consumer Faith. *Managed Healthcare.* 1999;16–21.

Walker LM. What Do Patients Really Want? *Health and Medicine for Physicians—Hippocrates.* 1999:23(8);34–9.

CHAPTER 36

School Issues

Renee Thomas; Nancy Y. Olson, MD; Susan J. Wright, OT;
and Laurie Ebner-Lyon, RN, APN.C.

In this chapter...

We describe the legal rights children have to an education and ways that parents can work with the school to get extra help for the child with juvenile myositis (JM), from getting around the building to obtaining services such as physical therapy or tutoring for children who cannot attend school. It is important to have clear communication between your child, her doctors, and school personnel. We also suggest ways to make school participation easier and safer for your child with JM.

From the family's point of view...

"Our child's teachers have been great, and the other kids look out for him, too. With a Section 504 plan, we were able to have his physical education (PE) classes adapted and to obtain physical therapy through the school system. We stay in constant contact with the PE teacher to discuss creative ways to keep him involved, and we set up other possible accommodations for his classroom—extra time to take tests, a beanbag chair for reading time, and help carrying his books to and from the bus, among other things. Luckily, with regular communication with the school, we haven't needed to use many of these accommodations, but they're there in case we do!"

When a child is diagnosed with juvenile myositis (JM), she wants to know that life will remain as normal as possible. It is very reassuring for a child to maintain a daily routine of going to school. Good school attendance is essential, although children with myositis may miss school for doctor appointments and occasional testing, treatment, or hospitalization.

When children are newly diagnosed, they face many challenges that can affect their school performance, such as tiredness, muscle weakness, a rash that causes embarrassment, and anxiety over changes in body image.

Fortunately, with early diagnosis and aggressive treatment, muscle weakness and fatigue generally resolve or improve dramatically in several weeks to months.

Therefore, most school accommodations may only be needed for a short time. Some children, however, have illness that is more difficult to manage and could require long-term school accommodations.

Children with juvenile myositis do very well in school with good planning, developing a supportive team, setting realistic goals, and reassessing needs as often as necessary. There is no perfect plan, and every child has unique and special needs due to age, personality, and academic ability.

What Does the Law Say About My Child's Rights?

Section 504 of the Rehabilitation Act of 1973 states, "No qualifying handicapped individual shall solely by reasons of his handicaps, be excluded from participation in, be denied the benefits of, or be subjected to discrimination under any program or activity receiving Federal financial assistance."

Section 504 establishes that students with disabilities have a right to a free, appropriate public education even if the disability does not interfere with his or her ability to learn. The law requires schools to develop a 504 plan allowing for accommodations in the regular classroom. Parents have the right to be included in the process of developing an Individualized Education Plan (IEP) or 504 Accommodation Plan and the right to due process if they disagree.

The Individuals with Disabilities Education Act provides children with special needs the right to a free, appropriate public education in the least restrictive environment with an IEP. Under this law a child is eligible only if the disability interferes with her ability to learn. For a child with JM to qualify under this law, she must be evaluated by a multidisciplinary team and designated as eligible for special education based on physical disability as "other health impaired" or "orthopedically impaired."

In addition to federally mandated laws, states have their own laws addressing special education, and each school district may have subtly different evaluation polices and financial and/or staff abilities that could limit what they would be able to provide. You can obtain a copy of your state's and school district's educational laws by contacting your school district or county department of special education.

Understanding the Process

To develop an IEP, first you must identify the child's academic goals and then develop a strategy to implement them that considers the child's medical and psychological needs. The goal is for your child to achieve academic success to the best of her ability. The parent, child, and school are partners in planning and implementing a program to address the goals using a team approach to ensure every opportunity for the child's success. Each partner bears some responsibility in causing that to happen.

Parents' Responsibility

You will need to become familiar with the laws and procedures and the specific forms you need to fill out for your school district and state.

Educate yourself and your child about her illness and be able to communicate this information.

Inform the school by phone and in writing concerning your child's diagnosis. (Sample letters are provided by The Myositis Association. See *To Learn More* at the end of this chapter.) Ask what the school's procedures and policies are and what documentation you or your physician will need to provide. A parent or legal guardian is required by the Health Insurance Portability and Accountability Act of 1998 (HIPAA) to sign a release of information form, allowing your medical team to communicate with the school nurse or any other school staff member and vice versa.

Because parents cannot be at school to serve as advocates for their child, identify someone at school who will be your child's advocate. It can be a nurse, teacher, guidance counselor, principal, or anyone who is willing to work with the child, family, and school staff.

After those steps are completed, your team will need to decide which steps to take next. These next steps will be determined on the basis of the disease activity and severity and the school's policies. First, decide whether you need a simple meeting among the teacher, school nurse, and principal or a full staff meeting. We recommend whenever possible that you ask for a full staff meeting, which is one that all school personnel who see your child on a regular basis attend. Include all of your child's teachers, relevant administrators, the school nurse, counselors, director of transportation, bus drivers, and/or whomever you feel is needed. This is the best way to ensure that everyone has the same information and that everyone understands what modifications or accommodations may be needed for your child. You have the right to bring a medical specialist and/or therapists to either an informal or formal meeting. Do *not* attend this or any formal meeting alone. It helps to have support—bring the other parent, an advocate, family member, or friend. Depending on your child's age and maturity, she can attend all or any appropriate part of the meeting. Be sure to explain to your child what you are doing and why. Based on this meeting, the team will determine whether an informal or formal process (an IEP or 504 Plan) will be necessary to provide services for your child. Some school districts do not permit any accommodations or services unless they are done through a formal process.

Child's Responsibility

Children need to have some control over their own lives. Children who are included in the decision-making process and have a voice are usually more compliant. Because the child is the focus of the planning, without her cooperation, no system will succeed.

Help your child develop language to communicate with the teacher. She should know the name of her disease, the name and dosage of her medications, and how the medications help her. She needs to be able to tell you, the teacher, or the nurse how she feels and what specifically is a problem.

Schoolwork should be a priority. Children with JM need to learn their physical limitations and the importance of not becoming too tired to do their classwork. Some children push themselves too hard in their struggle to fit in. You, your medical team, and your school team can help your child find the appropriate balance between school, play, physical education, extracurricular activities, and jobs.

School's Responsibility

The school must provide an equal opportunity for your child to learn, monitor your child's progress, notify parents of any problems as soon as possible, and, ultimately, ensure that your child is learning. If the school has entered into an accommodation agreement, it must also ensure that all modifications and accommodations are met. Ask the school to provide:

- A calendar of events, including class trips and special programs
- Weekly class schedule, who teaches each class, and locations of each class
- Bus schedule
- Copies of school forms (IEP, 504 Accommodation Plan)
- Educational rights information
- List of services the school provides (such as physical therapy, psychological counseling, medical services) and the name of the contact person for each service
- School policies and teacher's classroom policies (some may not be appropriate for your child)
- Medical release forms

Do We Need to Start a Formal or Informal Process?

Implementation of the process can be done formally or informally, and each has its benefits and drawbacks. In an informal arrangement, parents and school personnel informally discuss and mutually agree on accommodations. Changes can be accomplished by phone, email, notes, and informal meetings. An informal process is good when there are few and minor requests. Simple requests make it easier for the school and may involve fewer staff members. Your child's illness may change quickly, and accommodations can easily be made while the child still needs them.

The disadvantage of an informal process is that it is not binding and therefore may be inadequate, depending on the cooperation of the school district. There may be no recourse if the plans are not met. There is no accountability or mandatory time frame or system to ensure that recommendations are followed. Furthermore, without the thorough evaluation required in a formal process, your child may not qualify to receive additional services.

The formal process involves developing a 504 Accommodation Plan or IEP. The IEP or the individualized health plan (IHP) is used in some districts in place of a 504 plan. The benefits of a formal process is that your child will be evaluated to determine eligibility for special education or accommodations. This process involves parents and many experts from the school district. Accommodations will be provided on the basis of the evaluation. There are structures and time limits for every step of this process. The child's IEP or 504 plan is reviewed annually. Furthermore, it is the parents' responsibility to monitor and ensure that all accommodation plans are met. Unfortunately, this process can take a significant amount of time, and your child's needs may have already changed before the accommodations have been initiated and are in place.

Suggestions Concerning the IEP and 504 Plan

- An IEP is a legally binding document. Do *not* sign any form if you do not understand it or if you disagree with any recommendation in it. You can take it home, ask for a copy to review, or obtain consultation before signing.

- Make sure you understand the timetable for the evaluation process and when services and accommodations begin. Bring a calendar and document everything.

- Ask for a review of your child's IEP or 504 plan if her medical condition changes before the annual review.

- Keep the language open-ended; include words and phrases like "as needed" or "when the disease is more active."

- Keep good records of all phone calls and meetings, and always include the date and the person contacted. Follow up with a note to confirm what was discussed. If corresponding by email, keep copies of your notes and their responses.

- Set up communication systems for you and the school (teacher) regarding questions, problems, notification of disease activity changes, daily disease reports, etc. Find out what method is best (notes, email, calls, fax) and when the best time is.

Complaint Process

Request a copy of the school polices and your rights under the law concerning this issue. The complaint process can be time consuming and complicated. While managing disputes, your child might not receive services, although she still needs them. For example, a typical complaint might be that you do not agree with the results of the evaluation. Therefore, you have rights to further steps, such as requesting, in writing, an independent evaluation and other testing formats, which the school (or school district) should pay for. Another example: If the school has failed to comply with the agreed upon accommodations or has not provided them within the mandatory time, you should complain immediately. Call the school, and send documentation detailing your complaints by registered mail. The school should respond immediately, and a meeting should be set to resolve all problems. If problems are not resolved, you may contact your state board of education to clarify questions about your child's situation or choose to begin mediation, a due process hearing, or a court hearing.

Which Medical Issues Do We Tell the School About?

Suggested Medical Documents to Be Provided to the School

- Documentation of your child's disease—some schools may require a physician's signature.

- Medication list, including dosage, length of time, taken with or without food, and possible side effects (a physician's signature may be required).

- Occupational and physical therapists' recommendations, including a list of what your child can do and should not do and suggested alternative activities. This is important for physical education, recess, and classroom activities.

- Diet restrictions.

- Be sure to provide medical recommendations and reports from other specialists who see your child on a regular basis.

(See also Table 36.1, *General guidelines for formal letters and forms*, at the end of this chapter.)

Unpredictability and Variability of Disease

- Explain the unpredictability and chronic nature of juvenile myositis. Discuss any patterns your child's illness may exhibit, such as regular morning or afternoon tiredness.

- List the common triggers that may increase disease activity, such as susceptibility to infection.

- There are many common viruses in schools. Not all are a danger to your child. However, depending on your child's medication and state of myositis activity, it may be very important for you to inform your child's doctor when your child has come in contact with certain viruses. Discuss with the doctor which viruses require medical attention. Make sure the school nurse has a list of which viruses are of concern, and have her notify you immediately when other children get them. For example, if your child has not had chicken pox or been immunized, depending on your child's medication and condition, it could be important to be notified immediately (within 24 hours) by the school when other children have chicken pox. The risk can be lower if your child has had chicken pox or been vaccinated, but your child's doctor should be notified immediately. For further information on this topic, see *Chapter 29, Vaccines and Infection Protection.*

- Request that a letter be sent to all parents about the importance of not sending sick children to school. All children will benefit from this handout.

- Stress is another common trigger of disease activity. Explain that reducing stress by encouraging your child's development of good coping strategies can help manage the juvenile myositis. Stress over absences, tests, inability to finish school activities due to tiredness, or family changes can make the illness more difficult to manage.

- Excessive activity can also contribute to tiredness. Your child might be able to participate in only some physical activities during physical education (gym) class. Special arrangements will probably be needed so that your child can perform her own physical therapy exercises during the physical education class. Once your child is recovering, she may be allowed to participate in full physical education but will need to be allowed to rest if her muscles become sore or if she becomes tired.

Physical and Psychological Issues

Psychological stress can be induced by looking different (e.g., steroid-induced weight gain); not being able to keep up with classmates; having to discontinue sports; not being able to participate in physical activities, dating, or going to the prom; or not being invited to birthday parties. Mood swings caused by the disease, medications, and/or the onset of puberty are important topics to discuss with the school staff. Your child may have a difficult time with peers and maintaining a focus on academics during these times.

Your child needs a person at school whom she trusts and whom she can contact when a problem occurs. This person could be the nurse, counselor, principal, or even a secretary—someone who can intervene for the child before a problem becomes serious. Some students just need a brief coping break when they become stressed and need a person or place to help them regroup before going back to class. Sometimes a short rest in the nurse's office and a listening ear are all that are needed.

If the school, you, and your medical team determine that your child needs psychological counseling for an extended period of time, your child might qualify for this counseling under *Related Services.* If your school does not have a staff psychologist, ask your medical team for a recommendation.

It is important for your child to feel included in all activities whenever possible. Using "buddy systems" or peer helper programs can help ensure that your child is not isolated.

Many children who are different in some way (not just those with JM) are subjected to cruel teasing by other students. Such teasing can be very distressing, so it is helpful to counteract it in many ways. First, you can teach your child not to take it personally and help her develop ways to talk about her illness to her peers. Role-playing, practicing answers, and humor help your child cope with difficult situations. Teasing can occur because of ignorance and fear on the part of the teaser. You can work with teachers to alleviate this ignorance by educating your child's classmates about JM. For example, a teacher and your child could co-teach an informational class about juvenile myositis. Alternatively, your child could present a report or a show-and-tell. The class could engage in role-playing activities, or a health class could study a unit on autoimmune diseases or chronic illnesses. In addition, consider explaining to classmates—especially younger children—why your child may need to use assistive devices or adaptive equipment (wheelchair) at school.

Children do not like to be asked constantly how they feel and do not want attention drawn to them when their illness is active. Developing a code system is a subtle communication tool for your child to use in the classroom. This system works well when the illness is not visible. For example, a commonly used technique is a numerical scale placed at the corner of the teacher's desk. Your child can discreetly point to the appropriate number corresponding to her pain, weakness, or tiredness level when she enters the room. Ask your medical team and teachers for other suggestions.

Medication

Almost all schools have a zero tolerance drug policy, which means that no child may carry or take any medication independently. All medications must be administered by the school nurse or other designated person. Dispensing medicine may be set up as an informal process but usually must be part of a formalized plan. Formal plans ensure that systems are in place for your child to receive her medicine. Work with your medical team to try to have all medicines given at home whenever possible.

Other Issues to Consider

Sun Exposure and Rashes

Children and adults may be surprised to see a rash and can say things that can embarrass your child. With practice, your child can tell others that the rash is not contagious and that it is part of her disease. Describe for the school staff any problems the rash may cause; for example, itching or burning of the skin could cause lack of focus in the classroom. It is important for children with juvenile myositis to avoid trauma to the skin. They may need padding over areas such as elbows, knees, or buttocks to prevent pressure or trauma that can result in calcifications. Your child might need an accommodation if the fabric in school uniforms is irritating. For more information about skin issues, see *Chapter 16, Skin Rashes and Sun Protection.*

Moisturizers or Sunscreen

You should apply sunscreen at home before sending your child to school in the morning and send supplemental sunscreen to school. Ask for permission for your child to keep a moisturizer and sunscreen lotion accessible (children might not be permitted to keep lotion in their desk or locker or apply it any place other than the nurse's office). Teachers might not be permitted to apply lotion, so the school nurse will apply lotion if your child cannot. Inform the nurse if your child is allergic to latex gloves. Provide your child's school with sunscreen and sun protective clothing to be made available to her for all outdoor activities, e.g., recess, physical education, and field trips.

Physical Therapy or Other Special Services

Your medical team might recommend services, such as physical therapy, occupational therapy, or special tutors for your child. Most school policies require that your child be evaluated in order to qualify for such services to be provided by the school. Typically, these services are provided by the school only if it is determined that your child needs them for basic functioning or safety at school. Examples include therapy to avoid choking in the lunchroom or to prevent falling out of a chair or falling on stairs due to muscle weakness. The school is not required to provide these services to achieve basic mobility or normal activities. If the school recommends any of these services, be sure to consult and get approval from your medical team.

Transportation Issues

When possible, drive your child to school, instead of having her walk or wait for the bus, to help your child conserve energy for classes. If your child must ride the bus and needs assistance going up and down the steps of the bus, make arrangements for someone to help your child at school and at home. Bus drivers are not permitted to leave the wheel to help your child. Your school district might provide handicapped bus/van service, but this usually requires your child to ride a separate bus for handicapped students. Some school districts charge for this bus service. Busing within school district boundaries might be provided for private schools. Ask the bus company for last pick-up and first drop-off.

Parents can get a temporary or permanent handicap placard to obtain a parking space near the door of most public buildings. In some neighborhoods with only street parking, you can also get a handicapped parking space in front of your house.

Building Accessibility

You, your child, and ideally a physical therapist should evaluate the school, classroom, and grounds for accessibility issues. Determine the proximity of lockers, stairs, and bathrooms. Plan for the distance and time needed for walking between classes. Make plans for any physical accommodations and help that your child may need during emergency drills. Children who have difficulty walking up or down stairs may need adult assistance or be allowed to use an elevator. Your school might not permit staff to lift your child up or down the stairs, even if she only needs assistance temporarily. Lifting can be unsafe and cause injuries and is a liability issue. Your child may need to be bused to the nearest wheelchair-accessible school within your district if your school does not have an elevator and if your child requires long-term use of an elevator.

Physical Education (PE) and Sports

Whether to allow a child with myositis to participate in sports is a decision you and your medical team must make. Many children do participate but sit out temporarily when the disease is active. Although most states have mandatory PE requirements, these can be waived or modified with medical documentation and very specific plans for your IEP. Also find out whether your child's school has any existing PE accommodations, such as indoor sports or other programs for those who cannot participate in usual PE activities. Ask if your child can receive PE credit for her physical therapy or if she can do physical therapy exercises during PE class. Most children participate in regular PE with the option to self-limit activities. Many kids would rather participate in PE activities than receive physical therapy in school. Ask your child's PE teacher to suggest other ways your child can participate and still receive credit. For example, she could keep score, keep records, be a linesman, etc.

Once your child is recovering, she may want to participate in PE but also be able to stop and rest if she feels tired or if her muscles are sore. Your child should not be pushed too hard in PE and should set her own limits on the amount of exercise she can tolerate. This is important because many children cannot catch themselves when knocked off balance and can be injured—especially by hitting their head or breaking a bone. They should have their activities modified if there is a risk of other students knocking them down.

Getting Homework Assignments and Notes When School Is Missed

There are many ways to get homework assignments when school is missed. Many schools post them on web sites. You can also email most teachers or ask them to send written information.

You may need to remind teachers that not all children can do work when they are not well. Your child may be home but may be feeling ill or tired and, consequently, may be unable to do any work. Ask your teacher what is absolutely necessary for make-up work. Explain that when your child has missed many days, she may still be very tired, even though she has returned to the classroom. Attending classes may be all that your child can accomplish until she has completely recuperated. Completing current assignments may be a difficult task. Trying to complete many days of make-up work can cause overwhelming stress and often can add to recuperation time. Although your child's teacher plans the curriculum, the medical team, parent, and student should work with the teacher to ensure that the workload is appropriate.

Sometimes teachers will allow the grade your child had before the missed days to "stand" (especially if your child is an A or B+ student). Ask the teacher to permit your child *not* to have to make up reports, quizzes, or tests, with the understanding that you will help your child learn the missed classroom information. However, if you request this, there will be fewer grades to average, which could be a disadvantage.

Accommodation Suggestions for Weakness, Fatigue, or Pain

Pain and tiredness from muscle weakness are usually not visible. It is not enough just to state this. In order for teachers to help your child, provide examples of what behaviors your child may exhibit when she is in pain or very tired.

- Morning issues. Children need to attend classes. If necessary, start your daily routine earlier to help your child get to school on time.
- Children may require assistance from parents and at school with dressing and using the toilet at illness onset when weakness is moderate to severe.
- Your child may need clothing that is easy to put on, take off, and fasten.
- Younger children are often asked to sit on the floor during assemblies or in class. Bleachers or a chair should be provided. Remember to ask your child about what will work best for her.
- If your child is allowed to rest temporarily, she can avoid asking to go home. Ask if your child can rest in the nurse's office and then resume classes. Provide a pillow, snacks, book, or books on tape.
- Try to schedule non-academic classes for the end of the day in case your child must leave early because of tiredness.
- A seat at the rear of the classroom might be better so that your child can stand and move without disturbing the other children.
- Your child might need someone to help carry her lunch tray or open her milk.
- Your child might need to leave class early to get to the next classroom due to active myositis or fragile bones. This also helps prevent unnecessary bumping into the walls.
- Schedule classes to minimize distances between classrooms.

- Your child could be a line leader and set a slower pace for the group.
- Books could be too heavy for your child to carry. Ask for a second set of books for home or spare books to be kept in specific classrooms or additional lockers. Alternatively, other students could help carry books or your child could use a wheeled backpack.

Ways to Eliminate Unnecessary Hand Use and Handwriting Fatigue

With a little creativity, you and your child's teacher can find ways to reduce the amount of strain put on the hand and arms by writing. For example, answers on worksheets and tests can be circled instead of written out. Ask the teacher to find ways other than repetitive writing for learning spelling words and math facts, such as flash cards. Assure the teacher that you will help your child learn the spelling words and math facts. Allow the child to use a calculator, but make sure that your child does know her math facts and functions. Your child may not want to use one during class if no one else is using one. To avoid hand fatigue from typing, find a good voice recognition program for your computer.

Testing Modifications

If your child is having problems taking tests and is therefore receiving significantly lower grades than normal, ask your school about accommodations for testing. Discuss this with your child, because she might not want to be perceived as receiving "special privileges." However, doing well in school is very important, and if poor test results, due to myositis, are keeping grades low, then your child needs an accommodation, such as:

- A test administered in several sessions throughout the day or over several days
- Questions that can be checked or circled rather than ones that require answers in the form of long written sentences
- A teacher's aide, who will write the answers
- Increased spacing between questions, which gives the child more room to write
- Large print
- Oral exams
- Reduced number of items per page
- Untimed tests taken in a separate room
- Access to a tape recorder, computer, and/or calculator

Be sure to set accommodations in advance for major tests, such as the SAT, Iowa testing, mandatory state proficiency tests, etc.

Absenteeism

High schools mandate that students must attend a certain number of days in order to graduate. Ask for a waiver if the onset of myositis prevents your child from completing credits. If the onset of illness begins during the last part of the senior year and your child has missed more than the allowed number of days, find out whether your child can do a walk-through graduation ceremony and complete credits during summer school. If your school does not offer summer school, make arrangements with the reciprocating school within your district. (Transportation might not be provided.)

In many districts, homebound services are typically not provided until a student has missed two to three consecutive weeks of school, so ask for a copy of your school district's polces. As soon as you know that your child will be missing at least two weeks of school, call the school immediately, and make plans with the school advocate to try to have the policy waived to expedite quick services.

Students with chronic or severe juvenile myositis might miss a few days intermittently for illness flares. To provide homebound services during these periods, an IEP is required to classify a student as "other health impaired." Your medical team will provide documentation of disease flares. Your medical team can also help you and the school determine whether this accommodation is needed at disease onset or during prolonged treatments. In some cases children might find it more accommodating to be homeschooled until they are able to resume their normal activities, sometimes starting back to school on a half-day basis until they are physically able to attend full-day sessions.

Private School

There is no one answer to what is mandatory for private schools. You might need to find a compromise between what your child needs and what the school can provide. Some schools may not have the necessary facilities, staff, or funding to provide special services. Some districts may fund special services at private schools. If your child's needs are beyond your school's capability, your child may have to attend another school. However, some schools will make great efforts to do everything possible to help your child.

Table 36.1. General guidelines for formal letters and forms.

The school may require formal letters as documentation for their records. In all correspondence with schools and medical providers, be clear and courteous, thank those who help you, and keep the letter simple. Always make a copy for your records. Letters should be addressed to the principal and/or the appropriate person who is responsible for special education services. Provide copies for teachers, if appropriate.

Document names, dates, conversations, and be precise concerning complaint issues. Sometimes it might be best to hand deliver the letter. If you do, document the date and time in your notes, and get a receipt from the person to whom you delivered it. Sometimes it may be necessary to mail letters by registered mail, which gives you proof that the school received the letter.

Formal Processes That Require Letters

- Request for evaluation
- Independent evaluation
- Re-evaluation
- Review and revision of 504 Accommodation Plan
- Mediation
- Due process hearing
- Viewing or obtaining copies of your child's records

Medical Documentation Forms

Letters should be addressed to the principal and school nurse. Most schools and physicians will have their own forms for the following, due to privacy laws:

- Permission for shared information between school and physicians and allied health personnel (occupational or physical therapist's recommendations)

- Permission to take medicine

- Notification of medicine changes

- Notification of changes in myositis disease activity

- Notification of severe effects or behavioral changes caused by the illness or medication

- A current signed Health Insurance Portability and Accountability (HIPAA) consent form, which gives the medical healthcare team permission to communicate with the healthcare professionals at the school, such as the nurse or occupational, physical, or speech therapist. A separate school release needs to be signed by the parent to allow the medical team to communicate with non-medical personnel at the school, such as the teacher, PE instructor, or principal.

Table 36.2. Resources for educational rights.

- Other parents of children who have special education needs. Even if it is a different disease or disorder, parents may be very familiar with your school's policies and be able to give you help, support, and advice.

- Social workers.

- Local phone book and libraries. They may have information and addresses for services.

- State special education department. It should be able to provide all materials and answer questions for you. You may need to make an appointment before visiting its office for a consultation.

Key Points

- When your child is first diagnosed with JM, it can be overwhelming. You will have many things to learn and do, including informing your child's school and asking for special services from them. You will need to reassess your child's needs over time and inform the school of changes.

- Develop a partnership with your school, your child, and her medical team. Such partnerships can be formal or informal; each has advantages and disadvantages. Each partner also has responsibilities.

- Keep your child's school informed about her medical situation and physical and psychological needs. Provide the necessary documents, as well as additional information. Work with the teachers to educate your child's classmates about JM, to avoid teasing and cruelty.

- If necessary, make arrangements for physical education waivers, getting homework assignments, and homeschooling for extended absences.

- See Table 36.2, *Resources for educational rights*, for more helpful information.

To Learn More

The Myositis Association (TMA).

Your child and school. Available from: www.myositis.org/jmbookresources.cfm.
Sample letters to school officials, brochures written for teachers, and more.

Arthritis Foundation.

Arthritis in Children, Teens and Young Adults: Teachers & Students. Available from: www.arthritis.org/communities/juvenile_arthritis/children_young_adults.asp.
Articles and materials related to school, including information on education laws and school services for children with arthritis and related conditions.

Eurydice. Avenue Louise 240, B-1050 Brussels; Phone: 32-2-600-53-53; Internet: www.eurydice.org; Email: info@eurydice.org.

Information network on education in Europe; to boost cooperation by improving the understanding of educational systems and policies.

Family and Advocates Partnership for Education (FAPE). PACER Center, 8168 Normandale Blvd, Minneapolis MN 55437-1044; Phone: 952-838-9000; Internet: www.fape.org; Email: fape@fape.org.

Information on IDEA and other disability laws.

National Center on Education Outcomes (NCEO). University of Minnesota, 350 Elliott Hall, 75 East River Road, Minneapolis MN 55455; Phone: 612-626-1530; Internet: www.education.umn.edu/NCEO; Email: nceo@umn.edu.

Information on state accommodations, NCEO publications, and more.

National Dissemination Center for Children with Disabilities (NICHCY). P.O. Box 1492, Washington DC 20013; Phone: 800-695-0285; Internet: www.nichcy.org; Email: nichcy@aed.org.

NICHCY (formerly the National Information Center for Children and Youth with Disabilities), funded by the U.S. Department of Education and the Office of Special Education Programs, is a central source of information on the Individuals with Disabilities Education Act (IDEA); "No Child Left Behind," as it applies to those with special needs; and information based on research into effective education practices. Web site has pages just for children, research information, state resources, education publications, and more.

Parent Information and Resource Centers. Available at: www.pirc-info.net.

Funded by discretionary grant from U.S. Department of Education.

U.S. Department of Education.

A Guide to the Individualized Education Program. Available at: www.ed.gov/parents/needs/speced/iepguide/index.html.

State Contacts and Information. Available at: www.ed.gov/about/contacts/state/index.html?src=ln.

CHAPTER 37

Summer Camps

Ann S. Christiano, MS, ARNP; Dana Driesman-Klover, BSc OT, OT Reg. Ont.; Megan Perron, RN, BScN; Joyce L. Sundberg, RN; and Ilona S. Szer, MD

In this chapter...

We give parents the information they need to feel comfortable allowing their children with juvenile myositis (JM) to participate in the wonderful experience of summer camp.

From the family's point of view...

"Camp has opened my eyes. It's not just a place but a feeling. When I am having a bad day, I can go back in my mind to that feeling of love and belonging, and I can know that there are people out there who are going through the same things I am. I have met some of my best friends in the whole world by just stepping out of my car and spending one week at this place where everyone belongs and understands each other. Although this disease has been a burden in my life, it has also been a blessing. Thanks to my disease I have been able to experience a feeling that not many others have. This feeling cannot be named or described, but it does exist. It exists in anyone who has ever spent one minute, one day, one week, or even several weeks at camp.

"So after at least ten tie-dyed T-shirts, more than ten zips on the zip line or over one hundred times walking back and forth from the tent area to the dining hall, and over fifty morning stretches, I want to say thank you. Thank you for talking my parents into sending me to camp."

Summer brings hot dogs on the grill, swimming with friends, and lazy days just hanging out. For many children summer frequently includes going to camp. Some children may want to go to camp over a weekend or for a longer stay, and others may want to participate in a day camp that is close to home. However, when a child has a chronic illness, parents are often reluctant to allow their child to be away from home. Fortunately, summer camps for children with special needs have been available for many years. The first camps for children with diabetes were started in the 1920s. Now there are many camps for children with illnesses such as arthritis, muscular dystrophy, and juvenile myositis. Increasingly, healthcare providers are recommending camp as part of a comprehensive treatment program for children with chronic health conditions. Whether it is a day camp or an overnight camp, the camping experience gives children with JM the opportunity to meet new friends, learn new skills, and have fun swimming, fishing, sailing, and toasting marshmallows over an open fire.

How Does Summer Camp Benefit Children with Myositis?

The ideal camp experience provides an opportunity to experience a situation where everyone is accepted, where everyone belongs, and where no one is identified by her personal challenges. The environment is structured to allow everyone to participate to the fullest extent possible and to show that children of all abilities can contribute. Differences or disabilities are not overlooked, just taken as a fact of life from which to begin and enjoy the opportunities for fun. At camp everyone shares similar challenges; everyone appreciates each other's accomplishments. Success is measured in one's ability to face a challenge and decide how to overcome it.

Children with chronic health conditions know what it means to be misunderstood. It can be overwhelming living in a world that does not understand your challenges. Children with any chronic illness or disability may feel a variety of emotions, from the awkwardness of being different to feeling inadequate, isolated, or unhappy. The right camp is a way to bridge these difficulties by allowing children to participate, compete, develop skills and friendships, and make developmental progress in an environment where they are in the norm and no longer different because of their illness.

In addition to providing the experience of acceptance and belonging, camps enable children to learn new skills and information in a pressure-free environment. There are no grades and no tests. Children learn many things from each other, including new skills and insights about their own condition. Most medically-oriented camps provide children with JM an opportunity to have a typical camp experience with medical support available. Campers often learn through informal discussions with other campers and staff.

Some studies have looked at the effect of the camp experience. These studies suggest that first-time campers gained more knowledge about their illness than returning campers. Returning campers had improved self-esteem during the camp experience. Other studies reported a positive correlation between knowledge and self-concept. There are, therefore, benefits for both new and returning campers.

Other research found that the camp experience itself provides support for children. The camp program need not be heavily weighted with education or formal work on self-esteem. By simply providing children who share the same or a similar condition the opportunity to have a normal camp experience, children can make significant gains.

Given the freedom to stretch their limits, children will frequently demonstrate that they are capable of far more than their parents suspected. Perhaps the most surprising result of the camp experience is how much the child's own self-perception changes. The changes may not be apparent immediately, but in time they emerge. For example, several weeks after camp had ended, some children were interviewed and asked about their camp experiences. Their responses included:

- "I felt fully accepted; no questions asked."
- "I now have more confidence in myself."
- "I realize I have choices many times, all day long."
- "I realize I am accountable for my decisions."
- "I formed new, strong friendships that will last a lifetime."
- "I conquered home sickness."
- "I learned new activities like tie-dying, sports, and teamwork."
- "I have a better understanding of my diagnosis."
- "I will now be more responsible for my own medical treatment."
- "I know myself better."

Parental Concerns About Camp

It can be a frightening experience to send your child to camp because you are entrusting her care to strangers. It is even more frightening for the parents of a child with a difficult and unpredictable medical condition. At home, under the watchful eye of parents and family, children are well protected. It can be difficult for parents to feel comfortable with others taking care of their precious child and meeting her special needs. Parents are often more anxious about sending their children to camp than the children themselves are about going. By meeting or talking with the healthcare providers, counselors, staff, as well as other campers, parents can gain the confidence needed to permit their child to attend camp. There is no question that parents must feel secure that their child is receiving all needed medications and that knowledgeable healthcare providers are quickly available in case of an emergency. To ensure your peace of mind and a positive experience for your child, make sure the camp provides:

- A safe environment
- Experienced staff
- Adequate supervision
- Challenging and stimulating programs
- Well-organized, age-appropriate recreational activities
- Environment that encourages development of meaningful relationships
- Environment that fosters independence
- Staff who can help campers meet the challenges of daily living and solve problems as challenges arise
- Rest time and opportunities for quiet activities

How Do I Choose a Summer Camp?

When choosing a summer camp for your child, you can obtain information from a variety of sources. Ask your child's JM doctor if he or she has information about camps that might be appropriate. The Arthritis Foundation and Muscular Dystrophy Association sponsor camps for children with JM and other illnesses, and The Myositis Association and the Cure JM Foundation offer camp scholarships for medically approved camps. The American Camping Association provides information about camps for children with special needs, as well as suggestions about how to contact and interview camp directors. Below we discuss issues to consider when choosing a summer camp for your child with JM.

Type of Camp

Day camps allow children to participate in many activities and programs while still living at home, whereas overnight camps enable children to live away from home, with other children and adults. Camp sessions can be as short as a weekend or can extend to two weeks. To determine what is best for your child, ask: Has she ever been away from home before? Is the illness under enough control to allow her to have a positive experience? Are campers allowed to call home and parents allowed to call camp? What is the daily schedule like? Is there a choice of activities? Are there rest periods incorporated into the day? What time do they get up and go to bed? What are the evening activities?

Trained Staff

It is best for your child to attend a camp staffed by people who are knowledgeable about JM. Staffing numbers and qualifications will be important to assess. You need to know whether the camp can accommodate your child's special medical needs, including physical, emotional, and/or psychosocial aspects. Find out who will be providing care to your child while attending the camp. A camp affiliated with an organization such as the Arthritis Foundation or Muscular Dystrophy Association has physicians, nurses, and therapists on staff. Questions to ask include: What is the staff-to-camper ratio? Do staff members stay in the camper cabins at night? What is the medical back-up should a camper need more medical care than can be provided at camp?

It is important that someone with a medical background be available and knowledgeable about your child's condition in case she needs assistance with treatments or medicines. The staff should also be aware of the medications your child is taking and their potential side effects.

If there is not an appropriate medically oriented camp in your area, consider working with your local YMCA (or another organization known for excellent summer camps) and your child's doctor to help establish one. Most camps for children with chronic conditions have been the fruit of parental efforts with input from health professionals. Do not despair if one does not exist; consider starting one!

Accessible Facilities

It is extremely important to find out about the facilities that are available. You need to know how far away the cabins, bathrooms, and showers are located from the dining hall and from the area where most of the activities take place. Some campgrounds are hilly, which can present a problem for some children. They may choose not to participate in some of the activities because it is too difficult or too far for them to walk. If the distances or hills will be a problem for your child, find out whether there are other ways to transport campers. Some camps use golf carts and vans to transport campers who have difficulty walking, whereas others provide a walking buddy. Wheelchairs should, of course, be made available as needed.

Are the cabins and activity rooms wheelchair accessible? Are the grounds and outdoor activities accessible to your child? An accessible environment will make it easier for your child to function. It is important to let the camp know what your child's needs are so arrangements can be made before her arrival.

Activities

The camp should have a variety of activities from which your child can choose. The activities should be adaptable to your child's special medical needs. There should be staff available to ensure the safety of every camper in every activity. Be sure the camp you choose also allows for brief rest periods throughout the day. A room for supervised arts and crafts provides an ideal alternative activity for children who simply cannot remain physically active all day long.

Nutrition

It is important to know who will be providing and preparing the food at your child's camp and whether the facilities are flexible enough to meet your child's nutritional needs. Many children have specific dietary restrictions because of medication or allergies, or they need supplements because of poor food or fluid intake. You should also find out if someone will be available to provide dietary education, if necessary, to your child or the staff. Some camps make special arrangements with families ahead of time if a child requires a particularly restrictive diet, which can be sent to camp by the family.

Special Needs

Review your child's special needs with the camp coordinator, including the need to apply sunscreen regularly and to wear a hat and protective clothing. Find out whether they can accommodate the challenges your child may have. If your child is having emotional difficulty, for example, be honest about it so the staff can be sensitive to her moods. Let them know what those challenges are and how you are dealing with them presently, and find out if they are comfortable with them as well. Find out whether there is a social worker or psychologist available to the staff and campers.

Location

Availability of a camp may vary from state to state. You must decide how far you are willing to travel to enroll your child in a summer camp. If the cost of travel to camp is too expensive, there are resources available, such as Angel Flight, which is a group of private pilots who transport patients to and from medical appointments as well as chronic illness camps.

For those who cannot travel to overnight camps there might be day camps available in your community that can accommodate your child's needs. Schools often provide day camps during the summer, as do libraries, parks, and recreation centers.

Cost

If the cost of camp would prohibit your child from attending, try to find scholarship money or other funding options available to you. Speak to your social worker or other healthcare provider who may offer some assistance. The Myositis Association, Cure JM Foundation, Arthritis Foundation, and Muscular Dystrophy Association offer scholarships and opportunities for children to raise money to go to camp. See the organizations listed at the end of this chapter for contact information.

In summary, camp is a wonderful experience for children. Children with JM can benefit for many years to come once they are allowed to experience the camaraderie and fun of summer camp. Children need to experience the challenges of childhood before they can be productive adults. Camp allows even the most vulnerable children to feel accepted and valued.

Key Points

- Children with JM can benefit greatly from going to camp, including developing greater confidence, self-esteem, and taking responsibility.
- Parents need to do the proper research about potential camps to ensure that it will be a positive experience for their child and to reduce their own worries.
- In choosing a camp, consider how long it will be, whether it has enough qualified staff, the activities it provides, how accessible it is, whether it can accommodate the special needs of your child, as well as cost and location.

To Learn More

The Myositis Association.

Summer camps for JM. Available from: www.myositis.org/jmbookresources.cfm or 800-821-7356.

Information on scholarships to summer camps, including application and guidelines.

Cure JM Foundation. Phone: 760-487-1079; Internet: www.curejm.com; Email: info@curejm.com.

Information on scholarships to summer camps.

American Camping Association, 5000 State Road 67 North, Martinsville IN 46151; Phone: 765-342-8456; Internet: www.acacamps.org; Email: parents@ACAcamps.org.

Find a camp: search for camps for specialty clientele or those with special needs. Available from: http://find.acacamps.org/finding_special_needs.php.

Search for camps based on special needs, cost, location, age of child, and other criteria.

Arthritis Foundation.

Summer camps. Available from: www.arthritis.org/communities/juvenile_arthritis/about_ajao.asp or 800-568-4045.

Select Summer Camp option from the "About AJAO" page to view a list of the upcoming summer camps, their locations, and related information.

Easter Seals, 230 West Monroe Street, Suite 1800, Chicago IL 60606; Phone: 312-726-6200 or 800-221-6827; Internet: www.easter-seals.com.

Contact Easter Seals for more information on Camp without Barriers.

Muscular Dystrophy Association.

MDA summer camp. Available from: www.mdausa.org/clinics/camp.html or 800-572-1717.

General information on MDA camps, some of which are free.

MDA clinics/services zip code locator. Available from: www.mdausa.org/locate.

Contact your local MDA office for information on summer camps in your area.

Reports in the Medical Literature

Punnett AF, Thurber S. Evaluation of the asthma camp experience for children. *Journal of Asthma.* 1993;30(3):195–8.

Stefl ME, Shear ES, Levinson JE. Summer camps for juveniles with rheumatic disease: do they make a difference? *Arthritis Care and Research.* 1989 March;2(1):10–5.

CHAPTER 38

Searching the Internet for Reliable Information

Ann Kunkel, BS; Susan J. Wright, OT; Carol B. Lindsley, MD; and Jane G. Schaller, MD

In this chapter...

We offer suggestions about how you can get to reliable information from the Internet and avoid misinformation.

From the family's point of view...

"After our daughter was diagnosed with juvenile dermatomyositis, my husband and I scoured the Internet. Organizations' sites and children's online journals continued to comfort me as I read what to expect and how others had successfully met the challenges of JM. I am grateful to have found this priceless information."

Where Can I Find Internet Sources for Information on Juvenile Myositis?

By now you might have looked at some of the web sites listed in the *Resource Appendix* or at the end of other chapters (*To Learn More*). There are many useful web sites that contain reliable information, and a few selected sites are provided at the end of each chapter in this book. The web sites of organizations that provide support for patients with juvenile myositis (JM) and their families are a good place to start your search for information. Through these organizations, such as The Myositis Association, the Arthritis Foundation, and the Cure JM Foundation, you can find a wide variety of information about JM as well as links to other web sites, discussion boards, and chat rooms where you can ask questions and share information with others. Other sources of good information include government, university, or medical school web sites, as well as hospital, health system, and healthcare facility web sites. Among web sites with reliable information, there could be other web sites with unreliable information. How can you tell the difference?

If you search the Internet using a search engine, such as Google, Lycos, or Yahoo, you will find a lot of information, but it may or may not be reliable. You will have to evaluate its reliability yourself. However, if you search the Internet through the Health on the Net Foundation (HON) web site, you can search all medical and health web sites available or only those that are accredited by the HON Code of Conduct. The HON Code of Conduct defines a set of principles for web site developers to use in the presentation of information, so readers will be properly informed as to the source and purpose of the information they are reading. To help you evaluate the information you find on the Internet, compare it with other resources, such as this book, to see if the information is similar. If you find discrepancies, check with your doctor.

On the Internet, you will find many different types of information about JM, from simple definitions of what it is, to patients' journals, to technical information that has been simplified for the lay public, to technical information that the doctors share with each other. The latter type consists of research articles published in specialized medical journals. This is the information that your child's doctors read and sometimes write. You can access this cutting-edge research in several ways.

Many medical references can be found in electronic form on the Internet by using a searchable web site known as PubMed, which is supported by the U.S. National Institutes of Health. You can find articles in the PubMed database by typing in search terms, such as "juvenile myositis" or "juvenile dermatomyositis." The database can also be searched by a particular author, in a particular year, or based on the type of reference (review vs. article, English vs. other language, animal vs. human study). You will get a list of article abstracts, or summaries, which you can read. However, if you want to read the full article, you will probably have to look it up in the library of a university or medical school. Some journal articles are available in full text at no charge from PubMed Central (see *To Learn More*). Some of the journals using this site provide immediate full access to the articles, whereas other published research papers are available only on a delayed basis, after appearing first in their primary journal.

The National Institute of Arthritis and Musculoskeletal and Skin Diseases (NIAMS) web site also has helpful guidelines for finding health information on the Internet, as well as information about medical and health directories and services provided by the federal government. NIAMS also offers information about talking with your doctor, patient issues, choosing a doctor, obtaining personal health records, access and privacy laws, and links to other helpful web sites.

How Can I Be Sure the Information I Find Is Reliable?

One of the best ways to verify the reliability of information is to ask your child's physician. Remember that even though you can find reliable information on the

Internet, it might not apply to your child and could even be harmful. Each child's case is unique; what worked for one child might not work for another.

Out-of-date information may not be reliable because research advances result in changes in health information. Web sites that provide medical information should be updated frequently, and most sites will provide the last revision date.

When evaluating medical information, check to see that it is being provided by a medical professional and that references are provided to support the information; then, check with your physician. Often, commercial products and services may be offered on a web site, and the claims made for these should be supported by references as to the source of the information and the credibility of the claims made. Beware of web sites that offer "miracle cures." If the information sounds unbelievable, it probably is. Remember: Anyone can put information or misinformation on the Internet.

Key Points

- The Internet is a valuable tool that can help you find information about JM and related services and make contact with other families who are dealing with JM. It can also allow you to participate in chat rooms and discussion boards.

- Not all information on the Internet is reliable, and it is important to follow some guidelines for evaluating whatever information you find. Your child's physician is one of the best ways to verify the information you find on the Internet.

- Some good sources for information about JM are organizations that support the JM community, as well as government, university, medical school, and hospital or healthcare facility web sites.

- If you don't have a computer, you can still access the Internet through libraries that offer this service.

To Learn More

The Myositis Association (TMA).

Resources. Available from: www.myositis.org/jmbookresources.cfm.
   Links to helpful information and Internet sites, including support organizations, clinical trial information, and more.

National Institute of Arthritis and Musculoskeletal and Skin Diseases (NIAMS), National Institutes of Health (NIH).

How to Find Medical Information. Available at: www.niams.nih.gov/hi/topics/howto/howto.htm.
   Information on where to find reliable medical information both on and off the Internet.

National Institutes of Health (NIH).

PubMed Central. Available at: www.pubmedcentral.nih.gov.
   Free archive of biomedical and life science journal articles.

National Library of Medicine, NIH.

   MedlinePlus. Available at: www.medlineplus.com or www.nlm.nih.gov/medlineplus. Health topics, drug information, medical dictionary, and other resources.

   PubMed. Available at: www.pubmed.gov or www.ncbi.nlm.nih.gov/entrez. Search engine for published medical abstracts and articles.

For more information on these organizations, see Myositis-Specific Organizations *and* Government Resources *in the Resource Appendix.*

Additional Information:

Wood MS. *Health Care Resources on the Internet: A Guide for Librarians and Health Care Consumers.* NY: Haworth Press Inc; 2000.

CHAPTER 39

How We Learn About Juvenile Myositis

Daniel J. Lovell, MD, MPH, and Frederick W. Miller, MD, PhD

In this chapter...

We describe how we learn about juvenile myositis (JM) through different types of research studies and how the findings lead to the development of new treatments for myositis. We will explain why it is important for children with myositis and their parents to participate in research studies in order to develop better treatments and, ultimately, to find a cure for JM. We will also provide you with some guidelines for what you should do and ask when you or your child is considering taking part in a clinical research study.

From the family's point of view...

"Our daughter was not doing well with her current treatments, so her doctor suggested I consider involving her in a research study to learn more about her JM and to obtain a second opinion. It was an invaluable learning experience. We both asked a lot of questions and learned much more about JM than we ever expected—the way JM develops, what may be involved in bringing on the illness, the specific problems she was having, and what other treatment options we had. I hope that all parents consider including their children in research studies. The study not only helped our daughter tremendously but made us realize that participating in research is the only way for us to move forward and hope to cure or prevent myositis from developing in the first place!"

Research is a lengthy process: It can take years to find out answers to questions. Because of the limitations of how research on humans can be conducted, usually a single research study is not enough to answer a question completely. So when a research study reports a result, more studies are done to try to confirm or disprove the findings. Sometimes the other studies may produce different results due to slightly different patients being studied or different study methods, so more research questions arise to study.

Because research reports are technical in nature, it can be difficult for parents and children with myositis to understand all of the terms and conclusions. Most of the time, when studies seem to reach different conclusions, it is not because one study is wrong but because of differences in the way the studies were performed. It is best when you read a research report to discuss it further with your child's myositis doctor or other healthcare professionals to understand better the contents and conclusions. More "user-friendly" publications specifically for patients, such as the newsletters from The Myositis Association and Cure JM Foundation, can be very helpful to keep you updated about new research findings on JM.

What Types of Research Help Us Learn More About Juvenile Myositis?

To understand illnesses such as JM and to develop better treatments, it is necessary for scientists, doctors, patients, and healthy volunteers to be involved in research. There are three categories of research: basic, clinical, and translational research. We will describe each category of research separately, but one of the most dramatic changes recently is the integration of the categories of research to understand diseases and treatments more quickly and thoroughly.

Basic research seeks to better understand how the body, cells, or molecules within the cells function. It is conducted in the laboratory, on particular types of cells, tissues, proteins, or genetic material (such as DNA or RNA). The focus of basic research is to better understand basic processes, such as how molecules, cells, or tissues perform a particular function or how they relate to other tissues, not necessarily to develop new treatments or to understand any particular disease better.

Examples of basic research include trying to understand better what things influence the development of the muscles in growing animals or the effect that poor blood flow has on muscle function. An example of basic research in autoimmune diseases is the study of substances in the body that increase inflammation, such as tumor necrosis factor alpha (TNF-α) (see *Chapter 15, New Therapies on the Horizon*).

Clinical research involves human beings. Clinical research can be divided into two categories: observational and interventional.

Observational studies include studies in which data are collected from or about humans, but a new experimental treatment is not involved. Observational studies include studies that seek answers to questions such as, How often does JM occur? and, Is the frequency of JM higher or lower in certain groups, such as boys versus girls or blacks versus whites? Observational studies also describe the types of symptoms or complications patients may develop with a disease or group of diseases (such as JM) and how doctors can identify and treat them. Much of the information presented in this book, particularly about the characteristics of JM patients, is the result of observational studies.

It's also important to understand better whether there are particular traits or events that increase the risk of developing JM. The term for the type of research that systematically studies the nature and causes of a condition in a specific group of people or a population is "epidemiology." Epidemiologic studies help us better understand the extent and scope of the illness, which then allows us to design better clinical research studies. For example, epidemiologic studies have determined that certain forms of myositis are more common in girls and that in children there is a much greater frequency of dermatomyositis than other forms of myositis. This type of research can also show that certain patients are at greater risk for certain complications of JM or its treatment. Epidemiology studies also help in defining the genes and the factors from the surroundings or environment that may be important in explaining why certain children develop JM.

Another type of observational study is called a "natural history study" (also called "outcome" study). Natural history refers to the change of a disease over time in a given individual or a group of individuals. These studies are focused on the long-term clinical evolution and outcomes of JM. Natural history studies often look at the outcome of patients five, ten, fifteen, or twenty years after the beginning of the myositis to better understand how these illnesses affect individuals on a long-term basis.

An interesting fact to remember about these types of studies is that since our treatment of an illness often changes over time, the outcome of patients who began their treatment over ten years ago might not be the same as the outcome that will occur in patients who are just developing the illness today—particularly if our treatments are more effective, which we hope they are.

The third type of research is translational research, which is one of the newest and most exciting areas of research because it combines basic research and clinical research. Examples of *translational research* include studies that take products that have been shown to be important in basic research and put them into human studies, such as studies of the effect of blocking TNF-α in humans. Translational studies can take blood or tissues from humans and test them in the laboratory: for example, a study might place samples of blood or particular cells from children with JM in cultures of healthy tissue or animal models to see the effect the sample from the child with JM has on the functioning of the tissue culture or animal model. Translational research helps us to understand what is going wrong in the pathways or processes of JM (see *Chapter 3, The Pathways to Juvenile Myositis*). From the use of translational research to understand the illness process better, new blood and imaging tests have been developed to follow your child's recovery over time (see *Chapter 10, Charting Your Child's Progress*) and new treatments to be tested have been identified (see *Chapter 15, New Therapies on the Horizon*).

How Are New Treatments Tested?

The types of research described above are focused on understanding an illness; another form of research is focused on studying the treatment of an illness. These studies are called clinical trials, therapeutic trials, or interventional studies.

This type of research looks at whether a new treatment is effective and safe for people with JM or other illnesses. New treatments are not just drugs; they can also include biologic therapies, medical devices, activity or exercise programs, dietary supplements, and complementary therapies (also commonly called alternative therapies).

A drug is a chemical compound intended to diagnose, treat, cure, or prevent a disease by affecting the structure or function of the body. Examples of drugs used in the treatment of myositis include corticosteroids and methotrexate (see *Chapter 7, Treatment Possibilities in the Beginning* and *Chapter 12, Possible Medicines During the Course*).

A biologic therapy is a product, like globulin or antigen, made by cells in the body or in the laboratory, used to prevent, treat, or cure disease. These products are usually large proteins that are designed to mimic closely the structure of a particular protein in the body. Most biologic therapies are designed to have a specific effect, such as bind to a certain receptor or protein on the cells or tissues in the body (see *Chapter 15, New Therapies on the Horizon*).

A medical device is an instrument, machine, implant, or reagent used in the laboratory to diagnose, cure, treat, or prevent disease. Examples of some medical devices used by health professionals to treat myositis include electrical stimulators of muscle contraction and splints used to improve joint motion.

A variety of exercise programs have been used to improve both the motion and strength in children with myositis and are discussed in *Chapter 13, Rehabilitation of the Child with Myositis*.

Another category of treatment is called complementary medicines. These are also commonly referred to as alternative medicines. This form of therapy consists of diverse medical and healthcare systems, practices, and products not presently considered part of conventional medicine. Complementary and alternative treatments for myositis are discussed in *Chapter 14, Complementary and Alternative Approaches to Juvenile Myositis*.

New treatments for myositis and other illnesses are developed by testing the drugs, biologic therapies, medical devices, or complementary and alternative therapies in clinical trials. In the United States, the Food and Drug Administration (FDA) oversees the design and conduct of these different clinical trials and grants licenses to make and sell drugs, biologic therapies, and medical devices to healthcare providers to treat subjects. Other countries have similar regulatory agencies that oversee the ethical conduct of research studies and the safety of these new treatments. It's important to know that before any new treatment is given to humans, extensive testing is done in the laboratory and in several species of animals. This testing in animals is done to determine the short-term and long-term effects of the new treatment as well as how useful the medicine might be, the best dose to use, how long the treatment might affect the body, and if the treatment causes birth defects, cancer, or other unacceptable side effects. However, tests in animals cannot predict with 100% accuracy what will happen when the same treatment is given to human beings, so clinical trials are generally done gradually, using very few people to start and increasing the number if the treatment looks promising. Clinical trials are divided into four stages called Phase 1, 2, 3, or 4 trials.

Phase 1 studies involve the first use of a particular treatment in human beings. Their primary goal is to establish initial safety and tolerance of the drug in the dose range expected to be needed in later clinical trials and to give some indication of what side effects might occur. Phase 1 trials might also find out how a medicine is metabolized and cleared by the body. This first exposure of the new drug or biologic agent in humans is usually done in a small number of healthy adult volunteers and in adult patients with the illness that the medication or biologic agent is intended to help.

If the results from Phase 1 studies suggest that the treatment is safe, then Phase 2 studies are performed to establish evidence of effectiveness of the treatment in humans with the specific illness for which the treatment is intended. These studies define the types, frequency, and extent of the benefit of the treatment so that later larger clinical studies will be most informative. Phase 2 studies often involve gradual increases in the dose of the study medication, either in the same patient or in different groups of patients. They can range from small to moderate in size (for example, as few as five to as many as two hundred study subjects). Phase 2 studies are usually conducted on adult patients, but if the FDA has licensed the treatment for another disease, then Phase 2 studies can also be done on children.

In Phase 3 studies, the intent is to demonstrate that this new treatment is safe and effective in treating the disease being studied. These clinical trials must be scientifically well designed so that at the end of the study there will be a definite answer to the question of whether there is a true benefit from the new treatment compared with no treatment or compared with standard treatments. They also examine the safety of the treatment over a longer period of time (in rheumatic diseases, typically ranging from several months to two years). They often involve from one hundred to several thousand patients. Phase 3 studies are considered by the FDA to be the most critical for determining whether a new treatment will be approved and licensed for treating that illness. Usually, clinical trials will be started in children only after the drug or biologic agent has either been approved by the FDA for use in adults (licensed) or when Phase 3 studies are in process or completed and the treatment looks like a promising new therapy. This is so that children are not exposed to an agent that might not be safe or effective. Occasionally, important new therapies are tested in children during phase 2 studies, particularly if the treatment is known to be safe or for illnesses in which few or no effective treatments currently exist.

Phase 4 studies are called surveillance studies, and these studies are done after the FDA approves an agent for prescription use in a particular illness. The focus of these studies is to define more clearly the safety of treatments when they are used in combination with other standard treatments and in patients who might not have been eligible to participate in earlier trials. The other goal of Phase 4 studies is to include very large numbers of patients who are followed up for long periods of time to better understand rare complications or late complications from new treatments.

One way that clinical trials determine whether a treatment works is to compare the new treatment to a placebo. A placebo looks, smells, or tastes just like the new treatment, but the placebo does not have any ingredients that would cause the same change in a person as the treatment being tested, so the placebo is an inactive or ineffective treatment. In Phase 2 and 3 studies, some patients are given a placebo so that the researchers can statistically compare the treatment with the placebo and reliably determine what effects the new treatment has (good and bad) in human beings. It is necessary to include patients treated with a placebo in studies in order to see the real benefits and side effects of a new treatment in the study population. For example, in some studies of children with arthritis, up to 40% of the patients who are given the placebo show significant benefit over a six to twelve month period. In this case, any new treatment would need to be effective in over 40% of the children to show that the new treatment was better than the placebo. In most trials that use a placebo, neither the healthcare providers nor the patients are told who was given the placebo and who received the new treatment. This way, they continue to give all patients equal care and do not become biased. This is called a "double-blind" study. Commonly, these studies are performed in subjects who have not responded to standard therapies.

As important as it is to develop new, truly effective treatments, it's also important that your child's doctor does not prescribe treatments that only *seem* to be effective based on unclear studies. The most reliable way to eliminate the use of only seemingly effective therapies and to identify truly effective therapies is to perform well designed clinical trials. It is important to perform scientific evaluations of new treatments, including clinical trials, before they gain general acceptance into the standard treatment plan. Most studies that use a placebo are done when it is truly not clear who is better off—those who receive a placebo and standard therapy or those who receive standard therapy plus the new treatment. New study designs for clinical trials have been developed that limit as much as possible the time and number of individuals who receive placebo treatments. In addition, most clinical trials are designed so that all study subjects, including those who have received the placebo, are offered the opportunity to continue to receive the new treatment after the experimental portion of the clinical trial is finished, if it was truly effective.

Whenever possible, the FDA applies special regulations for testing new treatments in children (the "Pediatric Rules") that allow for smaller focused studies that limit or avoid placebo testing. These rules generally require that the disease in children be similar to the one in adults, in which the new treatment has been tested extensively, and that the results of clinical trials in adults demonstrate both acceptable effectiveness and safety.

Many drugs that have been used for years or decades to treat certain illnesses have never been tested against a placebo. Their effectiveness is based on accumulated experience that may or may not give true and accurate information about the actual clinical benefit of the treatment for a particular illness or patient. Of the drugs used to treat patients with JM, only prednisone is currently licensed by the FDA for use in myositis. Very few clinical trials have been conducted in myositis patients, and almost all of them have used adult subjects, not children. It is through this experience in adult patients and some observational studies in children with myositis that the drug treatments for JM have been developed (see *Chapter 12, Possible Medicines During the Course*). Therefore, it is important to support research into all forms of myositis since findings from one form are often applicable to other forms.

How Are Patients Protected When They Enroll in Research Studies or Clinical Trials?

Several agencies are responsible for protecting human subjects who are enrolled in observational studies or clinical trials. The National Institutes of Health (NIH) and private foundations, including The Myositis Association and Cure JM Foundation, fund many of the clinical research studies performed in persons with myositis. Before these studies can be done, they are reviewed by independent experts who critically assess their scientific importance and reliability. These same experts review study designs to make sure they follow all rules established by the NIH and other agencies to protect the safety of the human subjects involved in any type of clinical research supported by the NIH. Government agencies and local groups of experts at each hospital or medical center also evaluate clinical studies to ensure that they meet established standards for ensuring the safety of the subjects. No clinical research project will be given funding, no matter how important the scientific information might be, if there are concerns about inappropriate or incomplete care or questions about the safety of the human subjects involved.

Many clinical trials funded by the NIH and drug companies have a specific oversight committee, which reviews the data from that project in an ongoing fashion to determine whether the study should be stopped or altered in any way because of unexpected or excessive negative effects on the patients involved. These oversight committees are often called "Data Monitoring Committees." They can stop or alter the study to protect the safety of the subjects if there seems to be a problem or if there does not seem to be any evidence of benefit from the new treatment.

If researchers are trying to get FDA approval for a drug, biologic agent, medical device, or complementary or alternative therapy, that study is reviewed by the FDA, both before it starts and throughout the study. The FDA, before it approves even a Phase 1 study in humans, requires and reviews many basic research studies of the treatment's effects in cells or tissues and in animals. Only if these results suggest that the treatment is potentially safe and not likely to harm humans will it permit Phase 1 studies to be performed. The FDA reviews, in an ongoing fashion, the results of all studies in all phases. Only after it is satisfied that the Phase 1, 2, and 3 studies demonstrate that a treatment is effective and that the benefit for patients is much greater than the potential for side effects caused by the new treatment will it approve the drug or biologic agent to be licensed for the disease on which it is being tested. Once the FDA licenses the agent, doctors can then prescribe it to treat that disease.

In addition, at each university or hospital that performs a clinical research study involving patients or healthy volunteers, the study must be approved by a committee called the institutional review board (IRB). These IRBs are required to follow guidelines from the federal government. Each IRB reviews studies based on strict rules. The purposes of the IRB are to make sure that any study involving human beings performed at its institution is done in the most appropriate way to ensure safety, that useful information will result from the study, that the patients' rights and privacy are protected, and that the study is conducted in an ethical manner. In addition, if there are serious problems observed during the course of a clinical trial, such as intolerance to or side effects from the treatment, then the IRBs require that those problems be reported not only to them but also to all other healthcare providers involved in the study and to the FDA. If the problem is one that might change a patient's desire to continue to participate in a study or to start a study, then the IRBs require that this information be shared with all current and potential study subjects. In addition, the IRB oversees the writing of the consent form that all study subjects must understand and sign before they begin participation in the study. The IRB must make sure that this consent form describes in a complete, accurate, and easily understood fashion the activities involved in participating in the research, the potential side effects, and the potential benefit of participation in a research study. Only after both the study and the consent form are approved by the IRB can the researchers enroll subjects in the study.

What Should I Consider Before Having My Child Participate in Clinical Research or a Clinical Trial?

Before you or your child participates in a clinical study and before any aspect of a clinical study is done on you or your child, you should have the doctor or researcher explain the study to you very thoroughly. All of your questions should be answered, and you should feel that you fully understand what will be done during the study, including the potential benefits, potential risks, and the potential cost to you or your insurance company for participating in that study. Only after you have had all of those questions answered adequately should you sign the consent form. Moreover, no part of the study should be started before you have signed the consent form. Participation in any research study is fully voluntary. You have the right to determine whether you or your child will participate in a study, and you have the right to withdraw from a study at any time without being penalized in any way. Doctors and other personnel who are involved in the study are expected not to have any financial or other ties to the organization that is funding the study that might impair their ability to provide a fair and accurate assessment of the effects of the study treatment (for a clinical trial). Any person who has such close personal or financial ties to an institution is said to have a "conflict of interest" and should not be a participant in that particular study. As a potential study participant, you have the right to ask whether any study personnel has a conflict of interest. You also have the right to ask more general questions about the relationship of personnel involved in the study with the sponsor of the study.

Specific questions we suggest parents and children ask before participating in a clinical trial are shown in Table 39.1.

Table 39.1. Questions to ask before participating in a clinical study.

1. What is the purpose of the study?
2. How long will the study last?
3. What does the study require in number of visits, blood tests, and other types of tests?
4. How often and how long are the study visits?
5. Will we be paid for our travel and other expenses (for example, food or hotel costs) related to participating in the study?
6. What are the possible benefits for my child in participating in the trial?
7. What are the possible risks, and how likely are those risks to happen to my child if she participates in the trial?
8. If this is a new treatment, has it been used in children before? If so, how was it tolerated?
9. If the study involves a new treatment, how is it given?
10. What is the chance my child will receive a placebo (inactive treatment)?
11. If my child gets worse during the study, what will happen?
12. If my child improves with the new treatment, will she have to stop it at the end of the study, or will it be available for my child to continue the treatment?
13. If my child is in the study, what part of the medical visits and care will be paid by the study, and what will my insurance or I have to pay?
14. How will participation in the study affect my child's being treated by her other doctors and the use of other medicines, such as antibiotics or over-the-counter medicines?
15. What will happen if my child gets sick or injured from being in the study?

Modified from the American College of Rheumatology web site at http://www.rheumatology.org/public/factsheets/clinical_new.asp.

What Are the Potential Benefits and Disadvantages of Participation in Clinical Research?

There is little risk in participating in observational studies. All patients, current and future, can potentially benefit from the results of an observational study, namely, increased understanding of the illness process, manifestations, or outcomes. If a new method of assessing a particular problem is being tried out, you should ask whether there are any potential complications or side effects from your child undergoing examination by this new procedure or testing method.

Clinical trials can benefit the participant by:
- Allowing access to a new treatment long before it is available to the general public
- Getting certain examinations and laboratory tests free of charge and having the illness followed up very closely
- Providing compensation (in some cases) for travel and other expenses for participation in the trial
- Most importantly, determining whether new treatments are or are not helpful for individuals with the particular illness in question

The potential disadvantages of participating in a clinical trial include:
- The fact that in some trials study subjects are required to stop some of their treatments before they can begin the trial
- The potential for being treated for a period of time with a placebo instead of the active treatment
- The visits to the clinic are usually more frequent
- Generally, more laboratory tests, including blood tests, are done. In addition, in Phase 1 trials, there is often incomplete understanding of the type and frequency of side effects.

Summary

Many types of research are necessary to advance our understanding of all aspects of illnesses in humans, including their treatment. It is only through research that we have been able to make the advances that are used every day to improve the lives of children with myositis. Because of the increasing sophistication of basic and translational research findings, a new understanding of the possible causes of JM, the subtypes of JM, and how we can predict who will need more treatments is being developed. New treatments are also being developed in a much more focused and scientifically informed fashion than they have been in the past. The only way that we can determine whether these newly designed therapies are safe and effective in children with myositis, however, is to do time-consuming and expensive clinical trials in patients with JM and other forms of myositis. These new treatments, coupled with improved ways to conduct the research studies, as well as international collaborations to standardize clinical studies in myositis, should encourage all children affected by myositis and their parents that more effective and safer therapies will be developed in the near future. To stay updated regarding this rapidly advancing field, please see the resources at the end of this chapter.

Key Points

■ To make progress in understanding JM and developing new treatments, it is necessary for scientists, healthcare providers, patients, families, and healthy volunteers to participate in research.

■ Basic research in cells and tissues and in animals is needed to define how the body works in health and in illness and how a treatment might change the body.

■ Clinical research involving patients is needed to determine the nature of illnesses, how they progress over time, and what treatments work best in which patients.

■ Many agencies ensure that clinical trials are performed as safely, efficiently, and ethically as possible.

To Learn More

The Myositis Association (TMA).

Clinical Trials. Available from: www.myositis.org/jmbookresources.cfm.
　　List of ongoing research studies and clinical trials.

Published Research. Available from: www.myositis.org/jmbookresources.cfm.
　　List of published research articles on myositis.

TMA Research Grants and Fellowships. Available from: www.myositis.org/jmbook resources.cfm.
　　List of research projects TMA has funded.

American College of Rheumatology (ACR).

Research. Available at: www.rheumatology.org/research/index.asp?aud=mem.
　　Listing of research information for patients with adult and juvenile myositis and other autoimmune or rheumatic diseases.

Clinical Trials and Registries. Available at: www.rheumatology.org/research/other/ research.asp.
　　Information about clinical trials for patients.

Clinicaltrials.gov, a service of the National Institutes of Health (NIH). Available at: www.clinicaltrials.gov.

Regularly updated information on federally and privately supported clinical research in human volunteers.

The Computer Retrieval of Information on Scientific Projects (CRISP), National Institutes of Health (NIH) and U.S. Department of Health and Human Services. Available at: http://crisp.cit.nih.gov.

Searchable database of federally funded biomedical research projects at universities and other organizations.

Cure JM Foundation.

Research. Available from: www.curejm.com.
　　Foundation established to raise funds for research into JM.

For additional information, see the Resource Appendix.

Specific Research Organizations:

American College of Rheumatology (ACR) Working Group for Juvenile Myositis.

This Juvenile Myositis Group, made up of pediatric rheumatologists, meets annually to exchange information about JM research studies that are open for enrollment and any preliminary results from these studies; fosters collaborative research on JM throughout the United States, Canada, and Europe. Chair: Bianca A. Lang, MD, FRCPC.

International Myositis Assessment and Clinical Studies Group (IMACS). Office of Clinical Research, National Institute of Environmental Health Sciences (NIEHS), National Institutes of Health (NIH), 10 Center Drive, CRC, Room 4-2332, MSC 1301, Bethesda MD 20892-1301; Internet: https://dir-apps.niehs.nih.gov/imacs/home.htm.

A coalition of healthcare providers and researchers with experience and interest in all forms of myositis. Aims to discover better therapies through clinical and basic research by developing consensus and standards on the conduct and reporting of adult and juvenile myositis studies, performing collaborative therapeutic trials, and planning, facilitating, and conducting international collaborative myositis research. Internet site houses a listing of collaborative studies being conducted by IMACS members, assessment tools, educational materials, and meeting presentations for its membership. Families may access some of these materials for educational purposes. Coordinators: Lisa G. Rider, MD; Frederick W. Miller, MD, PhD; and David A. Isenberg, MD, FRCP.

Paediatric Rheumatology International Trials Organisation (PRINTO). IRCCS Istituto G. Gaslini, Divisione di Pediatria II—Printo, Largo Gaslini, 5, 16147 Genova Italy; Phone: 0039-010-38-28-54; Internet: www.printo.it or www.pediatric-rheumatology.printo.it; Email: printo@ospedale-gaslini.ge.it.

Facilitates the standardization, development, and reporting of controlled clinical trials and to study new therapeutic approaches for the treatment of rheumatic diseases. Web site lists available abstracts, papers, and ongoing projects, calling for participation from physicians who see children with juvenile rheumatic conditions. Composed of academic, clinical centres actively engaged in the research/clinical care of children with pediatric rheumatic diseases. Main focus is to study new therapeutic approaches for the treatment of these diseases. Coordinators: Nicolino Ruperto, MD, MPH, and Alberto Martini, MD, Prof., Divisione di Pediatria II.

Childhood Arthritis and Rheumatology Research Alliance (CARRA). Department of Pediatrics, 300 Pasteur Drive Room G310, Stanford CA 94305-5208; Phone: 650-724-7117; Internet: www.carragroup.info; Email: carrainfo@stanford.edu.

National organization of pediatric rheumatologists interested in research in childhood rheumatic diseases; fosters, facilitates, and conducts high-quality clinical research in the field of pediatric rheumatology by creating a multi-center network of pediatric rheumatology research centers across North America, increasing the number of children who participate in studies and reducing the time it takes researchers to reach valuable conclusions.

Network for Juvenile Dermatomyositis. A working group of the Paediatric Rheumatology European Society (PRES). Juvenile Dermatomyositis Research Centre, Institute of Child Health—University College London, 30 Guilford Street, London WC1N 1EH UK; Phone: 44-0-20-7905-2667; Internet: www.pres.org.uk; Email: info@pres.org.uk or c.pilkington@ich.ucl.ac.uk.

Consists of centers undertaking research and/or clinical work in juvenile dermatomyositis and other juvenile idiopathic inflammatory myopathies; facilitates collaborative research in these areas and provides a forum for discussion, information sharing, problem solving, and presentation of research proposals. Chair: Clarissa M. Pilkington, MD.

CHAPTER 40

How You Can Help: Raising Awareness and Funds for Research

Harriet Bollar; Patience H. White, MD, MA; Marco Herrera; and Bob Goldberg

In this chapter...

We provide information about how you can be your child's best advocate by helping to educate others about juvenile myositis (JM), to influence legislation, or to raise money for research.

From a child's point of view...

"The first annual Myositis Awareness Day was held on my birthday, September 21, 2001. I wanted to do something special to help other kids who also have JM. I decided I would ask for donations to organizations supporting JM instead of presents for my birthday. That first year, I raised $369! The following year, I raised about $300. In 2003 my mom printed out the invitations on the computer, but they didn't say that I wanted donations for JM instead of presents. She didn't expect me to want to do it again, but I insisted. I plan to ask for donations every year for my birthday until there's a cure. I don't want any other children to have to go through this, and this is one small way that I can help make sure that a cure is found."

From a parent's point of view...

"After a year of watching our son battle JM with such strength, courage, and fortitude, we decided it was time for us to turn our time worrying into action. With other families, we started a nonprofit foundation to increase public awareness and raise money for a cure. We have found it very helpful to become activists. It gives us a sense of control over a disease that is so unpredictable. It provides us with a positive outlet for our fears and our frustrations. It allows us to meet other families affected by JM and share our stories, our concerns,

> *and our triumphs. As parents of a child with JM, we should do everything we can within our power to help find the cure. If not us, then who?"*

> "Never doubt that a small group of thoughtful, committed citizens can change the world. Indeed, it is the only thing that ever has."
>
> ® by Margaret Mead (Courtesy of the Institute for Intercultural Studies, Inc., New York)

What Is Advocacy?

Through advocacy, you can change the world, one person at a time! An advocate is an informed spokesperson who fosters, protects, educates, and raises awareness on a given issue. Advocacy is perhaps the most effective way to bring about change. Every little bit of advocacy helps on many different levels.

Sharing information about JM with others, such as your child's teacher, principal, and school nurse, is a form of advocacy that can help your child now and other children with JM in the future. For example, you can use the information in this book to prepare fact sheets to give to teachers, family members, and friends to help them better understand JM. This is advocacy on a personal level, and if enough of us practice it every day we can foster a better understanding of this rare condition and its effects on our children.

How Can I Be an Advocate?

Depending on where in the disease course your child is and how much time you have, you can consider becoming an advocate for myositis at any of the following levels: personal, local, state, or national (Table 40.1). Use your own creativity to find a way to advocate that inspires you. You will be more successful by advocating for something you are passionate about and are committed to. You can address many advocacy issues with the aid of organizations that represent JM, such as The Myositis Association and Cure JM Foundation.

How Can Organizations Help You Become an Effective Advocate?

Although you may be new to advocacy, there are organizations combating JM with advocacy experience. Joining forces with them can make your efforts more effective than trying to do it alone, and working with others can be very rewarding. Through such organizations, you can make contact with other families with whom you can share information and ideas about how to advocate together effectively.

By working with these organizations you can increase public awareness in many ways, such as obtaining a proclamation from your state government to declare September 21 *Myositis Awareness Day*, which has been done in many states.

Myositis Awareness Day is a special day set aside to honor myositis patients and their families and to raise awareness about this rare condition. It was first established by families of myositis patients in Massachusetts and was recently recognized by the U.S. House of Representatives through a proclamation of National Myositis Awareness Day. It is a time for the families and friends of myositis patients to get together for fundraising events and to educate others. For more information about this special day and how you can help celebrate it, contact The Myositis Association.

Tips to Help You Be an Effective Advocate

Join forces with others through nonprofit organizations that represent JM patients. Focus on areas you are passionate about. Are you concerned about more access to specialists in your area, research funding, better access to schools, or

Table 40.1. Types of advocacy.

Personal Advocacy

- Help your child with juvenile myositis (JM) prepare an information sheet for friends, classmates, and teammates. You could use information from this book or The Myositis Association and Cure JM Foundation web sites.

- Become a member of existing myositis advocacy organizations. Connect with other parents through these organizations' Internet discussion boards and through their family support networks.

Raising Awareness of JM Locally

- Sponsor a booth at a health fair.

- Write an article for your local newspaper.

- Get involved locally to raise funds for organizations that sponsor juvenile myositis research, such as The Myositis Association and Cure JM Foundation.

- Get your employer to provide Flex Time for employees to make it easier to go to doctors' appointments.

Getting Your State Involved

- Propose to your state legislature that September 21 be proclaimed *Myositis Awareness Day*.

- Work with organizations and coalitions to influence legislators to get what you need or want (such as more funding for research, better facilities for people with disabilities, and better insurance coverage).

National Advocacy

- Work with organizations and coalitions to present your ideas to your federal representatives and senators.

- Work with lobbying groups to educate your congressional representatives about the importance of funding more basic and clinical research for myositis.

better insurance coverage? Do you want to educate the public about myositis, or do you want to focus on raising awareness in the medical community?

Learn as much as you can about JM, including the status of healthcare and care facilities for children with myositis. It would also be helpful to learn additional facts, such as the economic impact of the disease, cost of healthcare, current status and needs for research, access to education, and availability of drugs for children. As you become more aware, you will be able to deliver a powerful message to others.

Try to understand the audience you will be addressing as best you can, and present things in a manner that is most appropriate for them. Try to explain things in a simple manner that can be understood by everyone.

A successful advocate focuses on the long term and realizes that timing is critical. An issue that is not passed in one legislative year may pass the following year, as current events change how people perceive issues. Bills that are not passed need to be reintroduced each legislative session because bills are not carried over from one session to the next.

Never pass up an opportunity to tell others about JM.

How Can I Help Effect Change?

When your child is diagnosed with a condition such as JM, it often sparks a desire to bring about change in a certain area, such as research funding, medical care, education, or assistance for those with special needs. First, you must identify the areas you most want to change. Those areas are the ones in which you think or say, "It shouldn't be this way." Observe what you complain about the most and start there. Next, envision how it would look in an "ideal world," where your complaint would be "cured." What would have to shift, change, or be transformed to get the situation from where it is to where you want it to be? A good technique is to work backward from the desired outcome. For example, if you wanted to start a discussion group of parents who informed each other about the latest scientific findings on JM, imagine that you have the group together and that it is running smoothly. List all the things that would be involved, such as how often and where you would meet. How would the members find the scientific studies (on the Internet, in the library)? Who would run the meetings? Who could members contact if they didn't understand some of the science? And finally, who would you call and invite to join the group?

If you seek to make changes at the national level, this will require the ability to influence legislation. Patients and their families can influence policy at the state and federal levels by acting in unison and through nonprofit patient-based organizations formed to represent their interests, such as The Myositis Association and Cure JM Foundation. Because nonprofit organizations are prohibited from making financial contributions to campaigns of elected officials, their power and ability to influence legislators lie in the organizations' ability to bring together large numbers of patients and their families in order to make their collective voices heard. Patient organizations have done this effectively by forming coalitions (a combination of advocacy groups) and collaborating with each other through such groups as the American Autoimmune Related Diseases Association (AARDA).

It is often through collaboration and coalitions that patient groups are most successful. When new, promising medical advancements, such as stem cell research, have come along, patient groups have joined forces to form coalitions, such as the Coalition for the Advancement of Medical Research (CAMR) to advocate for appropriate funding and for the necessary regulatory environment to allow these new technologies to prosper.

As in any volunteer organization, patients and their families are crucial components of an effective grassroots advocacy network. Parents and families of children with JM can be advocates any time by taking advantage of every opportunity to share their stories and to educate others about the physical, emotional, and financial hardships that a diagnosis of JM brings into their lives. When you're part of an advocacy group, you can turn your despair and feelings of helplessness into the glue that binds you together and gives you the strength to help others, as well as yourself. No one can influence legislators more than the people who are hardest hit because most decisions are made on the basis of an emotional response rather than a rational one. When children are involved, this creates undeniable strength and often touches the hearts of legislators who are parents themselves.

Raising Money for Research

There is a great need for more research into the causes of JM and to find better treatments for these rare diseases. Research studies are very expensive, and although the government funds some research, it only selects a few studies to fund. Families and friends of patients can have a huge impact on the progress that is made by raising money for JM research. Participating in fundraising events can be very satisfying and is a way to do something positive to help your child and all children with JM. There are many ways to raise money for research, and one of the first steps you can take is to contact a nonprofit organization, such as The Myositis Association or Cure JM Foundation, and get information about how to organize fundraising events in your area.

Fundraisers are very effective when it comes to educating the community and raising awareness about JM. It is important to get other people involved. Invite family members and friends to help with these events. It is a way for them to show their support and to do something positive for people they care about. Such events are also very encouraging to children who are ill, showing them they are not alone and that everyone is making an effort to improve the situation. They are also a lot of fun!

The money you raise and donate to nonprofit organizations that fund JM research is then provided to scientists (such as many of the authors of this book) who apply for grants to conduct studies to find out about the causes of and possible treatments for myositis.

Here are some of the things you can do to raise money for research:

- Organize special events in your community, such as golf tournaments, walk-a-thons, dinner dances, garage sales, lawn mower races, and even old-fashioned lemonade stands. Small events may not seem worthwhile, but every dollar counts.

- Letter-writing campaigns to friends and associates, in which you tell your story and ask them to remember JM when they make charitable contributions, can raise considerable amounts of money and educate others about JM.

- Find out whether your employer has an employee matching gift program or accepts requests to distribute a portion of their yearly charitable contributions to organizations that are of special interest to their employees.

- Join forces with others through campaigns such as WAMO! (Working Against Myositis for Others). WAMO! is a program of The Myositis Association that recognizes volunteers in communities across the nation working to raise awareness and further understanding about myositis through local campaigns and events. Because people who have myositis often don't have the strength or energy to play a leadership role, The Myositis Association seeks the help of those who don't have the disease but are concerned and care deeply about those who do.

- Join Team JM, which is a volunteer group of the Cure JM Foundation. Families dealing with JM join together to raise awareness about juvenile myositis and funds for research. Everyone is welcome to participate, including patients and siblings.

Key Points

- Advocacy is one of the most effective ways to bring about change.

- You can be an advocate at any level, from personal to national.

- Patients and their families are crucial components of an effective advocacy network.

- Working with other families through an association that represents myositis patients can increase the probability of successfully bringing about change.

- Patients, families, and friends can be effective fundraisers and instrumental in educating others about juvenile myositis by organizing community events.

To Learn More

The Myositis Association (TMA), 1233 20th Street NW, Suite 402, Washington DC 20036; Phone: 202-887-0088 or 800-821-7356; Internet: www.myositis.org; Email: tma@myositis.org.

> Visit the "Juvenile Myositis," "Advocacy," "Newsroom," or "How to help" pages for more information.

Cure JM Foundation, 836 Lynwood Drive, Encinitas CA 92024; Phone: 760-214-4004; Internet: www.curejm.com; Email: info@curejm.com.

> Visit the "Fundraising," "Join Team JM," and "News Stories" pages for more information.

Glossary of Terms

Active myositis: When your child has clinical signs of weakness or rash or when the laboratory tests indicate that inflammation is still present. This is sometimes referred to as disease activity.

Activities of daily living: Tasks done in the course of the day considered essential for normal life, such as eating, bathing, going to the bathroom, walking. These everyday activities are part of your child's function and may be assessed by the healthcare team.

Adaptive physical education: Modified physical education classes for children with myositis. Often your child can even do her physical therapy exercises as part of adaptive physical education.

Alanine aminotransferase (ALT, also called SGPT): A protein found in many tissues, including muscle, which is often used to screen for liver problems. When involved tissues, such as muscle, are inflamed, the levels of this protein often increase in the blood.

Aldolase: A substance found in several tissues, especially in muscle and liver. When the muscle is inflamed, the contents of the muscle cells (including aldolase) can enter the blood. As more muscle injury occurs, the amount of aldolase in the blood increases.

Antibody: A protein made by your child's immune system that recognizes bacteria and viruses and other structures outside her body.

Antinuclear antibody (ANA): A protein or antibody produced by the immune system that binds to the nucleus of certain cells. The ANA is the most common autoantibody in patients with juvenile myositis.

Arthralgia: Pain in a joint.

Arthritis: Inflammation of joints, which may result in swelling, stiffness, limitation of motion, or pain.

Aspartate aminotransferase (AST, also called SGOT): A protein found in many tissues, including muscle and liver. When the muscle is inflamed, the levels of this protein increase in the blood.

Aspiration pneumonia: Infection in your lungs caused by breathing bits of food or liquid into your lungs.

Atrophy: Thinning or wasting away, as in muscle.

Autoantibody: A type of antibody made by your child's immune system that recognizes specific parts on the surface or inside of cells in her own body. Many autoantibodies recognize all cells, not just muscle cells.

Autoimmune disorder: A condition in which the immune system, which normally protects the body by attacking infections and other harmful exposures, does not work right and attacks part of your own body instead.

Autoimmunity: The presence of autoantibodies (proteins) or immune cells that recognize normal, healthy cells or tissues.

441

Avascular necrosis: A condition that cuts off the blood supply to the bone, causing part of it to die.

Axial: On an axis. Axial muscle groups include the muscles controlling the trunk, such as abdominals and those controlling the head.

Biologic agent: Product, like globulin or antigen, made by cells in the body or in the laboratory, used to prevent or treat disease. Often the product is directed against a specific target in the body or may replace a certain protein or provide cells to the body. A complementary and alternative biologic agent differs in that it uses substances found in nature that have biological activity to affect the body's function and symptoms; these do not prevent or treat disease.

Biopsy: Removal of a piece of tissue from the body to study its structure under the microscope. In children with juvenile myositis, a muscle or skin biopsy can help to define your child's condition.

Calcinosis: A condition in which hard lumps or sheets of calcium form under the skin and in the connective tissue.

Cataract: Clouding of a portion of the lens of the eye, sometimes resulting in blurred vision. Some children who receive corticosteroids develop a cataract.

Childhood Health Assessment Questionnaire (CHAQ): This questionnaire helps the healthcare team learn how the child with myositis actually functions in everyday life activities.

Childhood Myositis Assessment Scale (CMAS): A series of tests that evaluate muscle strength and endurance.

Chronic: Persisting for a long time.

Compression fracture: A loss of bone height, which can result in collapse and is caused by low bone calcium. It usually occurs in the spine, but it can occur in other places, such as the hip. It is often capable of being repaired with appropriate treatment for bone density and inflammation.

Contracture: Limited joint movement resulting from muscle weakness or inflammation in the connective tissue. Also, shortening of muscles and tendons, causing a joint to stay bent and not extend fully, or to stiffen in one position. The presence of calcinosis crossing joints may also result in contractures.

Corticosteroid: Also referred to as steroid, glucocorticoid, or prednisone therapy. An anti-inflammatory hormone made by the body. It is produced synthetically as a medication to treat severe inflammation or swelling.

Creatine kinase (CK): A protein found in muscle that is important for generating a quick source of energy for muscle. When muscles are inflamed or injured, CK spills into the bloodstream, so a higher amount in blood tests shows ongoing muscle inflammation. Also known as CPK.

Cushingoid: Side effects of a high dose of corticosteroid medication, including puffy "moon" face, weight gain, brittle bones, thin skin, and muscle weakness.

Cytokine: A protein made by one type of cell in the immune system that has effects on other immune cells; sometimes thought of as hormones of the immune system.

Dermatologist: Type of doctor who treats skin disorders, like the rash of juvenile dermatomyositis.

Dermatomyositis: An illness involving skin and muscle inflammation, which results in longstanding rash and muscle weakness. Adult dermatomyositis starts after age eighteen years.

Diabetes: A disease in which sugars in the body are not processed normally because of a defect in insulin metabolism. This leads to elevated blood sugar levels, frequent urination, and other problems if it is not controlled. Two different types can occur in juvenile myositis: in one, the body is not responding properly to the level of insulin. In another, the child also develops the autoimmune form (Type I diabetes).

Diagnosis: Identification of a specific illness or disease.

Dietician: A nutritional specialist.

Disease activity: The problems in the illness that are the direct result of the ongoing myositis and its associated inflammation. For your child myositis disease activity may include things like muscle weakness, elevated blood levels of muscle enzymes, skin rashes, arthritis, and/or a number of other active problems from the myositis.

Disease course: Development and duration of the illness. Change in the illness over time.

Disease damage: Long-lasting changes that are not caused by current inflammation. These changes are the result of previous disease activity or long-term side effects of the medicines used to treat juvenile myositis.

Distal: Furthest from the center of the body, below the elbows or knees. For muscle groups, this includes finger and hand muscles.

Dysphagia: Problems with swallowing; trouble moving food or liquid from your mouth to your stomach. Dysphagia can occur in any of the four stages of swallowing.

Dysphonia: Difficulty speaking because of problems in the voice box or tongue weakness. Dysphonia often leads to a weakened or abnormal voice.

Dyspnea: Difficulty breathing, or shortness of breath.

Electromyogram (EMG): A test that checks the electrical activity of muscles and the pattern of electrical activity. It is sometimes used to help confirm a diagnosis of juvenile myositis.

Endocrinologist: A doctor who specializes in the diseases of organs that make hormones. Endocrinologists take care of children with juvenile myositis who have problems such as growth abnormalities, developmental and other hormonal imbalance problems, thyroid disease, high blood lipids, diabetes, or lipodystrophy.

Endurance: The ability to engage in physical activity for a sustained period of time.

Environmental exposures/factors: Things in your surroundings that you come in contact with and that may play a part in what happens to you. These factors may include viruses, ultraviolet light from the sun, and toxins.

Erythema: Redness of the skin caused by inflammation.

Esophageal dysmotility: Difficulty in swallowing caused by problems with the esophagus.

Esophagus: Swallowing tube that passes food from the pharynx (back of the mouth) to the stomach.

Extra-muscular: Outside the muscles.

Factor VIII-related antigen (or von Willebrand factor antigen): A protein found on blood vessels that gets released into the bloodstream when the vessels are inflamed or injured. Some doctors test for this antigen to follow the progress of juvenile dermatomyositis.

Fatigue: Physical tiredness that is common in children with myositis. The muscles, when inflamed, can become fatigued easily.

Fibrosis: Scarring of a tissue resulting in damage.

First-line treatment: Medicine or treatment doctors try as the first therapy for your condition.

Flare: A return or increase of problems from increased myositis activity.

Flow cytometry: A blood test available at certain medical centers in which the number of different types of white blood cells is counted. Some doctors use parts of this test to see if your child's dermatomyositis is active and requires treatment.

Gastroenterologist: A doctor who diagnoses and treats diseases of the digestive tract (stomach and intestines).

Gastrointestinal (GI): Involving the digestive system. This can include the esophagus (swallowing tube), stomach, or intestines.

Gene: Inherited material inside your body's cells that give directions for your body to work as it should. Genes are made of DNA.

Generic drug: A medicine identical to a brand-name medicine but sold at a lower cost to the patient. Generic drugs have different names than brand-name medicines.

Gottron's papules: Red and raised or rough scaly patches present over the top of the joints, such as knuckles, elbows, knees, insides of the ankles, or even over the toe joints.

Heliotrope rash: Purple or red color over the upper eyelids. This may have associated eyelid swelling. Named after the color of the heliotrope flower.

Hyperlipidemia: Higher-than-normal blood levels of fats (lipids).

Idiopathic inflammatory myopathies: Medical term used to describe the group of illnesses where there is muscle inflammation and weakness with no known cause. Idiopathic means arising from an unknown cause; myopathy is a disorder of the muscle.

Immune response: The body's reaction to substances or antigens.

Immune system: A system of the body that normally protects you against infection but can cause problems in autoimmune diseases.

Immunosuppression: Treatments that alter your child's immune system and decrease the ability to fight infections or respond properly to vaccinations.

Immunosuppressive: Having the ability to slow down or suppress the immune system; an immunosuppressive drug is known as an immunosuppressant. Immunosuppressants lower the body's ability to fight off infection.

Inclusion-body myositis: A form of myositis involving slowly progressing weakness affecting distal muscles (hands and feet) and thigh muscles. This condition is rare in children.

Individualized Education Plan (IEP): A plan developed by a school to set educational goals and provide special services and adaptations for students who have special needs.

Inflammation: A condition characterized by redness, pain, or swelling where immune cells enter affected tissues. This can be caused by the body's response to an infection or injury or by an autoimmune response.

Infusion: Giving a solution through a vein.

Insulin: A hormone produced by the pancreas that aids in transport of sugar (glucose) to the muscles. Insulin resistance, which some children with juvenile myositis develop, is a condition in which the pancreas pumps extra insulin into the blood to try to keep the blood levels of glucose normal and steady.

Interstitial lung disease: Inflammation of the lung that sometimes causes scarring, making it harder for oxygen to get from the lung into the blood. This is uncommon in children with myositis.

Intravenous: Method of administering medicine through a needle directly into your vein.

Juvenile dermatomyositis (JDM): An illness involving skin and muscle inflammation, which results in rash and muscle weakness. Juvenile dermatomyositis first occurs before eighteen years of age.

Juvenile myositis (JM): A group of illnesses involving muscle inflammation and weakness that has onset during childhood. Juvenile dermatomyositis is the most common form of myositis in children.

Juvenile polymyositis (JPM): An illness involving muscle inflammation resulting in muscle weakness but without the characteristic rashes of juvenile dermatomyositis. Juvenile polymyositis has onset in children less than eighteen years of age.

Lactate dehydrogenase (LDH, LD): A protein found in many tissues including muscle. When muscle is inflamed, the levels of this protein increase in the blood.

Licensure/drug labeling: A process by which the Food and Drug Administration determines that a drug is safe and effective for a particular disease.

Lipid: A fat found in the blood. Lipids that may be checked in your child's blood include cholesterol and triglycerides.

Lipodystrophy: Loss of body fat tissue.

Lymphocytes: Specialized cells of the immune system that normally help protect against infection. In autoimmune conditions these cells can be involved in the illness process. There are two types of lymphocytes involved in myositis: B lymphocytes, which produce antibodies and autoantibodies, and T lymphocytes, which help in response to viral infection or may be overactive in autoimmune conditions such as myositis.

Magnetic resonance imaging (MRI): A method of creating an image of internal organs, including the muscles, which is done using a strong magnet and without the use of radiation. In muscle MRI, the STIR or T2-weighted images can see water or inflammation in the muscles. T1-weighted images see the muscle thinning and any scarring or fatty infiltration into the muscles.

Malar rash: A facial rash that covers the cheeks and bridge of the nose in a butterfly shape. This is often seen in children with juvenile dermatomyositis and systemic lupus erythematosus.

Manual muscle testing: A physical test used to measure muscle strength.

Mixed connective tissue disease: A condition with clinical signs of two or more of the following diseases: juvenile arthritis, systemic lupus erythematosus, juvenile myositis, or scleroderma. If a person has mixed connective tissue disease, he or she will have high levels of anti-RNP autoantibodies in his or her blood.

Muscle enzymes: Proteins found in the muscle tissue that can leak into the blood when the muscle is inflamed or injured. See also creatine kinase, aldolase, lactate dehydrogenase, alanine aminotransferase, and aspartate aminotransferase.

Muscle mass: Muscle bulk.

Muscle strength: How much force the muscles can move in a defined position. In juvenile myositis, the muscles are weak initially because of muscle inflammation. Later, loss of strength may be due to the muscles becoming thin (atrophied) or scarred.

Myalgia: Muscle pain.

Myopathy: Disease of muscle.

Myositis: A group of illnesses in which inflammation of muscle often results in general muscle weakness or discomfort.

Myositis-associated autoantibodies: Autoantibodies (proteins) present in myositis patients and in those with other autoimmune diseases.

Myositis-specific autoantibodies: Autoantibodies (proteins) seen only in myositis patients. Examples include anti-Jo1 and other t-RNA synthetases, anti-signal recognition particle, and anti-Mi-2.

Nailfold capillaries: The capillaries that form loops at the base of the fingernail. In juvenile dermatomyositis, these blood vessels become enlarged, distorted in shape, and may drop out. This symptom reflects the small blood vessel or capillary involvement that is also present in the muscle, skin, and other tissues. Some doctors examine these to follow your child's progress.

Neurologist: A physician who specializes in the diagnosis and treatment of disorders of the neuromuscular system.

Occupational therapist: A trained health professional who offers advice on how to plan and organize activities. They make splints, recommend assistive devices, and educate you in energy conservation and joint protection.

Occupational therapy: Treatment of a physical condition, such as juvenile myositis, using exercise, adaptive equipment, splinting, and energy conservation strategies.

Ophthalmologist: A physician who specializes in the diagnosis and treatment of diseases affecting the eye.

Orphan disease: A rare disease, defined in the United States for purposes of drug licensing policy as a disease diagnosed in fewer than 200,000 total persons. All forms of myositis are orphan diseases.

Osteoporosis: A condition that leads to thinning and weakening of the bones.

Overlap myositis: Myositis that occurs along with other autoimmune disorders or which may develop into another autoimmune disease.

Pathologist: A doctor who looks at changes in body tissues and fluids caused by different conditions.

Pediatric neurologist: A doctor who specializes in the care of children and adolescents with disorders of the neuromuscular system.

Pediatric rheumatologist: A doctor who specializes in the care of children and adolescents with rheumatic conditions.

Photoprotection: Protection from the sun.

Photosensitivity: Abnormal reaction of the skin to sunlight.

Physiatrist: A doctor who specializes in helping patients overcome the loss of physical abilities. Physiatrists supervise the rehabilitation team, develop initial goals and treatment plans, and monitor the treatment program.

Physical function: The ability of the muscles to do work. Function is usually decreased in those with juvenile myositis. Physical function measures may check on muscle endurance (the ability to sustain activities over time) and fatigue, as well as the ability to perform everyday life activities.

Physical therapist: A trained health professional who assesses mobility and gait patterns, joint range of motion, biomechanical integrity of joints, muscle strength, and pain. The physical therapist also recommends exercise programs, appropriate assistive devices, proper shoes for walking, heat treatments, and patient/family education.

Physical therapy: Also physiotherapy; treatment of a disease or condition using physical methods, including exercises, administration of heat or cold, and massage. These treatments are prescribed or administered by the physical therapist.

Polymyositis (PM): Chronic muscle inflammation causing muscle weakness, without the characteristic rashes of dermatomyositis. Adult polymyositis has onset after eighteen years of age.

Proximal: Toward the center of the body. Examples of proximal muscles are quadriceps (thigh) and biceps (upper arm).

Psoriasis: A common chronic skin condition in which red scaly patches form on the elbows, knees, scalp, and other body parts. It is often itchy. Some children with juvenile myositis develop psoriasis. Sometimes the rashes of juvenile dermatomyositis can be confused with psoriasis.

Psychiatrist: A physician who specializes in the treatment of mental or emotional disorders.

Psychologist: A health professional, usually a PhD, who specializes in evaluating mental abilities and providing appropriate treatment.

Puberty: The development of the child's sexual maturity.

Pulmonary: Involving the lungs.

Pulmonary function tests (PFTs): Breathing tests designed to measure the health and efficiency of the lungs. By having your child take a deep breath in and then out, the lung volumes can be examined. Part of this test, called DLCO, examines how the oxygen moves from the air tubes into the bloodstream.

Pulmonologist: A specialist who evaluates and treats lung, voice, and breathing problems.

Pulse therapy: Higher doses of medicine given over a short period of time through a needle in the vein. Sometimes corticosteroids are given as pulse therapy for juvenile myositis.

Range of motion (ROM) exercises: Type of exercise to keep flexibility and movement in joints. Stretching exercises are one type of range of motion exercise.

Refractory: Resistant or unresponsive to treatment.

Relapse: Return of symptoms after a period of remission or no disease activity. Also known as recurrence.

Remission: Absence of active myositis. Period of time when the patient shows no symptoms of the illness and is able to come off all medicines to treat myositis.

Respiratory: Relating to the lungs and breathing.

Rheumatic disease: Diseases involving joints, tendons, muscles, ligaments, and associated structures. Juvenile myositis is a rheumatic disease.

Rheumatologist: A doctor who specializes in diagnosis and treatment of rheumatic diseases.

Scleroderma (systemic sclerosis): A rare disease that affects the skin, other connective tissues, and sometimes other parts of the body, which causes a thickening and contraction of the affected areas.

Second-line drugs: Medicines chosen after symptoms do not improve after using first-line medicines.

Side effect: An unwanted reaction to a drug or treatment.

Sign: A finding of an illness or condition that is recognized on a physical examination performed by a health professional.

Social worker: A professional who refers people to resources and services to help them get the care and assistance they need.

Speech-language pathologist: A professional trained to diagnose and recommend treatment for problems of swallowing. Speech-language pathologists are trained to conduct certain tests to diagnose the specific reason for swallowing difficulties and will work with a dietician to plan the most appropriate diet for your child and consult with your child's physician and nurse for medical aspects of treatment.

Steroid myopathy: Muscle weakness resulting from corticosteroid treatment.

Strengthening exercises: Exercises prescribed by healthcare professionals with the goal of strengthening the muscles. Several different types of strengthening exercises are done in a graded way, as your child's strength improves.

Swallow study: Also known as a modified barium swallow study. In this test, various foods are coated with barium, or barium of varying textures is swallowed. Then X-rays or videotapes are taken to see how food passes from the mouth to the stomach.

Symmetrical: Affecting both sides of the body equally, e.g., weakness in both arms or both legs.

Symptom: Problems that a child experiences relating to an illness or condition.

Systemic: Affecting the whole body, not just a single area.

Systemic lupus erythematosus (SLE or lupus): An autoimmune disease that causes inflammation in many parts of the body, including the skin, joints, and sometimes internal organs.

Therapy: Treatment of a disorder through medicines, rehabilitation, and physical exercises, and/or other approaches.

Topical treatments: Medicine applied to the skin, such as steroids and tacrolimus, to treat the skin rashes of dermatomyositis.

Tumor necrosis factor (TNF) alpha (TNF-α): A protein, called a cytokine, produced by several kinds of cells, including inflammatory cells, that promotes inflammation. It is an important cytokine in the pathway contributing to some autoimmune diseases, including myositis.

Ulcer (also called an ulceration): A break in the surface of the skin or intestines that usually extends into deeper tissues, often due to blood vessel inflammation. Can be a sign of serious illness that requires intense therapy.

Vasculitis: Inflammation of the blood vessels. When it occurs under the skin, it can cause a visible rash.

Vasculopathy: Diseases associated with blood vessels.

von Willebrand factor antigen: See Factor VIII-related antigen on page 443.

Resource Appendix

Editors: Kathryn A. Spooner; Harriet Bollar; Clarissa M. Pilkington, MBBS

Contributors: Anne M. Connolly, MD; Peter B. Dent, MD; Laurie Ebner-Lyon, RN, APN.C.; Richard S. Finkel, MD; Adam M. Huber, MSc, MD; Ann Kunkel, BS; Carol B. Lindsley, MD; Barbara E. Ostrov, MD; Angelo Ravelli, MD; Nicolino Ruperto, MD, MPH; Jane G. Schaller, MD; Lori S. Wiener, DCSW, PhD; and Susan J. Wright, OT

In this appendix...

We provide a list of resources for possible services and support available to families, children, and other people impacted by the lives of children with juvenile myositis (JM). Many organizations relate to JM in general, whereas others specifically relate to a particular topic or chapter. Some organizations serve people around the world; some work mainly with those children and families located in a certain country or region. Check at the end of each chapter for more resources specific to the subject matter within that chapter.

This appendix is divided into six sections:

1. **Myositis-Specific Organizations** (page 449)

2. **Other Support Organizations** (page 451)

3. **Finding a Doctor or Specialist** (page 453)

4. **Books and Online Diaries** (page 458)

5. **Government Resources** (page 458)

6. **Resources for Children and Family Support** (page 459)

Myositis-Specific Organizations

The Myositis Association (TMA).

1233 20th Street NW, Suite 402, Washington DC 20036; Phone: 800-821-7356; Internet: www.myositis.org; Email: tma@myositis.org.

The Myositis Association is the only group in the United States solely dedicated to those suffering from all forms of the inflammatory myopathies. Its mission is to find a cure for the inflammatory and other myopathies, while serving those affected by these diseases. TMA is a nonprofit, 501(c)3 organization.

TMA realizes this mission through its many programs and services for adults and children with myositis, along with their families and friends. TMA focuses much attention on the JM community with uniquely designed programs to meet its special needs, challenges, and concerns. JM children and families can join the worldwide support group of families, along with regional groups that foster face-to-face meetings; participate in the JM-specific online message boards, allowing families to communicate with other families through a single message; become a part of the e-pals program for children to communicate with others close to their age; and connect with families at regional and annual conferences, with programs geared toward those affected by JM.

TMA publishes a quarterly newsletter, the *OutLook*, as well as the *JM Companion*, specifically for families affected by childhood forms of myositis, with special *Just for Me* pages for kids. Physicians and healthcare professionals receive the *Myositis Monitor*, an electronic publication with the latest research news and treatment updates, and other outreach materials. The Association provides written and online information to share with friends, doctors, or others interested in learning more; online bulletin boards for sharing ideas, suggestions, and encouragement; scholarships for children to attend summer camps; updates on current research and clinical trials; and more. TMA funds substantial research for all forms of myositis, with grant and fellowship monies earmarked for deserving JM studies.

The TMA Medical Advisory Board and Board of Directors include representatives from the JM community.

Cure JM Foundation.

836 Lynwood Drive, Encinitas CA 92024; Phone: 760-487-1079; Internet: www.curejm.com; Email: info@curejm.com.

The Cure JM Foundation is an all-volunteer, nonprofit 501(c)3 organization established by families of JM patients to promote awareness of and to find a cure for this rare disease. It is the only organization dedicated solely to children afflicted by JM, and their families.

The Cure JM web site offers helpful hints for parents, research information, photos of symptoms and treatment side effects, informal peer support, and a host of other resources for families of children suffering from JM.

Cure JM manages Team JM, a nationwide network of grassroots volunteers. Open to anyone with a passion to find a cure for JM, Team JM works locally and regionally to raise money for research while promoting community awareness of this disease. The Cure JM Foundation also supports those who want to organize a local event, to benefit JM research, by providing information, support from Team JM leaders, and free brochures, posters, and promotional items.

In addition to Team JM, the foundation also sponsors the Cure JM Family Support Network. This informal peer support group gives parents and other family members of children suffering from JM the ability to share their experiences and support each other. The Family Support Network offers a variety of resources for JM families, including regional support representatives, a "Bear Hugs" program for patients, and a Parent/Child network that matches parents and patients affected by JM with other families facing the same challenges.

The Myositis Support Group UK.

Les and Irene Oakley, 146 Newtown Road, Woolston, Southampton, Hampshire SO19 9HR UK; Phone: 023-80-449708; Internet: www.myositis.org.uk; Email: enquiries@myositis.org.uk.

The Myositis Support Group UK reaches out to those in the United Kingdom who suffer from all forms of myositis, including childhood forms. This group hosts a web site with information on the illnesses, links to other sites, a buddies list to find others in your area who also have myositis, a bulletin board, and more. They offer a free newsletter to all UK residents, either by mail or email, with a free email subscription to other people around the world.

Other Support Organizations

American Autoimmune Related Diseases Association (AARDA).

22100 Gratiot Avenue, E. Detroit MI 48021; Phone: 586-776-3900; Internet: www.aarda.org; Email: aarda@aol.com.

A national voluntary health agency and a member of the National Health Council (NHC) dedicated to eradicating all autoimmune diseases and alleviating the physical, emotional, and socio-economic suffering from these disorders. AARDA fosters collaboration in education, research, and patient services to better serve those affected by these conditions and sponsors physician conferences, research, legislative advocacy efforts, and a national awareness campaign.

American Juvenile Arthritis Organization (AJAO).

Arthritis Foundation (AF); P.O. Box 7669, Atlanta GA 30357-0669; Phone: 800-568-4045; Internet: www.arthritis.org/communities/juvenile_arthritis/about_ajao.asp.

Serves parents, health professionals, and young adults with myositis, arthritis, or other rheumatic disorders. Programs and services include an accessible web site with information on the illnesses they serve, including treatments, programs and national/local activities, newsletters, annual family conferences, support for summer camps throughout the country, and awareness, advocacy, and educational offerings throughout the year. Offers pamphlets on illnesses, medications, and specific topics like school issues, as well as training materials for parents and health professionals. Activities encourage those with rheumatic diseases to help each other through support groups, education, and initiating research efforts to find a cure.

Arthritis Foundation (AF).

P.O. Box 7669, Atlanta GA 30357-0669; Phone: 800-568-4045; Internet: www.arthritis.org.

Supports the more than one hundred types of arthritis and related conditions through advocacy efforts, programs and services, and research funding. Offers drug guides with information on medicines used to treat rheumatic conditions like myositis, along with other pamphlets focused on specific issues such as exercise and school. The American Juvenile Arthritis Organization (AJAO) is a council of the Arthritis Foundation, serving those with childhood rheumatic conditions and their families.

Easter Seals.

230 West Monroe Street, Suite 1800, Chicago IL 60606; Phone: 312-726-6200 (voice) or 800-221-6827; Internet: www.easterseals.com.

Services for people with disabilities and special needs, including summer camps, information on rehabilitation therapy, and equipment for those in need.

Muscular Dystrophy Association (MDA).

National Headquarters, 3300 E. Sunrise Drive, Tucson AZ 85718; Phone: 800-572-1717; Internet: www.mdausa.org; Email: mda@mdausa.org.

Publishes a bimonthly magazine, *Quest*, written for those affected by neuromuscular disease. Offers disease booklets and fact sheets through its web site for all diseases in its program, including myositis. This site allows patients to ask specific questions of an expert in the area. Information is available both in English and Spanish. Late-breaking news is available through email updates.

Medical services are available at many MDA clinics, which are located in most major and many other cities. Children up to age twenty-one may qualify for weeklong regional summer camps focused on children with neuromuscular conditions. Financing for adaptive equipment is available to those who qualify and have a doctor's prescription.

National Organization for Rare Disorders (NORD).

55 Kenosia Avenue, P.O. Box 1968, Danbury CT 06813-1968; Phone: 800-999-6673 (voice mail) or 203-797-9590; Internet: www.rarediseases.org; Email: orphan@ rarediseases.org.

Federation of voluntary health organizations helping those affected by rare "orphan" diseases, those disorders affecting fewer than two hundred thousand people in the United States, including JM. Committed to the identification, treatment, and cure of more than six thousand rare disorders through education, advocacy, research, and service. Provides an index of rare disorders, organizations, and support groups, along with information on medical assistance programs and other sources of assistance.

Paediatric Rheumatology International Trials Organisation (PRINTO).

IRCCS Istituto G. Gaslini, Divisione di Pediatria II—Printo, Largo Gaslini, 5, 16147 Genova Italy; Phone: 0039-010-38-28-54; Internet: www.printo.it or www.pediatric-rheumatology. printo.it; Email: printo@ospedale-gaslini.ge.it.

The Paediatric Rheumatology International Trials Organisation (PRINTO) is a non-governmental international network founded by Alberto Martini and Nicolino Ruperto in 1996. It initially included fourteen European countries (now forty-seven countries and more than two hundred centre worldwide), with the goal to foster, facilitate, and coordinate the development, conduct, analysis, and reporting of multi-centre international clinical trials, and/or outcome standardisation studies in children with paediatric rheumatic diseases. More information about PRINTO can be found at its web site.

With regard to juvenile myositis, PRINTO has developed a specific web site directed to families and health professionals (www.pediatric-rheumatology.printo.it) that contains three main sections. The first section gives families an up-to-date description on the characteristics of fifteen paediatric rheumatic diseases, including juvenile dermatomyositis. The second section provides a list of paediatric rheumatology centres, and the third, the contact information for the family self-help associations. The web site is currently available in more than fifty languages and is visited by one hundred thousand people monthly (more than three thousand per day) from 130 different countries.

The Shriners Hospitals for Children.

Shriners International Headquarters, 2900 Rocky Point Drive, Tampa FL 33607-1460; Phone: 813-281-0300, 800-237-5055 (referrals in the U.S.) or 800-361-7256 (referrals in Canada); Internet: www.shrinershq.org.

A network of pediatric specialty hospitals where children under the age of eighteen receive medical care free of charge.

Arthritis Society [Canada].

National Office, 393 University Avenue, Suite 1700, Toronto ON M5G 1E6 Canada; Phone: 416-979-7228; Internet: www.arthritis.ca; Email: info@arthritis.ca.

Web site features information on different types of conditions, including arthritis, polymyositis, and dermatomyositis; tips for daily living; programs and services offered; and resources.

Muscular Dystrophy Canada.

2345 Yonge St, Suite 900, Toronto ON M4P 2E5 Canada; Phone: 866-MUSCLE-8; Internet: www.muscle.ca; Email: info@muscle.ca.

Aims to provide relevant and current information about many types of neuromuscular disorders in an easy-to-understand format. Publications cover topics such as causes, symptoms, and treatments for these disorders. Informational articles can be downloaded from its web site, which also features program details, news and events, and chapters throughout the country providing support and information.

The Muscular Dystrophy Campaign UK (MDC).

Head Office, 7-11 Prescott Place, London SW4 6BS UK; Phone: 020-7720-8055; Internet: www.muscular-dystrophy.org; Email: info@muscular-dystrophy.org.

UK-wide charity that endeavors to create a world where muscle disease is not a barrier to quality or length of life. Invests over £1.5 million every year into research with the aim of finding treatments, cures, and better management for muscular dystrophy and related conditions. Provides support through information services, fact sheets, specialist medical services, grants for assistive equipment, and more.

Muscular Dystrophy Australia.

GPO Box 9932, Melbourne 3001 Australia; Phone: 61-3-9320-9555; Internet: www.mda.org.au; Email: info@mda.org.au.

Web site offers information on National Camp MDA, week-long camps throughout Southeastern Australia supported by MDA for those affected by neuromuscular conditions, as well as general information on disorders, coping as a parent or child, and more.

Finding a Doctor or Specialist

This section lists organizations and professional associations that can help in your search for a physician or specialist. You will often see "find a doctor/specialist" on the home page of these organizations' web sites; specific addresses are given below. Typically, it is best to find a specialist who has experience treating children with juvenile myositis. Where one is not available, you may be able to find specialists with experience treating children with other autoimmune diseases or pediatric specialists in general (see Chapter 5, Finding Help).

This section is divided by specialty: Finding a juvenile myositis doctor; Finding a pediatrician or family doctor; Finding a rehabilitation specialist; Finding an eye care specialist; Finding an endocrinologist; and Finding a specialist for other complications.

Finding a Juvenile Myositis Doctor

American College of Rheumatology (ACR).

1800 Century Place, Suite 250, Atlanta GA 30345-4300; Phone: 404-633-3777; Internet: www.rheumatology.org.

Professional organization of rheumatologists and associated health professionals dedicated to healing, preventing disability, and curing the more than one hundred types of arthritis and related disabling and sometimes fatal disorders of the joints, muscles, and bones. Members include practicing physicians, research scientists, nurses, physical and occupational therapists, psychologists, and social workers.

Find a rheumatologist. Available at: www.rheumatology.org/directory/geo.asp?aud=pat. Search by location or name. Choose a state or country, and check the box for "Pediatric or Pediatric Rheumatology Board Certified."

American Academy of Neurology (AAN).

1080 Montreal Avenue, St. Paul MN 55116; Phone: 800-879-1960; Internet: www.aan.com; Email: memberservices@aan.com.

Provides valuable resources for medical specialists committed to improving the care of patients with neurological diseases. More than eighteen thousand members look to the AAN for the most comprehensive professional development, career enhancement, and practice improvement opportunities available.

Find a neurologist. Available at: www.aan.com/public/find.cfm. Check with individual doctors to determine which are pediatric specialists.

American Academy of Dermatology (AAD).

P.O. Box 4014, Schaumburg IL 60168-4014; Phone: 888-462-DERM; Internet: www.aad.org; Email: memsrv@aad.org.

Largest dermatologic association, with a membership of more than fourteen thousand physicians worldwide. Dermatologists are especially helpful in treating skin rashes of JDM. Select "Pediatric Dermatology" in specialities when searching.

Find a dermatologist. Available at: www.aad.org/public/searchderm.html.

Canadian Rheumatology Association (CRA).

912 Tegal Place, Newmarket, ON L3X 1L3 Canada; Phone: 905-952-0698; Internet: www.cra.ucalgary.ca; Email: eteixeir@ucalgary.ca.

Rheumalotogists Directory. Available at: www.cra.ucalgary.ca/cra1/public_sqldb/ search.htm. Search by name, city, province, or other criteria.

Paediatric Rheumatology European Society (PRES).

Children's Hospital University of Würzburg Josef-Schneider-Str. 2 97080 Würzburg Germany; Internet: www.pres.org.uk; Email: info@pres.org.uk.

List of Paediatric Rheumatology Centres within Europe. Available from: www.printo.it/ pediatric-rheumatology.

Finding a Pediatrician or Family Doctor

American Academy of Pediatrics (AAP).

National Headquarters, 141 Northwest Point Blvd, Elk Grove Village IL 60007-1098; Phone: 847-434-4000; Internet: www.aap.org; Email: kidsdocs@aap.org.

Organization of sixty thousand pediatricians committed to the attainment of optimal physical, mental, and social health and well-being for all infants, children, adolescents, and young adults.

Find a pediatrician. Available at: www.aap.org/referral.

American Academy of Family Physicians (AAFP).

11400 Tomahawk Creek Parkway, Leawood KS 66211-2672; Internet: www.aafp.org; Email: email@familydoctor.org.

One of the largest national medical organizations, representing more than ninety-four thousand family physicians, family medicine residents, and medical students nationwide.

Find a family doctor. Available at: http://familydoctor.org/cgi-bin/memdir.pl.

American Medical Association (AMA).

515 N. State Street, Chicago IL 60610; Phone: 800-621-8335: Internet: www.ama-assn.org.

Aims to be an essential part of the professional life of every physician and an essential force for progress in improving the nation's health.

Doctor Finder. Available at: http://dbapps.ama-assn.org/aps/amahg.htm.

Canadian Paediatric Society.

2305 St. Laurent Blvd, Ottawa ON K1G 4J8 Canada; Phone: 613-526-9397; Internet: www.caringforkids.cps.ca; Email: info@cps.ca.

> *Find a Doctor.* Available at: www.caringforkids.cps.ca/resources/finddoc.htm. Search for individual doctors or children's hospitals by province/territory.

National Health Service (NHS), United Kingdom.

Quarry House, Quarry Hill, Leeds LS2 7UE UK; or Richmond House, 79 Whitehall, London SW1A 2NS UK; Phone: 0113-254 5000 (Leeds) or 020 7210 4850 (London); Internet: www.nhs.uk; Email: dhmail@doh.gsi.gov.uk.

> *Find Your Local Doctor (England).* Available at: www.nhs.uk/england/doctors/default.aspx.

Finding a Rehabilitation Specialist

Physical Therapists

American Physical Therapy Association (APTA).

1111 North Fairfax Street, Alexandria VA 22314-1488; Phone: 800-999-2782, Internet: www.apta.org or www.pediatricapta.org (Section on Pediatrics); Email: pediatrics@apta.org.

> Professional organization representing more than sixty-three thousand members. Fosters advancements in physical therapy practice, research, and education. Provides families with general physical therapy information.

> *Find a pediatric PT in my area.* Available from: www.pediatricapta.org/cnsmr/index.cfm.

Canadian Physiotherapy Association (CPA).

2345 Yonge Street, Suite 410, Toronto ON M4P 2E5 Canada; Phone: 416-932-1888 or 800-387-8679; Internet: www.physiotherapy.ca.

> *Find a Physio.* Available at: www.physiotherapy.ca/findaphysio.htm.

United Kingdom Chartered Society of Physiotherapy (CSP).

14 Bedford Row, London WC1R 4ED UK; Phone: 011-020-7306-6666; Internet: www.csp.org.uk.

> Information about physiotherapy and therapists within the United Kingdom; the professional body for all physiotherapists within the UK.

> *Find a Private Physiotherapist.* Available at: www.csp.org.uk/director/physiotherapy explained/physio2u.cfm.

Occupational Therapists

American Occupational Therapy Association, Inc. (AOTA).

4720 Montgomery Lane, P.O. Box 31220, Bethesda MD 20824-1220; Phone: 301-652-2682 or 800-377-8555 (TDD); Internet: www.aota.org.

> Professional association of approximately thirty-five thousand occupational therapists, occupational therapy assistants, and students. Provides general occupational therapy information and information on pediatric therapists experienced in the care of children with rheumatologic conditions.

> *Finding an occupational therapist.* Available at: www.aota.org/featured/area6/links/LINK03.asp. Search by state occupational therapy associations.

Canadian Association of Occupational Therapists (CAOT).

CTTC Building, Suite 3400, 1125 Colonel By Dr, Ottawa ON K1S 5R1 Canada; Phone: 613-523-CAOT (2268) or 800-434-CAOT (2268); Internet: www.caot.ca or www.otworks.ca (Canada's Occupational Therapy Resource Site).

General information about physiotherapy in Canada, where it can be accessed, and possible costs.

OT Finder. Available at: www.otworks.ca/otfinder.cfm.

Physiatrists

American Academy of Physical Medicine and Rehabilitation.

One IBM Plaza, Suite 2500, Chicago IL 60611-3604; Phone: 312-464-9700; Internet: www.aapmr.org; Email: info@aapmr.org.

Find a PM&R Physician. Available at: www.e-aapmr.org/imis/imisonline/findphys/find.cfm.

Association of Academic Physiatrists.

National Office, 1106 N Charles Street, Suite 201, Baltimore MD 21201; Phone: 410-637-8300; Internet: www.physiatry.org; Email: aap@physiatry.org.

Promotes excellence in education, research, and the practice of physical medicine and rehabilitation within the academic arena. Physiatrists specialize in physical medicine and rehabilitation and often work with those having musculoskeletal conditions like myositis.

Find a Physiatrist. Available from: www.physiatry.org/field/index.html. Search by state or other countries.

Finding an Eye Care Specialist

American Academy of Ophthalmology.

P.O. Box 7424, San Francisco CA 94120-7424; Phone: 415-561-8500; Internet: www.aao.org; Email: aaoe@aao.org.

Find an ophthalmologist. Available at: www.aao.org/aao/find_eyemd.cfm.

American Optometric Association.

243 N. Lindbergh Blvd, 1st Floor, St. Louis MO 63141; Phone: 800-365-2219; Internet: www.aoa.org.

Dr. Locator. Available from: www.aoadrlocator.org.

Finding an Endocrinologist

American Association of Clinical Endocrinologists.

1000 Riverside Avenue, Suite 205, Jacksonville FL 32204; Phone: 904-353-7878; Internet: www.aace.com.

AACE Physician Finder. Available at: www.aace.com/resources/memsearch.php.

Hormone Foundation.

8401 Connecticut Avenue, Suite 900, Chevy Chase MD 20815-5817; Phone: 800-HORMONE; Internet: www.hormone.org.

Public education affiliate of the Endocrine Society.

Find an Endocrinologist. Available at: www.endo-society.org/apps/FindAnEndo/index.cfm.

Lawson Wilkins Pediatric Endocrine Society.

Internet: http://lwpes.org; Email: secretary@lwpes.org.

Find a doc. Available at: http://lwpes.org.

National Committee for Quality Assurance.

2000 L Street NW, Suite 500, Washington DC 20036; Phone: 202-955-3500; Internet: www.ncqa.org.

> *Physician Directory and Search.* Available at: http://recognition.ncqa.org. Select "Diabetes Physician Recognition Program."

Finding a Specialist for Other Complications

Gastroenterologists (Stomach)

American Gastroenterological Association.

4930 Del Ray Avenue, Bethesda MD 20814; Phone: 301-654-2055; Internet: www.gastro.org.

> *GI Locator Service.* Available at: https://secure.gastro.org/GILocator/locator.asp. Find a physician specializing in disorders of the digestive tract by U.S. state, Canadian province, or other country.

Swallowing Specialists

American Speech-Language-Hearing Association (ASHA).

10801 Rockville Pike, Rockville MD 20852; Phone: 800-638-8255; Internet: www.asha.org; Email: actioncenter@asha.org.

> Professional, scientific, and credentialing association for more than 115,000 audiologists, speech-language pathologists, and speech, language, and hearing scientists.
>
> *Find a professional.* Available at: www.asha.org/proserv. Search by city, state, zip code, country, age of patient, and/or language of practitioner.

American Gastroenterological Association. See *Gastroenterologists (Stomach).*

Specialists for Nutrition

American Dietetic Association (ADA).

120 South Riverside Plaza, Suite 2000, Chicago IL 60606-6995; Phone: 800-877-1600; Internet: www.eatright.org.

> *Find a Nutrition Professional.* Available at: www.eatright.org/cps/rde/xchg/ada/hs.xsl/home_4874_ENU_HTML.htm.

Voice

American Speech-Language-Hearing Association (ASHA). See *Swallowing Specialists.*

Voice Foundation.

1721 Pine Street, Philadelphia PA 19103; Phone: 215-735-7999; Internet: www.voicefoundation.org.

> World's leading organization dedicated to solving voice problems.
>
> *How to Find a Voice Physician.* Available at: www.voiceproblem.org/resources/howtofind.asp. Tips on finding a voice physician in your area.

American Academy of Otolaryngology and Head and Neck Surgery.

One Prince Street, Alexandria VA 22314-3357, Phone: 703-836-4444; Internet: www.entnet.org; Email: info@entnet.org.

> Information on ears, nose, throat, and related structures of the head and neck.
>
> *Find an otolaryngologist.* Available at: www.entnet.org/ent_otolaryngologist.cfm.

Books and Online Diaries

For more print and online books about juvenile myositis and related issues, visit The Myositis Association web site at www.myositis.org and the Cure JM web site at www.curejm.com. See also Chapter 9, Coping with Myositis As a Family, for books that might be helpful for every member of your family.

Julia's JDMS Diary, by Ralph Becker (father) with contributions from Julia.

Available from: www.ralphb.net/jdms. Online book created to chronicle the events surrounding one girl's diagnosis and treatment of juvenile dermatomyositis (JDM) and to give other children and their families in the same situation some much-needed information and support.

Fenton, J (ed). ***Living with Myositis: Facts Feelings and Future Hopes.*** London: Thoughtful Publications; 2003. [B]

With humor, compassion, and common sense, London dermatomyositis patient and TMA member Jenny Fenton wrote and edited this resource for everyone dealing with myositis.

Kilpatrick JR. ***Coping with a Myositis Disease.*** Athens (TX): Kilpatrick Publishing Company; 2000. [B]

The four types of myositis have individual case reports from patients with the diseases, telling how the disease affected them, their families, and their work.

Government Resources

Centers for Disease Control and Prevention (CDC).

Public Inquiries/MASO Mailstop F07, 1600 Clifton Road, Atlanta GA 30333; Phone: 800-311-3435; Internet: www.cdc.gov.

Recognized as a leading federal agency for protecting the health and safety of people at home and abroad, providing credible information to enhance health decisions, and promoting health through strong partnerships. Serves as the national focus for developing and applying disease prevention and control, environmental health, and health promotion and education activities designed to improve the health of the people of the United States.

National Institutes of Health (NIH).

9000 Rockville Pike, Bethesda MD 20892; Phone: 301-496-4000; Internet: www.nih.gov; Email: nihinfo@od.nih.gov.

Part of the U.S. Department of Health and Human Services (www.hhs.gov), NIH is one of the world's premier medical research centers and funding agencies. Strives to foster fundamental creative discoveries and research strategies; to develop, maintain, and renew scientific resources in order to prevent disease; to expand the knowledge base in medical and associated sciences; and to exemplify and promote the highest level of scientific integrity, public accountability, and social responsibility in the conduct of science. Responsible for directing and supporting federal research related to complementary and alternative therapies.

The different institutes and centers within NIH host web sites with current information on topics in their field of study; publications, information packages, and handouts on health topics; and more. Some that may be of special interest to those affected by JM are:

National Institute of Arthritis and Musculoskeletal and Skin Diseases (NIAMS). Office of Communications and Public Liaison, NIAMS, NIH, Bldg. 31, Room 4C02, 31 Center Drive—MSC 2350, Bethesda MD 20892-2350; Phone: 301-496-8190; Fax: 301-480-2814; Internet: www.niams.nih.gov; Email: niamsinfo@mail.nih.gov.

> For free publications and information packages: http://catalog.niams.nih.gov or 877-226-4267.

National Institute of Neurological Disorders and Stroke (NINDS). P.O. Box 5801, Bethesda MD 20824; Phone: 800-352-9424 or 301-496-5751; Internet: www.ninds.nih.gov.

> To request free mailed brochures: https://ice.iqsolutions.com/ninds/orderpubs.asp.

National Institute of Environmental Health Sciences (NIEHS): Internet: www.niehs.nih.gov.

National Eye Institute (NEI). Phone: 301-496-5248; Internet: www.nei.nih.gov; Email: 2020@nei.nih.gov.

NIH Clinical Center (CC). Internet: http://clinicalcenter.nih.gov.

National Institute of Allergy and Infectious Diseases (NIAID). Phone: 301-496-5717; Internet: www.niaid.nih.gov/publications (see Autoimmune Diseases).

The NIH National Center for Complementary and Alternative Medicines (NCCAM). NCCAM Clearinghouse, P.O. Box 7923, Gaithersburg MD 20898; Phone: 888-644-6226 or 301-519-3153; Internet: http://nccam.nih.gov/health/clearinghouse/index.htm; Email: info@nccam.nih.gov.

Office of Dietary Supplements at NIH (focuses on products that are marketed as dietary supplements). Phone: 301-435-2920; Internet: http://dietary-supplements.info.nih.gov; Email: ods@nih.gov.

Office of Rare Diseases. Internet: http://rarediseases.info.nih.gov.

U.S. Food and Drug Administration (FDA).

5600 Fishers Lane, Rockville MD 20857; Phone: 888-INFO-FDA (888-463-6332); Internet: www.fda.gov.

> Responsible for protecting the public health by ensuring the safety, efficacy, and security of human and veterinary drugs, biological products, medical devices, our nation's food supply, cosmetics, and products that emit radiation, including complementary and alternative medicines. Also responsible for advancing the public health by helping to speed innovations that make medicines and foods more effective, safer, and more affordable; and helping the public get the accurate, science-based information they need to use medicines and foods to improve their health.

Resources for Children and Family Support

Band-aides and Blackboards.

Fairfield University, Lehman College, Bronx NY 10468; Internet: www.lehman.cuny.edu/faculty/jfleitas/bandaides; Email: fleitas@optonline.net.

> Sections geared for parents, children, and teenagers to answer the question, "What's it like to have medical problems?" Developed by Joan Fleitas, EdD, RN, Associate Professor of Nursing at Fairfield University.

Give Kids the World (GKTW).

210 South Bass Road, Kissimmee FL 34746; Phone: 800-995-KIDS; Internet: www.gktw.com; Email: dream@gktw.org.

GKTW Village provides accommodations, event tickets, and meals for children whose requests have been answered by wish-granting organizations. Its site publishes a list of organizations from around the world that grant wishes for children with life-threatening or life-altering conditions.

Hugs and Hope.

P.O. Box 56, Harshaw WI 54529; Internet: www.hugsandhope.org; Email: sockinabox@aol.com.

A 501(c)3 charity dedicated to helping sick children by giving encouragement and sponsoring special projects. Provides support for parents via their support network.

KidsHealth, Nemours Foundation.

Internet: www.kidshealth.org.

Web site featuring in-depth articles, games, and resources for families, with different sections designed for parents, teens, and kids. Kids' pages offer recipes, games, and general information on specific conditions, how to cope with difficult situations, and more. Teens' section gives advice on dealing with social and emotional issues that face most teenagers and young adults.

Make-A-Wish Foundation.

3550 North Central Avenue, Suite 300, Phoenix AZ 85012-2127; Phone: 602-279-WISH (9474) or 800-722-WISH (9474); Internet: www.wish.org.

As its name suggests, the Foundation is a wish-granting organization, helping countless children with life-altering illnesses realize their dreams. Founded in 1980 to help one boy who dreamed of becoming a police officer, the Foundation has touched over 110,000 children worldwide. Through granting wishes, Make-A-Wish aims to change the lives of those whose lives have been impacted by chronic illness. Wishes can come true by referring a child and following a short process to determine eligibility, identify a wish, and create the wish for each child. The Foundation's mission is to "share the power of a wish" with every child possible.

Starbright World.

Starlight Starbright Children's Foundation, 1850 Sawtelle Blvd, Suite 450, Los Angeles CA 90025; Phone: 800-315-2580; Internet: www.starlight.org.

Starlight Starbright Children's Foundation is a nonprofit organization that aims to transform the lives of seriously ill children and their families through imaginative programs that educate, uplift their spirits, foster a sense of community, and help alleviate the pain and fear of prolonged illness.

Starbright World helps teens overcome isolation by providing an online community where they can meet peers from all over the country without ever leaving their beds. This interactive community, geared toward children seven to eighteen years of age, is a monitored, secure site where children can chat with other children in supervised chat rooms, learn more about their illnesses, instant message, post to bulletin boards, and create their own blogs.

Starlight Starbright's programs empower children to cope better with the social and emotional challenges they face daily, addressing such issues as pain, fear, loneliness, and depression. For more information, talk to the social worker, child life therapist, or recreation therapist at your medical center or visit Starlight Starbright online.

Index

Acanthosis nigricans 299
Activities of daily living 173, 174, 178, 354, 441
Adaptations (*see also Physical adaptations*)
  home safety 100
Adaptive physical education 185, 441
Alleles 35–36
Allergies 116
Amblyopia 316
American Academy of Pediatrics 328, 334, 362
Americans with Disabilities Act (ADA) 357, 380
Amyopathic dermatomyositis 17
Antibodies, myositis-associated (*see Autoantibodies*)
Antigen presenting cells 33
  B lymphocytes 33
  dendritic cells 33
  macrophages 33
Antigen reactive cells 33
  NK cells 33
  T cells 33
Arthritis 12, 16, 19–20, 32, 38, 46, 48, 50, 74, 78, 98, 116, 128, 130, 140, 146, 186, 321, 324, 428
  definition of 269, 441
  juvenile idiopathic 272
  juvenile rheumatoid 15, 37, 87, 88, 175, 207, 305
  small joint 101
Arthritis Foundation 380, 414, 416, 419
Arthropathy 269–274
  classification 269
  damage 272
  definition 269
  duration 272
  frequency 270–271
  in juvenile myositis 269
  onset 271
  pauciarticular 271
  polyarticular 271
  treatments 272

Aspiration 242
  silent 243
Assessments 127–137 (*see also Disease activity, Disease damage, and specific assessment tools listed throughout index*)
  assessing muscle strength, endurance, and function 139–149
    importance of 142
  core set measures 132
  definition of improvement (response criteria) 132
Asthma 116
Atherosclerosis 299
Atrophy
  definition 441
  muscle 19, 67, 128, 173, 181, 254
  skin 222
Autoantibodies 14, 18–19, 32, 211, 292, 323, 325, 441
  anti-Mi-2 18, 19, 37, 347
  anti-RNP 32, 324
  anti-SRP 18, 19, 32
  anti-synthetase 18, 19, 271, 272, 292, 347, 349
  myositis-associated 18–19, 72, 446
  myositis-specific 18–19, 72, 156, 271, 347, 349, 446
    more common in adults 20
Autoimmune disease 10, 17, 213, 322
  definition 1, 32, 441
  organ-specific 32
  systemic 15, 32, 447
Autoimmunity 10, 35, 441
Avascular necrosis 270, 273, 442

Biopsy 64, 68, 442
  muscle 69–71, 347
Breathing problems 291–295
  causes 291–293
  detecting 292–293

respiratory 37, 162, 286, 292, 294, 334, 447
treatment 293–294

Calcinosis 16, 20, 59, 128, 131, 136, 140, 186, 218, 231–240, 270, 299, 306, 323, 336, 343, 345–347, 367
  appearance 232
  causes 233
  circumscripta 232
  composition 235
  defined 231, 442
  detection of 233
  exoskeleton 232
  in polycyclic course 344
  planar 232
  reducing risk of 346
  treatment 236–237
    medications 237
    physical therapy 238
    surgery 238–239
  tumoral 232, 236
Calcium 28, 276, 278
Catheter 90
Celiac disease 17, 255, 322, 324
Centers for Disease Control and Prevention (CDC) 328, 337
Chicken pox 328, 332
  shingles 332
Childhood Health Assessment Questionnaire (CHAQ) 134, 142, 144, 146–147, 442
  modified version 147
  scoring 146
Childhood Myositis Assessment Scale (CMAS) 134, 142, 144–147, 442
  scoring 145
Chimerism 35–36
Clinical trials 426, 429–434
  benefits 432
  participation in 430
  patient protection 429–430
  Phase 1 studies 427
  Phase 2 studies 427

Phase 3 studies 427
Phase 4 studies 427
Complementary and alternative
    medicine (CAM) 191–207, 426
  acupuncture 192, 195
  biologic therapies 198–199
  definition of 191
  mind-body interventions 197
  naturopathic medicine 195
  regulations 195
  safety 196
  side effects 198
  traditional Chinese medicine 192
  uses 192
Compression fractures 103, 442
Computed tomography (CT) 66,
    233, 277, 293, 323
Contractures 176, 178, 188, 232,
    442
  hand 186
  joint 48, 136, 140, 179–180, 187,
    236, 270, 273
  preventing development of 174
  tendons 179
Coping 109–125
  child's perspective 115
  effect on family 118–119
  grieving process 109
  living with 121–125
  parent's perspective 110–115
    emotional difficulty 110
    financial burden 110
    reaction 110
  peer reaction 119–121
  separation or divorce 119
  sibling's perspective 115
Corticosteroids 60, 78, 86, 154,
    157, 173, 238, 242, 265, 278,
    281, 314–315, 324–325, 327,
    330, 333, 426
  administration of 79
    tapering 80
  definition of 78, 442
  dosage 310, 345
  effectiveness of 78–79, 87
  impact on nutrition 255–256
  intravenous 80, 82, 159, 294
    frequency of 81
    pulse therapy 79, 81, 86, 87,
      165, 234, 265, 294, 325, 345,
      447
  methylprednisolone 79, 159, 315
    dosage 81
  prednisolone 79

prednisone 27, 79, 85–86, 103–
    104, 153, 157, 159, 234, 271,
    273, 276, 301, 313, 315, 342,
    346, 366–367, 369, 371, 429
  dietary restrictions 118
  dosage 157
  taken during pregnancy 369
  reducing 161
  results 82
  side effects 83–84, 159, 161, 184,
    270, 315, 348
    acne 160
    cataracts 160, 442
    cushingoid 85, 442
    decreased protection from
      infection 84
    diabetes 160
    effect on appearance 115, 120,
      121
    effect on development 266
    effect on growth 262
    elevated blood pressure 84
    excessive body hair growth 160
    fluid retention 84
    gastrointestinal effects 86
    glaucoma 160, 317
    high blood pressure 160
    impact on growth 265
    impact on nutrition 256
    increased appetite 257, 259
    metallic taste 84
    mood swings 83, 86, 117
    osteoporosis 160
    skin problems 85
    steroid myopathy 160, 448
    thrush 255–256
    weight gain 85
  topical 90, 223, 334, 447
Coxsackievirus 36
Crohn's disease 32, 169
CT scan 68
Cure JM Foundation 6, 112, 380,
    414, 416, 419, 429, 436
  newsletter 424
  Team JM 440
  website 59
Cushingoid 85, 442
Cytokines 38, 442

Dental care 259
Dermatologists 222–223, 442
Dermatomyositis 26
  definition of 9, 442
  symptoms of 9

Development 265–267, 361–366
  alcohol and drug use 366
  delayed 266
    treatment for 266
  effect on development 266
  impact of thyroid function 267
Diabetes 15, 32, 50, 116, 299, 301,
    322, 325, 442
Digestive tract
  effect of anxiety 250
  medications 249
  parts of 241
  problems in myositis 242, 248
  tests for 249
    barium swallow 249, 448
    upper endoscopy 249
Disease activity 128, 160, 178, 181,
    443
  assessing 131, 132
Disease Activity Score 134, 210
Disease damage 128, 443
  assessing 131, 134
Dual X-ray absorptiometry (DXA)
    74, 136, 277–278, 310
Duchenne muscular dystrophy 36
Dysphagia 242, 243, 245, 443
Dysphonia 283, 287, 443

ECMO (extra corporeal membrane
    oxygenation) 82
Education for All Handicapped
    Children Act 379
Electromyography (EMG) 26, 64,
    68, 443
Endocrinologist 261, 266, 268, 297,
    300, 301, 303, 305, 309, 310,
    312, 443
Enzymes 13, 129, 445
  alanine aminotransferase (ALT)
    13, 441
  aldolase 13, 66, 129, 441
  aspartate aminotransferase (AST)
    13, 441
  creatine kinase (CK) 13, 19, 129,
    198, 442
  lactate dehydrogenase (LDH) 13,
    129, 445
Epidemiology 425
Exercises 24, 90, 102–103, 105,
    426 (see also Rehabilitation)
  breathing 293
  conditioning 182
  effect of JM on aerobic fitness
    148
  fitting into schedule 182

frequency of 183
location 185–186
  clinic and rehabilitation hospital 185
  home 185
  school 185
range of motion 178–180, 447
role of parents 184
side effects 184
strengthening 181–182
  isometric 181
  isotonic 181, 183
stretching 180
treatments 178
Eye exams 313
Eye problems 313–320
  cataracts (see side effects in Corticosteroids)
  glaucoma (see side effects in Corticosteroids)
  inflammation 314
  medications, side effects of 314

Family and Medical Leave Act 378
Fatigue 45, 129, 147, 173, 181, 183, 184, 186, 395, 405–406, 443
Feeding tube 247
Fibrosis 67, 168, 292, 444
Finding help 53–61
  finding the right doctor 54
  specialists, questions for 55–56, 58–59
Flare 12, 158, 243, 361, 444
  detection 131
  indicators 12
Food and Drug Administration (FDA) 196, 207, 391, 426–427
Fundraising 439

Gastroesophageal reflux disease (GERD) 245, 255, 257
Gastrointestinal 16, 45, 47, 49, 81, 87, 91, 164, 165, 167, 251, 257, 260, 277, 347, 348, 444
Gastroparesis 254, 257
Genes 10, 34–37, 347
  definition of 10, 444
Global activity assessment 134
Glucocorticoids (see Corticosteroids)
Gottron's papules 11, 13, 16, 44, 59, 217, 323, 444
Group A Streptococcus 36
Growth 262–268
  catch-up 262

growth hormone 262, 264
impact of juvenile myositis 262
monitoring 262

Hashimoto's thyroiditis 267
Health Insurance Portability and Accountability Act 378, 397
Heliotrope 11, 13, 16, 44, 217, 323, 444 (see also Rashes)
HIV 363–365
HMOs 54
Human Leukocyte Antigens (HLA) 34, 444
Hyperlipidemia 299, 309, 444
  detecting 299–300
  treatment 302

Idiopathic inflammatory myopathies 9, 444
IMACS 132, 134
Immunosuppressive therapy 334, 444
Individualized Education Plan (IEP) 185, 354, 396, 404, 444
  developing 396–400
Individuals with Disabilities Education Act 356, 380, 396
Infection 36–37, 335
  risk of 335
  reducing 336
Influenza 36, 336 (see also influenza in Vaccines)
Infusion 79, 86, 88, 159, 164–165, 167, 210, 211–213, 335, 444
Insulin 298, 325, 444
Insulin resistance 299, 307–308
  detecting 299–300
  treatment 301
Integrative medicine 192
Interferons 38
Internet 59, 100, 104, 221
  reliability of 420
  searching 419–422

Joint protection 189
Joints (see Arthritis, Arthropathy, Contractures)
Juvenile dermatomyositis (JDM) 1, 4, 10, 16, 32, 43, 78, 131, 141, 186, 210, 217, 231, 255, 264, 267, 305, 342, 368
  definition of 25, 445
  diagnosis of 48–49, 63

diagnostic criteria 63
mortality 348
outcomes 341–349
  chronic continuous course 344, 347
  monocyclic course 342–343, 347
  polycyclic course 343, 345, 347
  predicting 346
relapse 342, 447
sine myositis 17
treatment 346 (see also Corticosteroids, Medications)
Juvenile myositis (JM) 4–5, 16, 109
  advocacy 436
  age 10
  aspects of 2
  calf pain 102
  causes of 10, 37
  definition of 9–22, 25, 445
  diagnosis 12–13
  diagnostic criteria 63
  distinguishing from other illnesses 14
  effect on muscles 139–140
  environmental factors 37, 442
    infection (see Infection)
    silica 38
    ultraviolet light exposure 37
    virus 36–37
  explaining 23–29, 116
  identifying 14
  indicators of severity 156
  joints (see Arthropathy, Arthritis)
  laryngeal problems (see also Voice problems)
  less common forms 17
  mortality 48, 79
  not contagious 10, 31
  outcomes (see Outcomes)
    course of illness 60
  pathways to 31–41
  rarity 11–12
  role of inheritance in 34–36
  skin involvement 217–218 (see also Rashes)
  symptoms 11–12, 38–41, 43–51
    calcifications 48
    change in voice 48
    fever 48
    muscle aches and pains 43
    muscle weakness 11
    other 12
    rashes 11
    treating 12
    weakness 43–46

treatment goals 56
types of 16
understanding of 4
Juvenile polymyositis (JPM) 4, 10, 17–18, 44, 78, 212, 219
 definition 25, 445
 diagnosis of 49, 63
 outcomes 349 (see also Outcomes)
  chronic continuous course 349
  polycyclic course 349

Larynx 284 (see also Voice problems)
Legal protection 377–381, 396
Leptin 307
Lipodystrophy 16, 20, 234, 305–312
 causes 307
 definition of 305, 445
 detection 309
 generalized 306, 309
 partial 305
 problems 307
 treatment 310
Lupus erythematosus (see Systemic lupus erythematosus)
Lyme disease 336

Magnetic resonance imaging (MRI) 14, 25, 66, 73, 130, 233, 310, 445
Malabsorption 248
Manual Muscle Testing (MMT) 134, 142–143, 445
Medical insurance 383–389
 complaints 387
 health maintenance organizations (HMO) 384–385
 indemnity or fee for service 383
 Kidcare 385
 Medicaid 384, 391
 point of service (POS) 384–385
 preferred provider organization (PPO) 384
 state supported supplemental insurance (SSI) 385
Medications 24, 26, 77–93, 153–172, 272, 402
 acyclovir 332
 adjusting 157
 antiviral 333
 azathioprine 161, 166–167, 170, 366, 371

side effects 167
biologic agents 208, 210–211, 333, 442 (see also new therapies in Medications; Monoclonal antibodies)
bisphosphonates 280
 side effects 281
chloroquine 318
 side effects 318
combinations 170
corticosteroids (see Corticosteroids)
costs 390–393
cyclophosphamide 167–168, 170, 266, 294, 335, 372
 benefits 167
 side effects 167
cyclosporine 161, 165, 170, 301, 371
 benefits 165
 dosage 165
 side effects 166
diltiazem 237
 side effects 237
fenofibrate 311
following directions 27, 91
for treating calcinosis 237
gemfibrozil 311
hydroxychloroquine 87–88, 159, 161, 314, 317, 371
 administration 88
 side effects 89
injections 26
intravenous immune globulin (IVIG) 82, 87, 89, 161, 163–164
 benefits 164
 dosage 164
 side effects 164
mesna 168
metformin 301, 310
methotrexate 82, 87, 153–154, 159, 161–163, 170, 238, 325, 366, 371, 426
 administration of 88
 side effects 88, 162–163
mycophenolate mofetil 169, 170
 benefits 169
 dosage 169
 side effects 169
new therapies 207–215 (see also biologic agents in Medications; Monoclonal antibodies)
 anti-B lymphocyte agents 211
 anti-complement agents 212
 anti-T lymphocyte agents 212

anti-TNF agents 210
 research studies 208
 side effects 208
 stem cell therapy 213
new treatments 425–429
nonsteroidal anti-inflammatory drugs (NSAIDs) 371
omeprazole 287
oral 26, 27
pioglitazone 310
prednisone 27, 325
ranitidine 287
risk-to-benefit ratio 157
rosiglitazone 310
second-line 154, 161–162, 310, 447 (see also specific medications under Medications)
side effects (see individual medications listed throughout index)
statins 311
supportive measures 90
tacrolimus 169–170
 benefits 169
 side effects 169
 taken during pregnancy 370
thiazolidinediones 301
topical 90, 223–224
Metabolic myopathies 50
Mixed connective tissue disease (MCTD) 16, 45, 324, 445
Modified barium swallow exam 47, 73, 245, 448
Monoclonal antibodies 208, 210, 213
 Campath 1H 212
 eculizumab 212
 infliximab 209, 218, 221, 247, 372
 rituximab 211
Multiple sclerosis 32
Muscle mass 70, 276–277, 445
Muscle strength, endurance, and function 139–151, 141–143
 definitions 443, 445, 446
 isometric dynamometry 144
 manual muscle testing 142–143
 myometer 144
Muscular dystrophy 50
Muscular Dystrophy Association 99, 414, 416
Myopathy 9, 445

Myositis *(see also Juvenile myositis)*
  adult 10, 20–22
  cancer-associated 18, 20
  care of 2
  classification 9
  definition of 1, 43, 446
  eosinophilic 17
  first described 35
  focal 17
  inclusion body 17, 20
  macrophagic 17
  orbital 17
  pronunciation 1, 9
  rarity 1
Myositis Association, The 4, 6, 112,
    159, 220, 380, 397, 414, 416,
    419, 429, 436, 438
  newsletters 424
  WAMO! (Working Against Myositis
    for Others) 440
  website 59
Myositis Awareness Day 435, 436
Myositis Damage Index 134
Myositis Disease Activity Assess-
    ment Tool 134
Myositis Disease Activity Score
    (DAS) 147

Nasal reflux 243
Nasendoscopy 285
National Committee for Quality
    Assurance (NCQA) 301, 385
National Institute of Arthritis and
    Musculoskeletal and Skin
    Diseases (NIAMS) 37, 420
National Institutes of Health (NIH)
    191, 420, 429
Neurologist 55, 64, 111, 386, 446
Nutrition 253–260
  avoiding salt 258
  avoiding sugar 258
  eating healthy 254, 258
  effect of inflammation 254
  impact of corticosteroids 255–
    256
  impact of JM on diet 254–255
  impact of medications 256
  importance of 249, 253–254
  improving 256–260
  in summer camps 415
  probiotic bacteria 257
  vitamin supplements 259

Occupational therapists 174, 186,
    446
Occupational therapy 107, 178,
    210, 387, 403, 446
Ophthalmologists 89, 313, 315,
    317, 319, 446
Orthotics 187–188
  functional 187
  purposes of 187
Osteoblasts 275
Osteoclasts 275
Osteoporosis 136, 184
  causes 276–277
  definition of 275–276, 446
  diagnosing 277–278
  preventing 278
  treatment 279–281
Outcomes 60, 341–342, 345
  course of illness 60
  flare *(see Flare)*
  recovery 24, 27
  relapse 60, 95, 130, 153–154,
    161, 164, 447
  remission 12, 154, 447
  unpredictable course 109
Overlap myositis 16–18, 44, 70–71,
    231, 255, 272, 321–326, 446
  treatment 325

Pancreatitis 309
Panniculitis 310
Paronychia 85
Physiatrists 174, 446
Physical adaptations 95
  physical assistance 102
    changing positions 97
    dressing 102
    eating 102
    head support 97
    moving a child 97
    obtaining equipment 100
    sitting up 97
    using a hoist 97
    using the toilet and shower 98
    walking 98, 103
    wheelchair 99–100
  physical effects 173–174, 176–
    178
  physical limitations 95–109
  play activities 100, 104
Physical therapists 174, 186, 446
Physical therapy 12, 129, 155, 173,
    232, 260, 271, 272, 387, 402,
    409, 415, 416, 447
Placebos 428

Plasma exchange 82
Pneumonia 47, 162, 242–244, 293–
    294, 336
  aspiration 243, 292, 441
Polymyositis (PM) 20, 26, 32, 447
Pregnancy 367–375
  breastfeeding 372
  outcomes 369
PRINTO 132, 134
Professional care, importance of 5,
    25
Pronation 188
Proximal 11, 63, 129, 447
Psoriasis 38, 45, 219, 325, 447
Psychologist 112, 117, 250, 401,
    415, 447
PubMed 4, 420

Rashes 1, 9–12, 14–15, 17, 19–20,
    24–25, 27, 38, 43–44, 46, 48,
    58, 60, 66, 71, 78, 80, 82, 89,
    128, 130, 134, 154, 158, 186,
    217–219, 402
  causes 219
  coping with 222
  Gottron's papules *(see Gottron's
    papules)*
  heliotrope *(see Heliotrope)*
  itching 221
  malar 45, 218–219, 323, 445
  periungual telangiectasia 218
  poikiloderma 222
  severe 218
  shawl sign 45, 218
  treatment 85, 89–90, 157, 161–
    162, 164–165, 167, 169, 212,
    222–225
  V-sign 45, 218
Raynaud's phenomenon 324
Rehabilitation 173–190 *(see also
    Exercises, Occupational therapy,
    Physical adaptations, Physical
    therapy)*
  exercises 177
    goals of 177
    importance of 177
  team 174
    assessments and treatments
      175–176
    educational programs 188
  Thera-bands® 181
  treatments 174, 176, 185
    assistive devices and mobility
      aides 186

heat and cold 185
massage therapy 186
Rehabilitation Act 355–356, 379, 396
Research 423
basic 424
clinical 424
translational 425
Resorption 236, 275–276, 279
Response criteria 132
Rheumatologist 55, 64, 96, 111, 154, 219, 346, 347, 358–359, 364, 378, 386, 446, 447

School issues 395–410
absenteeism 407
accommodations 405
attendance 61
building accessibility 404
complaint process 399
documentation 400
homework 404–405
physical and psychological issues 401–402
physical education 404
physical therapy 403
private school 407
transportation 403
Scleroderma 16–17, 38, 45, 72, 219, 305, 321–322, 324, 447
Sclerosis 15, 38, 231
Sexuality 361–365
birth control 363–364
sexually transmitted infections 364–365
Social worker 53, 55, 97, 112, 113, 115, 117, 118, 120, 250, 380, 391, 415, 416, 448
Speech-language pathologists 245, 286–287, 448
Sports 95, 117, 147, 173, 176, 318, 404
allowable 104
participation in 60, 183–184
Steatosis 309
Summer camps 411–417
benefits of 412–413
choosing 414–419
parental concerns 413

Sun protection 24, 28, 88, 219–222, 402
clothing 221
importance of 119, 223
sun blocks 220
sunscreens 220, 403
UV-protective automobile film 221
Swallowing problems and difficulties 46–48, 242, 245–246, 256
esophageal dysmotility 254, 443
Systemic lupus erythematosus (SLE) 15–16, 17, 32, 38, 45, 89, 136, 169, 305, 321, 323, 448

T-score 277
Tenosynovitis 270
Tests for juvenile myositis 13, 25, 60, 63–76, 128–131
antinuclear antibody test (ANA) 71, 441
blood tests 13, 24, 26, 64, 74, 129, 136
complete blood cell count 70
echocardiogram 73
electrocardiogram, EKG 73
EMG 13
eye exams 74
flow cytometry 72, 131, 236, 444
hemocult test 73
imaging studies 136 (see also CT scan, Magnetic resonance imaging, Ultrasound)
muscle biopsy 13
muscle enzyme tests 66
muscle imaging tests 66
nailfold capillary studies 71, 446
neopterin 72, 131, 236
other 14
pulmonary function tests 74, 447 (see also Breathing problems)
troponin level 74
urine analysis 71
von Willebrand factor antigen 72, 131, 236, 443
Thyroid disease 15, 17, 50, 261, 267, 305, 325
Tracheostomy tube 247
Transition 351–360
definition of 351

failure of 352
goal of 352
medical care 357
planning 353, 358
post-secondary education 353–355
services 354
workplace 355
Travel 336
Tuberculosis (TB) 328
Tumor necrosis factor alpha (TNF-α) 38, 234–235, 347, 424–425, 448
gene 234
tumor necrosis factor alpha–308 (TNF-α–308) 35

Ulcers 20, 218, 238, 248, 336, 347, 448
Ultrasound 66–67, 131, 180, 233, 245, 277

Vaccines 328
and immunosuppressive therapy 334
benefits and risks 328
FluMist 333
inactivated 328
influenza 328, 330, 333
live viral 330
live-attenuated 328
MMRII 330
Varicella-zoster immune globulin 332
Vasculitis 73, 248–249, 314, 372, 448
Vasculopathy 81, 448
Vitamin D 28, 86, 276, 278
Vocational Rehabilitation Act 380
Voice problems 283–289
laryngeal problems 286–287
laryngitis 286
laryngopharyngeal reflux 286
vocal fold nodules and polyps 286
treatment 287–288

West Nile virus 336